Mastering Geriatric Surgery

Kok-Yang Tan
Daniel Jin-Keat Lee • Priscilla Ng
Editors

Mastering Geriatric Surgery

Managing Frailty, Sarcopenia, and other Geriatric Issues in Surgery

Springer

Editors
Kok-Yang Tan
General and Colorectal Surgery
Khoo Teck Puat Hospital
Singapore, Singapore

Daniel Jin-Keat Lee
General and Colorectal Surgery
Khoo Teck Puat Hospital
Singapore, Singapore

Priscilla Ng
Department of Geriatric Medicine
Khoo Teck Puat Hospital
Singapore, Singapore

ISBN 978-981-95-0664-4 ISBN 978-981-95-0665-1 (eBook)
https://doi.org/10.1007/978-981-95-0665-1

This Springer imprint is published by the registered company Springer Nature Singapore Pte Ltd.
The registered company address is: 152 Beach Road, #21-01/04 Gateway East, Singapore 189721, Singapore

Preface

We gathered authors with years of domain expertise in the field of geriatric surgery and conceived this book. It aims to provide a comprehensive guide to the principles and practice of geriatric surgery. It can serve as a resource for surgeons, anaesthetists, geriatricians, nurses and allied health professionals. With this book, we hope to provide professionals with a deeper understanding of the critical issues that surround surgery in older persons and thus bridge the gap between surgical expertise and the holistic care that must accompany it.

The chapters reflect a transdisciplinary approach for geriatric surgical care, and the topics not only explore the physiology of ageing but also the technical aspects of surgery and broader decision-making when dealing with an older surgical patient.

We hope that this book inspires thoughtful, person-centred surgical care that will be good enough for our parents.

Singapore, Singapore — Kok-Yang Tan
Singapore, Singapore — Daniel Jin-Keat Lee
Singapore, Singapore — Priscilla Ng

About This Book

With rapidly ageing populations, surgical and perioperative care teams are presented with patients of increasing median ages. These teams correspondingly must deal not only with the pathology of the surgical issues but also with the changing physiology of the ageing person within which the surgical pathology resides. Current surgical practice must incorporate management of geriatric issues for a holistic and effective surgical care where value is captured by the patient. Surgical practice incorporating geriatric care management is thus a concept that is increasingly embraced by experts worldwide.

This book is a comprehensive textbook that will put together current principles and practice of integrating geriatric management within surgical and perioperative care. The book will discuss the science of ageing and how this impacts surgery and surgical consideration. It will focus on the concepts of frailty and sarcopenia accompanying surgical patients. It will also provide insights into the optimal model of care for surgical patients with reduced functional reserves and specific considerations on what should be considered optimal outcomes and how to achieve them.

This book will be essential information for the practicing surgeon and the perioperative care physicians, nurses and allied health professionals that will provide the multifaceted care demanded by the modern surgical patient.

Contents

Understanding the Older Person Who Needs Surgery

1

Priscilla Ng

1.1 Introduction

The proportion of the global population aged 60 and over is projected to double by 2050 (World Health Organisation 2021). Neoplastic and degenerative conditions increase with age, many of which are amenable to surgical treatment. Constant advancements in medical science also generate more therapeutic options to offer patients. It is thus no surprise that in many surgical specialities patients aged 65 and above account for a majority of the caseload (Etzioni et al. 2003).

The unique challenges of surgery in older patients encompass the physiology of ageing, a decline in physiological reserve and an increase in comorbid conditions. Understandably, the prudent surgeon wishes to tread cautiously. But since we cannot reverse the tide of a complex, ageing surgical population, the only way out is through mastery of the challenge. Familiarity with frailty and multimorbidity, and empowerment by evidence and the backing of a multidisciplinary team will enable our older patients to benefit from the full spectrum of our skill and care.

1.2 Geriatric Syndromes

Geriatric syndromes or "geriatric giants" were coined to describe the unique constellations of health challenges in older persons, such as impaired cognition, instability (falls) leading to immobility, incontinence, inanition, iatrogenesis, and the overarching frailty syndrome (Inouye et al. 2007). In 2017, the geriatric 5Ms were launched as a dynamic way of reframing the traditional geriatric syndromes for wider accessibility beyond the geriatric speciality (Molnar et al. 2017). Certain fields such as gastroenterology (Kochar et al. 2022) and rheumatology (Buehring

P. Ng (✉)
Geriatric Medicine, Khoo Teck Puat Hospital, Singapore, Singapore

K.-Y. Tan et al. (eds.), *Mastering Geriatric Surgery*,
https://doi.org/10.1007/978-981-95-0665-1_1

et al. 2024) have adapted it to their own context. For the first time, we will explore the relevance of perioperative issues in depth using this updated framework, summarised in Table 1.1.

Awareness and systematic screening must necessarily precede identification and management of geriatric syndromes. The American College of Surgeons National Surgical Quality Improvement Programme and the American Geriatrics Society, in the best practices guideline 'Optimal preoperative assessment of the geriatric surgical patient', recommend routine brief evaluation of domains such as cognition, mood, function and frailty (Chow et al. 2012). A positive screen of multiple or significant abnormalities should prompt further evaluation, such as a comprehensive geriatric assessment. Comprehensive geriatric assessment is defined by Rubenstein as 'a multidimensional, interdisciplinary diagnostic process to determine the medical, psychological and functional capabilities of a frail older person in order to develop a co-ordinated and integrated plan for treatment and long-term follow up' (Rubenstein et al. 1991). This multidimensional assessment by trained staff is followed by a multifactorial intervention implemented by members of a multidisciplinary team. When applied as an intervention in the perioperative setting, comprehensive geriatric assessment has been shown to improve outcomes such as complications and length of stay (Partridge et al. 2014).

Table 1.1 The geriatric 5Ms in the perioperative context

Geriatric syndrome	Relevance in perioperative context
Mind	Dementia • Establishing cognitive baseline • Mental capacity for informed consent Delirium • Risk counselling, screening, prevention, early detection • Perioperative cognitive disorders spectrum Depression • Impact on participation and surgical outcomes
Mobility	Function • Prognostic for surgical decision-making • Functional outcome as a key measure • Prehabilitation Falls • A preventable cause of geriatric trauma
Medications	Polypharmacy Medication optimisation as an intervention Perioperative medication management for delirium prevention
Multicomplexity	Frailty Sarcopenia Multimorbidity Biopsychosocial
Matters most	Individual values Shared decision-making Advance care planning Resuscitation status in the perioperative period

1.2.1 Mind

1.2.1.1 Dementia and Delirium

The relevance of cognitive assessment as part of the preoperative evaluation is multifold. Establishing the baseline cognitive function and screening for previously undiagnosed cognitive impairment allows prognostication of the risk of postoperative delirium, a major concern in undertaking surgery in older patients. This in turn facilitates risk counselling, prevention and early detection and intervention. Significant baseline cognitive impairment may also have a bearing on mental capacity and the ability to give informed consent for surgery.

Postoperative delirium is a syndrome of acute fluctuating alteration in cognition, conscious level and attention which occurs after anaesthesia and surgery. The incidence is cited as ranging from 15–53% of older patients after surgery, with patients undergoing emergency, cardiothoracic, vascular and hip fracture surgery at higher risk, to 70–87% of those requiring intensive care. The sequelae of postoperative delirium include increased length of hospital and intensive care stay, increased 30-day mortality, higher rate of discharge to an institution, functional decline and increased healthcare costs (Jin et al. 2020).

Postoperative delirium is part of a broader spectrum of perioperative cognitive disorders, ranging from emergence excitation or delirium; postoperative delirium; delayed neurocognitive recovery up to 30 days post procedure; postoperative mild or major neurocognitive disorder up to 12 months post procedure and segueing into standard mild or major neurocognitive disorder beyond 12 months (Evered et al. 2018). Preoperative cognitive screening is thus useful to establish that the deficit was not pre-existent. The odds ratio for developing dementia following postoperative delirium was 6.08 in a meta-analysis (Huang et al. 2021). The nature of the relationship is bidirectional: patients with diminished cognitive reserve are naturally at higher risk of developing delirium, while delirium itself is a cognitive insult increasing the long-term risk of cognitive decline in both cognitively intact and impaired patients.

Multiple societies and guidelines have recognised the importance of detection and prompt management of postoperative delirium, which starts with proactive screening for the condition. For example, the American Society of Anaesthesiologists (ASA) Perioperative Brain Health Initiative recommends delirium screening for older surgical patients prior to emergency surgery, before recovery room discharge, then until at least the fifth postoperative day (Peden et al. 2021). Preferred validated screening tools include the Confusion Assessment Method (CAM) (Inouye et al. 1990), CAM-ICU (Ely et al. 2001), or the 4 'A's Test (4AT) (Bellelli et al. 2014), all of which assess the features of acute fluctuating change, inattention, cognitive disturbance and altered consciousness as based on the Diagnostic and Statistical Manual of Mental Disorders, Fifth Edition (DSM-5) criteria for delirium.

Having identified the patient with delirium, the mainstay of management is a bundle of non-pharmacological multicomponent interventions. These vary between institutions but generally comprise early mobilisation, nutrition, analgesia, orientation, sensory support, sleep hygiene and medication review, originating in principles from the Hospital Elder Life Programme (Inouye et al. 2000), one of the first care models designed to prevent functional and cognitive decline. Proactive geriatrics consultation also reduces incidence and severity of delirium (Marcantonio et al. 2001). Guidelines from the American Geriatrics Society (American Geriatrics Society Expert Panel on Postoperative Delirium in Older Adults 2015), the Perioperative Quality Initiative (POQI) (Hughes et al. 2020) and the European Society of Anaesthesiology and Intensive Care Medicine (ESAIC) (Aldecoa et al. 2024) cover the non-pharmacological, pharmacological and systems-based management of delirium with only minor differences.

1.2.1.2 Depression

The 3Ds of geriatric cognition—dementia, delirium and depression—are interlinked. Dementia and depression are risk factors for the development of delirium. Delirium and depression are risk factors for future cognitive decline. Depression may produce cognitive impairment confounding the diagnosis of dementia ('pseudodementia'), or be a response to insight into early cognitive deficits, or be a true neuropsychiatric complication of dementia (Byers and Yaffe 2011).

Patients with a serious surgical diagnosis may experience reactive low mood. Conversely, a patient with pre-existing depression may have impaired judgement when weighing the benefits and risks of surgery. Depression is a predictor of acute and chronic postsurgical pain and, unsurprisingly, poorer patient satisfaction and health-related quality of life. Depression negatively impacts functional outcomes, presumably by impacting participation in prehabilitation and rehabilitation. Depression is even associated with increased postoperative infections and overall mortality, likely mediated by neurohormonal effects on immunity (Ghoneim and O'Hara 2016).

Psychological interventions have been studied as a component of balanced multimodal prehabilitation, although they tend to impact patient-reported outcome measures, including symptoms, psychological measures and quality of life rather than morbidity and mortality (Tsimopoulou et al. 2015).

1.2.2 Mobility

1.2.2.1 Function

Premorbid function of surgical patients is highly predictive of the functional prognosis at 1 year following major surgery. Functional status at baseline predicts the speed and completeness of postoperative recovery (Stabenau et al. 2018). Functional measures such as the Eastern Cooperative Oncology Group Performance Status (ECOG-PS) correlate well with survival after curative surgery and hence may be factored into treatment decisions in surgical oncology (Hanaoka et al. 2022).

Functional recovery is often rated as having higher importance by older patients compared to traditional outcome measures of mortality or progression-free survival (Hofman et al. 2015). This underscores the importance of assessing function and other patient-reported outcome measures (PROMs) alongside conventional metrics.

The idealised concept of postoperative recovery as described by Allvin encompasses 'a return to a state of normality and wholeness defined by comparative standards, regaining control over physical, psychological, social and habitual functions, returning to preoperative levels of independency/dependency in activities of daily living, and regaining one's optimum level of well-being' (Allvin et al. 2007).

A low physical activity level, which is also a component of the frailty phenotype, is associated with reduced aerobic capacity and physiological reserve to withstand the stress of major surgery. Patients experience an acute drop in functional capacity immediately following surgery, followed by recovery and rehabilitation. Prehabilitation aims to buffer physiological reserve preoperatively to facilitate a more rapid and complete recovery, and crucially, to prevent functional capacity from falling below the critical threshold needed to maintain functional independence and quality of life, particularly in the event of any unexpected complications (Tew et al. 2018).

1.2.2.2 Falls

Falls are a major contributor to the geriatric surgical caseload in the form of hip and other fragility fractures and head trauma. The global burden of hip fractures alone is estimated at 4–14 million annually and is projected to double by 2050, accompanied by significant morbidity and mortality (Sing et al. 2023). Geriatric 'silver trauma' patients sustain serious and often life-changing injuries with relatively low-impact trauma relative to younger patients. Moreover, they are at risk of under-triage due to the apparently minor mechanisms of injury, necessitating greater awareness and research in this area (Alshibani et al. 2021).

As falls are potentially preventable, clinicians at every level of the healthcare system from the primary care setting upwards may intervene by identifying patients at high risk of falls and referring them for assessment and multifactorial intervention. Similarly, pre-emptive osteoporosis screening and treatment may reduce the risk of fractures for patients who do fall. Patients who present with fragility fractures should be referred for prompt osteoporosis treatment for secondary prevention.

Identification of falls and mobility issues in the preoperative assessment of a surgical patient is pertinent due to the functional implications which present challenges as well as targets for prehabilitation and rehabilitation. Even in elective general surgical patients unrelated to trauma, a prior history of falls in the 6 months preceding surgery was associated with increased postoperative complications, discharge to an institution and 30-day readmission (Jones et al. 2013).

A combined model of orthogeriatric care has long been recognised as the standard of care for hip fractures. It established a standardised approach, including prompt surgery, analgesia and anaesthesia, early mobilisation, multidisciplinary management and setting of audit standards (National Institute for Health and Care Excellence 2023). The application of these principles has been broadened to become the forerunner of geriatric perioperative services in many other surgical disciplines.

1.2.3 Medications

Polypharmacy is a major contributor to the geriatric syndrome of Iatrogenesis. Older patients have more chronic conditions, necessitating the prescription of multiple medications, which in turn give rise to interactions and side effects, the number of which rises exponentially with the number of drugs involved. At the same time, pharmacokinetic effects, including decreased volume of distribution, decreased hepatic metabolism and decreased renal excretion, increase the susceptibility of the older person to medication effects. Polypharmacy is an independent risk factor for falls, hospitalisation and delirium (Hein et al. 2014).

Medication review and rationalisation is an important intervention offered by the geriatrician and is one of the suites of interventions recommended for frailty. Guidance for medication optimisation includes the American Geriatrics Society Beers Criteria for potentially inappropriate medication use in older adults (By the 2023 American Geriatrics Society Beers Criteria® Update Expert Panel 2023) and the STOPP/START criteria for potentially inappropriate prescribing in older people (O'Mahony et al. 2023).

The anaesthetist plays a key role in intraoperative and immediate perioperative medication management. Some of the evidence-based pharmacological interventions recommended for reduction of postoperative delirium include multimodal opioid-sparing analgesia, minimising of benzodiazepine use and dexmedetomidine as a preferred sedative. Conversely, pharmacological interventions which have not been shown to reduce delirium include a preference for a particular mode of anaesthesia (general versus regional), and most single agents such as cholinesterase inhibitors and melatonin, with the possible exception of antipsychotics (Swarbrick and Partridge 2022; Li et al. 2021).

1.2.4 Multicomplexity

1.2.4.1 Frailty

The frailty phenotype was described by Fried in 2001 as a clinical syndrome comprising three or more of unintentional weight loss, self-reported exhaustion, weakness (grip strength), slow walking speed and low physical activity (Fried et al. 2001). The consensus definition most relevant to the perioperative context is 'a medical syndrome with multiple causes and contributors that is characterized by diminished strength, endurance, and reduced physiologic function that increases an individual's vulnerability for developing increased dependency and/or death [when exposed to a stressor]' (Morley et al. 2013). Major surgery undeniably constitutes such a stressor. The impact of frailty on postoperative outcomes has been well documented, including increased morbidity and mortality, readmissions, length of stay and discharge to an institution rather than home (Hewitt et al. 2018; Lin et al. 2016).

The Society for Perioperative Assessment and Quality Improvement (SPAQI) recommendations for the preoperative management of frailty include frailty screening as part of the perioperative evaluation of older patients undergoing major elective surgery (Alvarez-Nebreda et al. 2018). Patients who screen positive are recommended for a diagnostic evaluation, preferably a comprehensive geriatric assessment. Over 20 validated frailty instruments are in use in surgical populations, based on variations of the two main models of frailty: the phenotype model by Fried and the cumulative deficit model by Rockwood in the Canadian Study of Health and Aging (CSHA) (Rockwood et al. 2005).

The corollary to surgery as a stressor is that elective surgery is a stressor which will be delivered in a predictable time and manner, offering a window of opportunity for pre-emptive mitigation. Multimodal prehabilitation may be considered to improve the prognosis (Alvarez-Nebreda et al. 2018). An individualised care approach is preferred for the surgical patient with frailty. The Centre for Perioperative Care (CPOC) and British Geriatrics Society (BGS) have also proposed a guideline for the Perioperative Care of People Living with Frailty with underpinning principles of Iterative shared decision-making; streamlined communication and documentation; comprehensive geriatric assessment and optimisation; and multispeciality, multidisciplinary working (Centre for Perioperative Care 2021).

1.2.4.2 Sarcopenia

Sarcopenia was first defined by Rosenberg in 1988 as the loss of skeletal muscle mass in the context of ageing (Rosenberg 1997). However, it is now recognised as being most commonly but not exclusively found in older persons, with implications for younger surgical patients as well. According to the updated European Working Group on Sarcopenia in Older People (EWGSOP) definition, a probable diagnosis of sarcopenia is made when low muscle strength is identified. The diagnosis is confirmed by the presence of low muscle quantity or quality, and the condition is considered severe when low physical performance is also present (Cruz-Jentoft et al. 2019). Sarcopenia in surgical patients is associated with increased complications, mortality at up to 5 years, length of stay and discharge to institutional care (Knoedler et al. 2023).

Frailty and sarcopenia share a significant overlap. The original frailty phenotype as described by Fried includes reduced grip strength, gait speed and weight loss, which correspond to reduced muscle strength, physical performance and muscle mass, respectively. Nevertheless, a differentiation is maintained, with sarcopenia being a disease of muscle and frailty a broader geriatric syndrome.

1.2.4.3 Multimorbidity

Multimorbidity is defined as the coexistence of multiple chronic health conditions in an individual, most frequently using a cut-off of two or more (Johnston et al. 2019). In the perioperative context, scales such as the age-adjusted Charlson comorbidity index, originally developed in medical populations, have been validated in surgical populations for prognostication of morbidity and mortality (Bhattacharjee et al. 2023).

Multimorbidity and frailty are frequently coexistent but distinct. A large study of older hospital patients found that 33.6% had both multimorbidity and frailty, 14.7% had multimorbidity only, 19.9% had frailty only and 31.8% had neither.

Multimorbidity and frailty had an additive effect on readmissions and a multiplicative effect on mortality and length of hospital stay (Lujic et al. 2022). However, in a cohort of older emergency surgical patients, while the prevalence of multimorbidity was as high as 74%, it did not appear to impact outcomes in contrast to the undifferentiated hospital population (Hewitt et al. 2016).

Specific optimisation of medical conditions is described in guidelines such as optimal preoperative assessment of the geriatric surgical patient: a best practices guideline from the American College of Surgeons National Surgical Quality Improvement Programme and the American Geriatrics Society (Chow et al. 2012); the American College of Cardiology/American Heart Association guidelines for cardiovascular optimisation (Thompson et al. 2024) and guidelines from various societies on perioperative diabetes management (Crowley et al. 2023), among many others.

As with frailty, an overarching patient-centred approach is warranted. One such guideline by the American Geriatrics Society Expert Panel on the Care of Older Adults with Multimorbidity focuses on five domains: patient preferences, interpreting the evidence, prognosis, clinical feasibility and optimising therapies and care plans (American Geriatrics Society Expert Panel on the Care of Older Adults with Multimorbidity 2012).

1.2.5 Matters Most

Finally, but certainly not least important of the 5 'M's, is what matters most to the patient, the raison d'être of all the other assessments. In all aspects of care of the older person, but particularly in the contemplation of high-stakes major surgery, the decision should be informed by the patient's values and priorities and psychosocial context. Patient-centred care is also the core underlying principle of dealing with the multicomplexity presented by frailty and multimorbidity.

There is a distinct age-related difference in patient priorities, with older patients placing more value on functional limitations and social functioning, and less on morbidities and pain experience (Hofman et al. 2015). In a study of older patients with life-limiting illness, most would not opt to receive a life-saving treatment if there was a likelihood of significant functional or cognitive impairment. A significant minority would not opt even for a treatment which would restore current function, if the treatment burden was high (Fried et al. 2002). An alternative mode of expression of patient values is in terms of valued life activities which patients hope to be able to resume following elective surgery. These domains include recreational activities, mobility, activities of daily living, instrumental activities of daily living and social activities (Kata et al. 2019).

A comprehensive geriatric assessment provides background information on cognition, function and social support and also helps build rapport for a more detailed exploration of the patient's understanding and thoughts regarding their diagnosis and the proposed surgery. An example of a simple framework to facilitate a shared decision-making discussion is Choosing Wisely UK's four 'BRAN' questions:

What are the Benefits? What are the Risks? What are the Alternatives? What Happens If I Do Nothing? (Barnett and Swart 2021). The significant life moment of major surgery may also present an opportunity for advance care planning, a process that goes beyond the making of a directive and involves a journey of reflection by the patient about their values and wishes, discussion with clinicians and designation of a representative (Keon-Cohen et al. 2025).

Due to the prevalence of chronic or potential life-limiting conditions among older patients, patients may also present with an existing 'do not attempt cardiopulmonary resuscitation' order in place which requires decisions by the team regarding its perioperative management. One audit noted that less than a third of such orders were formally suspended at the time of anaesthesia and surgery. Such patients fortunately comprised only 6% of those who required perioperative cardiopulmonary resuscitation. Of these, just over half achieved return of spontaneous circulation, although the eventual survival to discharge was about one in five (Nolan et al. 2024). These data may help inform treatment decisions.

1.3 Interventions

While the interplay of geriatric syndromes and the perioperative state is complex, the interventions need not be so. Fortuitously, there is an overlap of recommended interventions in two areas: between prehabilitation and the interventions for frailty and sarcopenia, and between enhanced recovery after surgery protocols and delirium guidelines.

1.3.1 Prehabilitation and Interventions for Frailty and Sarcopenia

Aerobic and strength exercise and protein–calorie nutrition are the mainstay of prehabilitation and interventions for frailty and sarcopenia due to the common mechanisms underlying the building of physiological reserve.

Prehabilitation: Exercise as an individual intervention has been shown to reduce postoperative pulmonary complications and overall morbidity in elective surgical patients (Heger et al. 2020), while nutritional interventions reduce length of stay (Gillis et al. 2018). Combining the modalities in multimodal prehabilitation reduces length of stay, complications and emergency department reattendance, and improves function (Molenaar et al. 2022; Skořepa et al. 2024). Strength and nutrition are interdependent, as a malnourished patient in a catabolic state would not be expected to build muscle.

Sarcopenia: The recommendation for nutrition in sarcopenia is balanced protein and energy supplementation as part of a multimodal approach. Older persons in fact require a higher protein intake of 1–1.5 g/kg/day compared to younger persons due to reduced metabolic efficiency in protein synthesis. There may be some data for specific nutrients such as leucine-enriched balanced amino acids and creatine. This is in combination with resistance and aerobic exercise for 20–30 min three times a week, and vitamin D supplementation for all levels short of the toxicity threshold (Morley et al. 2010).

Frailty: Physical activity, particularly resistance training, nutrition intervention and multicomponent interventions, had the potential to reduce frailty in meta-analyses. Other interventions which have been studied for frailty include comprehensive geriatric assessment, cognitive training and various geriatric care models (Sun et al. 2023).

1.3.2 Enhanced Recovery After Surgery Protocols and Non-pharmacological Delirium Prevention and Management Recommendations

Enhanced recovery after surgery (ERAS) is a multidisciplinary approach designed to promote recovery by reducing the inflammatory stress response to surgery. Using elective colorectal surgery as a representative example, the postoperative items from the ERAS Society recommendations (Gustafsson et al. 2019) are presented in Table 1.2 alongside the multicomponent non-pharmacological interventions performed by an interdisciplinary team for the prevention and management of delirium, respectively, from the American Geriatrics Society abstracted clinical practice guideline for postoperative delirium in older adults (American Geriatrics Society Expert Panel on Postoperative Delirium in Older Adults 2015).

It can be seen that multimodal opioid-sparing analgesia, adequate nutrition, early oral nutrition where feasible, promotion of gastrointestinal motility and early mobilisation are key features of ERAS and delirium prevention or management. To take a maximally reductionist approach, the simplified goal of drinking, eating and mobilising (DrEaMing) delivered as a bundled intervention with the aim of being able to DRink free fluids, EAt a soft diet and Mobilise with the maximum assistance of one person within 24 h of surgery, has been shown to shorten the length of hospital stay and postoperative complications after major non-cardiac surgery (Oliver et al. 2022).

Although not specified as such in the delirium guidelines, early removal of tubes and lines is likely to reduce delirium by eliminating the tethering effect which increases distress and serves as a barrier to mobilisation. Similarly, promoting sleep hygiene is likely to reduce the inflammatory stress response in a well-rested patient, good glycaemic control may decrease potential medical precipitants of delirium, and thromboprophylaxis is of additional benefit in a delirious patient with reduced mobility. It can thus be seen that the ERAS, traditionally in the surgical domain, and multicomponent interventions for delirium, traditionally the province of the geriatrician, dovetail across the majority of their components.

Finally, what ties it all together is the multidisciplinary team. Among those caring for older persons undergoing surgery, there are different areas of expertise but a common aim, and the evidence-based interventions across different domains also

Table 1.2 Comparison of enhanced recovery after surgery protocol and multicomponent non-pharmacological interventions for delirium

ERAS	Delirium prevention	Delirium management
Multimodal opioid-sparing analgesia	Pain management	
Neutral fluid balance Postoperative resumption of oral intake	Nutrition and fluid repletion	Maintenance of nutrition and hydration
Early mobilisation	Early mobility and/or physical rehabilitation	Mobility/exercise/physical therapy
Multimodal prevention of ileus	Prevention of constipation	
No routine nasogastric tubes		
Removal of urinary catheter after 1–3 days		
Thromboprophylaxis		
Glycaemic control		
	Cognitive reorientation	Reorientation, therapeutic activities, cognitive stimulation
	Sleep enhancement	Sleep enhancement
	Vision and hearing adaptation	Vision and hearing adaptation
	Appropriate medication usage	
	Adequate oxygenation	
		Nursing education and interventions
		Geriatric consultation

overlap significantly. Multimodal interventions necessitate delivery by a multidisciplinary team, comprising the surgeon, anaesthetist, geriatrician, cardiologist, internist, nurse, nurse clinician, physiotherapist, dietitian, pharmacist, medical social worker and others, with the patient at the heart of it (Whiteman et al. 2016).

Moving beyond multidisciplinary to transdisciplinary, a truly integrated team has open communication, collaborative assessment, management and decision-making, and is motivated to anticipate and facilitate each other's jobs. Thus, in our team, we have the surgeon ambulating the patient, the physiotherapist highlighting the patient's postural hypotension, the surgical intern taking a cognitive history, the geriatrician handing over an unplanned ICU admission to the intensivist and the nurse clinician coordinating and communicating. The goal of this book is to inspire and inform potential team members around the globe by developing further upon these concepts in the following chapters.

References

Aldecoa C, Bettelli G, Bilotta F et al (2024) Update of the European Society of Anaesthesiology and Intensive Care Medicine evidence-based and consensus-based guideline on postoperative delirium in adult patients. Eur J Anaesthesiol 41(2):81–108. https://doi.org/10.1097/EJA.0000000000001876

Allvin R, Berg K, Idvall E et al (2007) Postoperative recovery: a concept analysis. J Adv Nurs 57(5):552–558. https://doi.org/10.1111/j.1365-2648.2006.04156.x

Alshibani A, Alharbi M, Conroy S (2021) Under-triage of older trauma patients in prehospital care: a systematic review. Eur Geriatr Med 12(5):903–919. https://doi.org/10.1007/s41999-021-00512-5

Alvarez-Nebreda ML, Bentov N, Urman RD et al (2018) Recommendations for preoperative management of frailty from the Society for Perioperative Assessment and Quality Improvement (SPAQI). J Clin Anesth 47:33–42. https://doi.org/10.1016/j.jclinane.2018.02.011

American Geriatrics Society Expert Panel on Postoperative Delirium in Older Adults (2015) American Geriatrics Society abstracted clinical practice guideline for postoperative delirium in older adults. J Am Geriatr Soc 63(1):142–150. https://doi.org/10.1111/jgs.13281

American Geriatrics Society Expert Panel on the Care of Older Adults with Multimorbidity (2012) Guiding principles for the care of older adults with multimorbidity: an approach for clinicians. J Am Geriatr Soc 60(10):E1–E25. https://doi.org/10.1111/j.1532-5415.2012.04188.x

Barnett G, Swart M (2021) Shared decision making for high-risk surgery. BJA Educ 21(8):300–306. https://doi.org/10.1016/j.bjae.2021.03.006

Bellelli G, Morandi A, Davis DH et al (2014) Validation of the 4AT, a new instrument for rapid delirium screening: a study in 234 hospitalised older people. Age Ageing 43(4):496–502. https://doi.org/10.1093/ageing/afu021

Bhattacharjee HK, Kaviyarasan MP, Singh KJ et al (2023) Age adjusted Charlson comorbidity index (a-CCI) AS a tool to predict 30-day post-operative outcome in general surgery patients. ANZ J Surg 93(1–2):132–138. https://doi.org/10.1111/ans.18178

Buehring B, van Onna M, Myasoedova E et al (2024) Understanding the multiple dimensions of ageing: 5Ms for the rheumatologist. Lancet Rheumatol 6(12):e892–e902. https://doi.org/10.1016/S2665-9913(24)00230-3

By the 2023 American Geriatrics Society Beers Criteria® Update Expert Panel (2023) American Geriatrics Society 2023 updated AGS Beers Criteria® for potentially inappropriate medication use in older adults. J Am Geriatr Soc 71(7):2052–2081. https://doi.org/10.1111/jgs.18372

Byers AL, Yaffe K (2011) Depression and risk of developing dementia. Nat Rev Neurol 7(6):323–331. https://doi.org/10.1038/nrneurol.2011.60

Centre for Perioperative Care (2021) Guideline for perioperative care for people living with frailty undergoing elective and emergency surgery. https://cpoc.org.uk/guidelines-resources-guidelines/perioperative-care-people-living-frailty

Chow WB, Rosenthal RA, Merkow RP et al (2012) Optimal preoperative assessment of the geriatric surgical patient: a best practices guideline from the American College of Surgeons National Surgical Quality Improvement Program and the American Geriatrics Society. J Am Coll Surg 215(4):453–466. https://doi.org/10.1016/j.jamcollsurg.2012.06.017

Crowley K, Scanaill PÓ, Hermanides J et al (2023) Current practice in the perioperative management of patients with diabetes mellitus: a narrative review. Br J Anaesth 131(2):242–252. https://doi.org/10.1016/j.bja.2023.02.039

Cruz-Jentoft AJ, Bahat G, Bauer J et al (2019) Sarcopenia: revised European consensus on definition and diagnosis. Age Ageing 48(1):16–31. https://doi.org/10.1093/ageing/afy169

Ely EW, Inouye SK, Bernard GR et al (2001) Delirium in mechanically ventilated patients: validity and reliability of the confusion assessment method for the intensive care unit (CAM-ICU). JAMA 286(21):2703–2710. https://doi.org/10.1001/jama.286.21.2703

Etzioni DA, Liu JH, Maggard MA et al (2003) The aging population and its impact on the surgery workforce. Ann Surg 238(2):170–177. https://doi.org/10.1097/01.SLA.0000081085.98792.3d

Evered L, Silbert B, Knopman DS et al (2018) Recommendations for the nomenclature of cognitive change associated with anaesthesia and surgery-2018. Br J Anaesth 121(5):1005–1012. https://doi.org/10.1016/j.bja.2017.11.087

Fried LP, Tangen CM, Walston J et al (2001) Frailty in older adults: evidence for a phenotype. J Gerontol A Biol Sci Med Sci 56(3):M146–M156. https://doi.org/10.1093/gerona/56.3.m146

Fried TR, Bradley EH, Towle VR et al (2002) Understanding the treatment preferences of seriously ill patients. N Engl J Med 346(14):1061–1066. https://doi.org/10.1056/NEJMsa012528

Ghoneim MM, O'Hara MW (2016) Depression and postoperative complications: an overview. BMC Surg 16:5. https://doi.org/10.1186/s12893-016-0120-y

Gillis C, Buhler K, Bresee L et al (2018) Effects of nutritional prehabilitation, with and without exercise, on outcomes of patients who undergo colorectal surgery: a systematic review and meta-analysis. Gastroenterology 155(2):391–410.e4

Gustafsson UO, Scott MJ, Hubner M et al (2019) Guidelines for perioperative care in elective colorectal surgery: enhanced recovery after surgery (ERAS®) society recommendations: 2018. World J Surg 43(3):659–695. https://doi.org/10.1007/s00268-018-4844-y

Hanaoka M, Hino H, Shiomi A et al (2022) The Eastern Cooperative Oncology Group Performance Status as a prognostic factor of stage I-III colorectal cancer surgery for elderly patients: a multi-institutional retrospective analysis. Surg Today 52(7):1081–1089. https://doi.org/10.1007/s00595-021-02412-4

Heger P, Probst P, Wiskemann J et al (2020) A systematic review and meta-analysis of physical exercise prehabilitation in major abdominal surgery (PROSPERO 2017 CRD42017080366). J Gastrointest Surg 24(6):1375–1385

Hein C, Forgues A, Piau A et al (2014) Impact of polypharmacy on occurrence of delirium in elderly emergency patients. J Am Med Dir Assoc 15(11):850.e11–850.e15

Hewitt J, McCormack C, Tay HS et al (2016) Prevalence of multimorbidity and its association with outcomes in older emergency general surgical patients: an observational study. BMJ Open 6:e010126. https://doi.org/10.1136/bmjopen-2015-010126

Hewitt J, Long S, Carter B et al (2018) The prevalence of frailty and its association with clinical outcomes in general surgery: a systematic review and meta-analysis. Age Ageing 47(6):793–800. https://doi.org/10.1093/ageing/afy110

Hofman CS, Makai P, Boter H et al (2015) The influence of age on health valuations: the older olds prefer functional independence while the younger olds prefer less morbidity. Clin Interv Aging 10:1131–1139

Huang H, Li H, Zhang X et al (2021) Association of postoperative delirium with cognitive outcomes: a meta-analysis. J Clin Anesth 75:110496

Hughes CG, Boncyk CS, Culley DJ et al (2020) American Society for Enhanced Recovery and Perioperative Quality Initiative Joint Consensus Statement on postoperative delirium prevention. Anesth Analg 130(6):1572–1590. https://doi.org/10.1213/ANE.0000000000004641

Inouye SK, Van Dyck CH, Alessi CA et al (1990) Clarifying confusion: the confusion assessment method. A new method for detection of delirium. Ann Intern Med 113:941–948. https://doi.org/10.7326/0003-4819-113-12-941

Inouye SK, Bogardus ST Jr, Baker DI et al (2000) The Hospital Elder Life Program: a model of care to prevent cognitive and functional decline in older hospitalized patients. Hospital Elder Life Program. J Am Geriatr Soc 48(12):1697–1706. https://doi.org/10.1111/j.1532-5415.2000.tb03885.x

Inouye SK, Studenski S, Tinetti ME et al (2007) Geriatric syndromes: clinical, research, and policy implications of a core geriatric concept. J Am Geriatr Soc 55(5):780–791. https://doi.org/10.1111/j.1532-5415.2007.01156.x

Jin Z, Hu J, Ma D (2020) Postoperative delirium: perioperative assessment, risk reduction, and management. Br J Anaesth 125(4):492–504

Johnston MC, Crilly M, Black C et al (2019) Defining and measuring multimorbidity: a systematic review of systematic reviews. Eur J Pub Health 29(1):182–189. https://doi.org/10.1093/eurpub/cky098

Jones TS, Dunn CL, Wu DS et al (2013) Relationship between asking an older adult about falls and surgical outcomes. JAMA Surg 148(12):1132–1138. https://doi.org/10.1001/jamasurg.2013.2741

Kata A, Dutt M, Sudore RL et al (2019) What matters? The valued life activities of older adults undergoing elective surgery. J Am Geriatr Soc 67(11):2305–2310. https://doi.org/10.1111/jgs.16102

Keon-Cohen Z, Loane H, Romero L et al (2025) Advance care planning and goals of care discussions in perioperative care: a scoping review. Br J Anaesth 134(5):1318–1332. https://doi.org/10.1016/j.bja.2025.01.031

Knoedler S, Schliermann R, Knoedler L et al (2023) Impact of sarcopenia on outcomes in surgical patients: a systematic review and meta-analysis. Int J Surg 109(12):4238–4262. https://doi.org/10.1097/JS9.0000000000000688

Kochar B, Ufere NN, Ritchie CS et al (2022) The 5Ms of geriatrics in gastroenterology: the path to creating age-friendly care for older adults with inflammatory bowel diseases and cirrhosis. Clin Transl Gastroenterol 13(1):e00445. https://doi.org/10.14309/ctg.0000000000000445

Li X, Wang Y, Liu J et al (2021) Effects of perioperative interventions for preventing postoperative delirium: a protocol for systematic review and meta-analysis of randomized controlled trials. Medicine (Baltimore) 100(29):e26662

Lin HS, Watts JN, Peel NM et al (2016) Frailty and post-operative outcomes in older surgical patients: a systematic review. BMC Geriatr 16:157. https://doi.org/10.1186/s12877-016-0329-8

Lujic S, Randall DA, Simpson JM et al (2022) Interaction effects of multimorbidity and frailty on adverse health outcomes in elderly hospitalised patients. Sci Rep 12(1):14139. https://doi.org/10.1038/s41598-022-18346-x

Marcantonio ER, Flacker JM, Wright RJ et al (2001) Reducing delirium after hip fracture: a randomized trial. J Am Geriatr Soc 49(5):516–522. https://doi.org/10.1046/j.1532-5415.2001.49108.x

Molenaar CJ, van Rooijen SJ, Fokkenrood HJ et al (2022) Prehabilitation versus no prehabilitation to improve functional capacity, reduce postoperative complications and improve quality of life in colorectal cancer surgery. Cochrane Database Syst Rev 5(5):CD013259

Molnar F, Huang A, Tinetti M (2017) Update: the public launch of the geriatric 5Ms. Can Geriatr Soc J CME. http://canadiangeriatrics.ca/wp-content/uploads/2017/04/UPDATE-THE-PUBLIC-LAUNCH-OF-THE-GERIATRIC-5MS.pdf

Morley JE, Argiles JM, Evans WJ et al (2010) Nutritional recommendations for the management of sarcopenia. J Am Med Dir Assoc 11(6):391–396. https://doi.org/10.1016/j.jamda.2010.04.014

Morley JE, Vellas B, van Kan GA et al (2013) Frailty consensus: a call to action. J Am Med Dir Assoc 14(6):392–397. https://doi.org/10.1016/j.jamda.2013.03.022

National Institute for Health and Care Excellence (2023) Hip fracture: management: clinical guideline 124. NICE, London

Nolan JP, Soar J, Kane AD et al (2024) Peri-operative decisions about cardiopulmonary resuscitation among adults as reported to the 7th National Audit Project of the Royal College of Anaesthetists. Anaesthesia 79(2):186–192. https://doi.org/10.1111/anae.16179

Oliver CM, Warnakulasuriya S, McGuckin D et al (2022) Delivery of drinking, eating and mobilising (DrEaMing) and its association with length of hospital stay after major noncardiac surgery: observational cohort study. Br J Anaesth 129(1):114–126. https://doi.org/10.1016/j.bja.2022.03.021

O'Mahony D, Cherubini A, Guiteras AR et al (2023) STOPP/START criteria for potentially inappropriate prescribing in older people: version 3. Eur Geriatr Med 14(4):625–632. https://doi.org/10.1007/s41999-023-00777-y

Partridge JS, Harari D, Martin FC, Dhesi JK (2014) The impact of pre-operative comprehensive geriatric assessment on postoperative outcomes in older patients undergoing scheduled surgery: a systematic review. Anaesthesia 69(Suppl 1):8–16

Peden CJ, Miller TR, Deiner SG et al (2021) Improving perioperative brain health: an expert consensus review of key actions for the perioperative care team. Br J Anaesth 126(2):423–432. https://doi.org/10.1016/j.bja.2020.10.037

Rockwood K, Song X, MacKnight C et al (2005) A global clinical measure of fitness and frailty in elderly people. CMAJ 173(5):489–495

Rosenberg IH (1997) Sarcopenia: origins and clinical relevance. J Nutr 127(5 Suppl):990S–991S. https://doi.org/10.1093/jn/127.5.990S

Rubenstein LZ, Stuck AE, Siu AL et al (1991) Impacts of geriatric evaluation and management programs on defined outcomes: overview of the evidence. J Am Geriatr Soc 39(9 Pt 2):8S–16S; discussion 17S–18S. https://doi.org/10.1111/j.1532-5415.1991.tb05927.x

Sing CW, Lin TC, Bartholomew S et al (2023) Global epidemiology of hip fractures: secular trends in incidence rate, post-fracture treatment, and all-cause mortality. J Bone Miner Res 38(8):1064–1075. https://doi.org/10.1002/jbmr.4821

Skořepa P, Ford KL, Alsuwaylihi A et al (2024) The impact of prehabilitation on outcomes in frail and high-risk patients undergoing major abdominal surgery: a systematic review and meta-analysis. Clin Nutr 43(3):629–648. https://doi.org/10.1016/j.clnu.2024.01.020

Stabenau HF, Becher RD, Gahbauer EA et al (2018) Functional trajectories before and after major surgery in older adults. Ann Surg 268(6):911–917. https://doi.org/10.1097/SLA.0000000000002659

Sun X, Liu W, Gao Y et al (2023) Comparative effectiveness of non-pharmacological interventions for frailty: a systematic review and network meta-analysis. Age Ageing 52(2):afad004. https://doi.org/10.1093/ageing/afad004

Swarbrick CJ, Partridge JSL (2022) Evidence-based strategies to reduce the incidence of postoperative delirium: a narrative review. Anaesthesia 77(Suppl 1):92–101. https://doi.org/10.1111/anae.15607

Tew GA, Ayyash R, Durrand J et al (2018) Clinical guideline and recommendations on pre-operative exercise training in patients awaiting major non-cardiac surgery. Anaesthesia 73(6):750–768. https://doi.org/10.1111/anae.14177

Thompson A, Fleischmann KE, Smilowitz NR et al (2024) 2024 AHA/ACC/ACS/ASNC/HRS/SCA/SCCT/SCMR/SVM guideline for perioperative cardiovascular management for noncardiac surgery: a report of the American College of Cardiology/American Heart Association Joint Committee on Clinical Practice Guidelines. Circulation 150(19):e351–e442. https://doi.org/10.1161/CIR.0000000000001285

Tsimopoulou I, Pasquali S, Howard R et al (2015) Psychological prehabilitation before cancer surgery: a systematic review. Ann Surg Oncol 22(13):4117–4123. https://doi.org/10.1245/s10434-015-4550-z

Whiteman AR, Dhesi JK, Walker D (2016) The high-risk surgical patient: a role for a multi-disciplinary team approach? Br J Anaesth 116(3):311–314. https://doi.org/10.1093/bja/aev355

World Health Organisation (2021) Ageing and health. World Health Organisation, Geneva. https://www.who.int/news-room/fact-sheets/detail/ageing-and-health

Frailty in the Context of Surgery

2

Amanda Goh and Terence Ong

Take-Home Messages

- Frailty is a multidimensional condition marked by reduced physiological reserve which increases the risk of complications after surgery.
- Frailty requires proactive identification with tools, such as the Clinical Frailty Scale (CFS), and tailored frailty-targeted interventions to improve outcomes.
- A comprehensive frailty pathway across the person's surgical journey requires investment in resources, education and collaboration among healthcare teams.

2.1 Introduction to Frailty

Frailty is a state of increased vulnerability in which the body's capacity to respond to external stressors, even seemingly minor ones, is reduced which increases the risk of adverse outcomes (Clegg et al. 2013). Although it is commonly seen among older people, frailty is not a consequence of ageing. Rather, it reflects a cumulative decline across several interrelated physiological systems which leads to an accelerated decrease in physiological reserve. The pathophysiological process driving this remains incompletely understood. A complex interplay involving chronic inflammation, cellular senescence, mitochondrial dysfunction, dysregulated nutrient sensing, hormonal changes and environmental factors has been proposed as drivers to the development and progression of frailty (Clegg et al. 2013; Kim and Rockwood

A. Goh
Geriatric Medicine Unit, Universiti Malaya Medical Centre, Kuala Lumpur, Malaysia

T. Ong (✉)
Department of Medicine, Faculty of Medicine, Universiti Malaya, Kuala Lumpur, Malaysia
e-mail: terence.ong@ummc.edu.my

K.-Y. Tan et al. (eds.), *Mastering Geriatric Surgery*,
https://doi.org/10.1007/978-981-95-0665-1_2

2024). This has given rise to the hypothesised 'frailty cycle', in which a downward spiral of decline is seen. Hence, frailty can present across a spectrum where it could be mild, moderate or severe. Several risk factors are associated with frailty, such as increasing age, obesity, malnutrition, physical inactivity, smoking, multimorbidity and cognitive impairment (Dent et al. 2023).

The prevalence of frailty varies across different regions, population cohorts and clinical settings. Its prevalence among community-dwelling older adults range from 4% to 59% (Collard et al. 2012). The prevalence of frailty was noted to be higher among individuals who were disabled, hospitalised or institutionalised. This could go to as high as 80% (Joseph et al. 2014). With ongoing population ageing, the number of people living with frailty is expected to increase significantly in the coming years.

A common misconception among healthcare professionals is that frailty can be easily identified through a person's outward appearance, physical expression, or end-of-bed assessment (Hubbard and Story 2015). This often leads to the assumption that someone who appears thin, weak or vulnerable must be frail. In reality, frailty is a complex and multidimensional syndrome that is not reliably identified based solely on physical appearance. It encompasses a range of factors, including diminished strength, endurance and physiological reserves, as well as cognitive and psychological components. Features that may not be immediately observable. As a result, someone who appears physically healthy may still be frail, while someone who is acutely unwell may appear 'frail-looking' (Rockwood and Theou 2020).

Two different models of frailty have been described. The first is the 'phenotype' or physical frailty model (Fried et al. 2001). This frailty phenotype model (Table 2.2) has been conceptualised as a biological condition, linked to, yet distinct from ageing and disability. It proposed five criteria (unintentional weight loss, self-reported exhaustion, low energy expenditure, slow gait speed and weak grip strength). Individuals with three or more of these criteria would be considered frail, and those with one or two considered 'pre-frail' (Fried et al. 2001). The second frailty model is known as the cumulative deficit model which views frailty as the result of an accumulation of deficits across various domains, which includes cognitive, medical, functional and social domains. In this model, the number of deficits indicates frailty, with more deficits an individual has indicating greater frailty severity. Disability and comorbidities are viewed as parts of frailty, rather than separate conditions that are caused by frailty (Rockwood and Mitnitski 2007).

2.2 Frailty in the Surgical Setting

The number of older people undergoing surgery is increasing. This growth exceeds what is seen in other age groups. Hospital administrative data from England reported an almost twofold increase in the number of people aged 75 years or more undergoing surgery between 1999 and 2015 (Fowler et al. 2019). A US national anaesthesia registry reported that 34% of all surgeries performed over 3 years from 2010 onwards involved a person aged 65 years or more. The majority of these surgeries were orthopaedic and ophthalmology surgeries (Deiner et al. 2014). Projections estimate that by 2030, one in five surgical procedures will be performed on someone over the age of 75 years (Fowler et al. 2019).

Frailty is prevalent among 31% of older people on surgical wards (Doody et al. 2022). However, it varies across surgical specialities due to differences in patient characteristics, surgical complexity, elective or emergency setting, and variations in frailty assessment tools used (Table 2.1). For example, 23% of patients undergoing elective orthopaedic surgery were diagnosed as frail compared to 53% among those presenting with acute hip fractures (Van de Ree et al. 2019; Johnson et al. 2019). In oncology, frailty affects 25% of those undergoing elective cystectomy, and 39% of those requiring emergency general surgery for cancer complications (Khan et al. 2019; Chappidi et al. 2016). In vascular surgery, the incidence of aortic aneurysms and peripheral arterial disease rises with age, and approximately 52% of elective vascular patients being frail (Partridge et al. 2015).

Table 2.1 Prevalence of frailty across surgical specialities (all observational studies)

Surgical speciality	Author (year)	Country	Types of surgery	Total participants (*N*)	Mean age (years ± SD)	Gender (%) (M:F)	Frailty measure	Prevalence of frailty
Vascular surgery	Visser et al. (2019)	The Netherlands	Open aortic surgery (15%) Endovascular procedures (33%) Carotid surgery (25%) Peripheral bypass surgery (18%) Elective major limb amputation surgery (transfemoral, through knee disarticulation and transtibial) (9%)	630	71.8 ± 6.8	77.6:22.4	Groningen Frailty Indicator (GFI)	22.3%
	Mandelbaum et al. (2021)	The United States	Carotid endarterectomy (85%) Carotid artery stenting (15%)	1,426,343	70.9 ± 9.7	58.6:41.4	Johns Hopkins Adjusted Clinical Groups (ACG)	4.2%

(continued)

Table 2.1 (continued)

Surgical speciality	Author (year)	Country	Types of surgery	Total participants (*N*)	Mean age (years ± SD)	Gender (%) (M:F)	Frailty measure	Prevalence of frailty
Cardiac surgery	Afilalo et al. (2012)	The United States/ Canada	Isolated CABG (60%) Valve replacement/repair (18%) Valve + CABG (22%)	152	75.9 ± 4.4	66:34	Cardiovascular Health Study (CHS) Frailty Scale	20.0%
	Ahuja et al. (2024)	Australia/ New Zealand	CABG (58.2%) Valvular heart surgery (31%) CABG + valvular (10.8%)	46,928	68.6 ± 10.8	75.8:24.2	Clinical Frailty Scale (CFS)	6.7%
Orthopaedic surgery	Chen et al. (2019)	Taiwan	Surgery for hip fracture: Percutaneous cannulated screws (6%) Sliding hip screws (6%) Intra-medullary nail (proximal femoral nail (46%) Bipolar hemiarthroplasty (42%)	245	78.0 ± 11.0	32:68	Chinese-Canadian Study of Health and Aging Clinical Frailty Scale (CSHA-CFS)	22.4%
	Sun et al. (2021)	China	Elective orthopaedic surgery	313	73.9 ± 7.2	30:70	Clinical Frailty Scale (CFS)	29.7%
	Ninomiya et al. (2023)	Japan	Total hip arthroplasty	518	73.6 ± 5.9	9.3:90.7	Fried's modified phenotype	11.4%
	Flexman et al. (2016)	The United States	Elective/semi-elective spine surgery: Lumbosacral procedure (66%) Thoracic procedure (1.6%) Cervical procedure (32.4%)	52,671	56.1 ± 14.5	52:48	Modified Frailty Index (mFI)	4.0%

Table 2.1 (continued)

Surgical speciality	Author (year)	Country	Types of surgery	Total participants (*N*)	Mean age (years ± SD)	Gender (%) (M:F)	Frailty measure	Prevalence of frailty
Colorectal surgery	Niemeläinen et al. (2021)	Finland	Open surgery (24.2%) Laparoscopic (66.5%) Conversion (9.3%)	161	84.5	40:60	Clinical Frailty Scale (CFS)	26.9%
General surgery	Parmar et al. (2021)	The United Kingdom	Emergency laparotomy: Adhesiolysis (25%) Small bowel resection (21%) Stoma formation (17%) Right colectomy (16%) Hartmann's procedure (15%) Others (6%)	937	76.0 ± 6.8	43:57	Clinical Frailty Scale (CFS)	20.0%
Ophthalmology surgery	Varadaraj et al. (2021)	The United States	Cataract surgery	557	76.0	42:58	Fried's Frailty Score	11.0%
Urology surgery	Chappidi et al. (2016)	The United States	Radical cystectomy	2679	68.7 ± 10.9	81:19	Modified Frailty Index (mFI)	24.6%

SD standard deviation, *CABG* coronary artery bypass graft, *M:F* male:female

2.3 Clinical Burden of Frailty in Surgery

The clinical burden of frailty in surgery is substantial as it significantly impacts both immediate and long-term outcomes. People living with frailty have low physiological reserve which makes them more vulnerable to unfavourable surgical outcomes regardless of whether the surgery is elective or emergency. A meta-analysis of 16 studies with 444,885 patients who were identified as frail reported that frailty was an independent risk factor for poor outcomes across various surgical specialities, such as gastrointestinal, vascular, orthopaedic, urogenital, head and neck, emergency, neurological, oncological, cardiothoracic and general surgery (Panayi et al. 2019). Frailty was associated with a fourfold increased risk of 30-day mortality. It also significantly increased the risk for surgical complications, including major complications (Clavien-Dindo grade >III), wound-related complications, discharged to institutional care and hospital readmission (Panayi et al. 2019).

Additionally, complications and adverse surgical outcomes were more prevalent in patients with severe frailty (Panayi et al. 2019; George et al. 2021). For instance, rates of pulmonary complications such as pneumonia and respiratory failure following emergency abdominal surgery were 12%, 39% and 52% among those not frail, frail and severely frail, respectively. Cardiac and renal complications were more common in frail groups. Rates ranged from 7% to 21% for cardiac issues (e.g. cardiac arrest, arrhythmia, heart failure) and 5% to 18% for renal issues (e.g. acute kidney injury, dialysis, electrolyte abnormalities) across the frailty spectrum (Snitkjær et al. 2024). In addition to organ-specific complications, surgical site infections (SSIs) were also a common postoperative issue among frail older adults. For instance, frailty in orthopaedic patients undergoing total hip or knee arthroplasty is strongly associated with an elevated risk of SSIs, particularly deep SSIs like joint infections, rather than superficial ones (Wu et al. 2024). These postoperative complications contribute to slower recovery, greater rehabilitation needs and an extended time to regain independence in activities of daily living resulting in longer hospital stays compared to non-frail patients.

Among frail adults who underwent non-cardiac surgery, frailty increased 30-day mortality by 3–9 times, and 7–34 times among those classified as very frail, depending on the type of surgery. Ninety-day mortality was 3–9 times higher among those frail, and 6–36 times among those severely frail (George et al. 2021). Even in patients undergoing major emergency abdominal surgery, mortality rates rose steeply with increasing levels of frailty. Thirty-day mortality rates were 18.3% and 33.3%, respectively, among frail and severely frail patients. By 90 days, the mortality rates increased further to 26% among those frail and 46% in those severely frail (Snitkjær et al. 2024) (Fig. 2.1).

Delirium, characterised by acute confusion, fluctuating consciousness and impaired attention, is more prevalent among frail older adults after surgery. Delirium contributes to longer hospital stays and can impede recovery following surgery. A systematic review of 20 cohort studies involving 4568 patients reported that frailty conferred a threefold higher risk of postoperative delirium (Liu et al. 2022). Furthermore, postoperative delirium among frail older adults were associated with

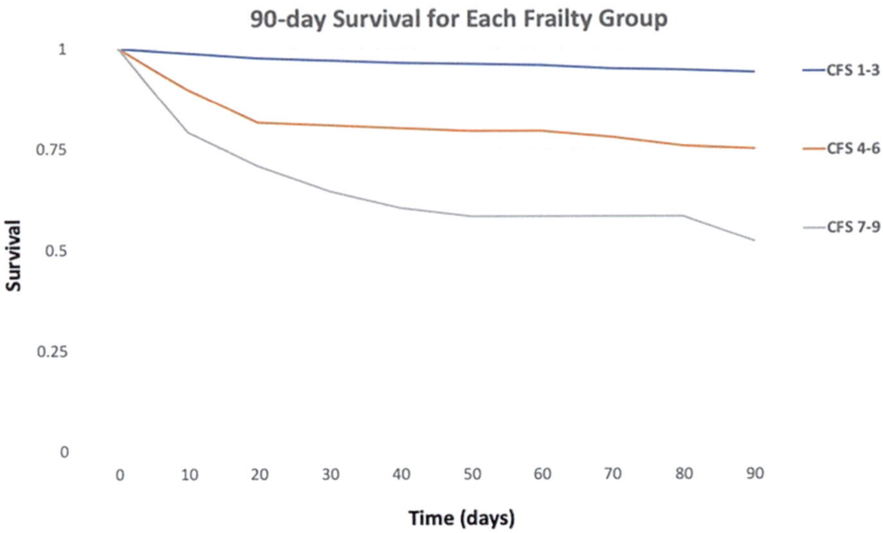

Fig. 2.1 Survival curves showing the 90-day survival for each frailty group among patients after major emergency abdominal surgery. CFS 1–3, not frail; CFS 4–6, frail; CFS 7–9, severely frail. *CFS* Clinical Frailty Scale. (Adapted from Snitkjær et al. 2024)

a reduction in mobility, more so than just frailty alone (Gandossi et al. 2023). This deterioration can result in temporary or permanent disability and dependency, often necessitating in the need for care at home or in a care facility. In one study, frailty was associated with care home admission among people after vascular surgery, such as aneurysm repairs and bypasses (Arya et al. 2016). Similar findings were observed in cardiac surgery patients, where both frail and pre-frail older adults were five times more likely to require intermediate care post-discharge (Lee et al. 2021).

2.4 Identification and Assessment of Frailty

Frailty is common among older adults undergoing surgery and is strongly associated with poorer outcomes. Hence, its identification is integral to the surgical management of the patient. Identifying those with or at risk of frailty enables surgical teams to stratify risk, facilitate shared decision-making and tailor intervention appropriately to the individual's need. Frailty assessments capture the complex interplay between physical, cognitive and functional ability of the older adult. It also reflects underlying physiological reserve. This provides a more comprehensive evaluation of the person's health beyond conventional variables such as chronological age or the American Society of Anesthesiologists (ASA) grade. For certain outcomes like mortality, studies have reported that frailty was a better predictor than either age or ASA grade (Farhat et al. 2012). All this contributes towards a more informed discussion with the individual of the potential benefits, risks and treatment options (surgical, non-surgical, or different surgical approaches).

For many older adults living with frailty, they may also have co-existing conditions and geriatric syndromes, such as cognitive impairment, sarcopenia, cachexia, polypharmacy and multimorbidity. Hence, identifying frailty would not only initiate frailty-targeted intervention but also trigger detection of these other co-existing conditions for further management. Numerous frailty assessment tools have been developed. For instance, one systematic review identified 42 different tools have been used in vascular surgery alone (Welsh et al. 2023). Some frailty tools identify physical manifestations of frailty (e.g. Fried Frailty Criteria which measures unintentional weight loss, hand grip strength, fatigue, slow gait and physical activity), utilise a pictorial infographic, or visual scale (e.g. Clinical Frailty Scale), are in the form of a questionnaire (e.g. FRAIL scale, Groningen Frailty Index or Edmonton Frailty Scale) or are data-driven where data is collated from medical records (e.g. Hospital Frailty Risk Score or electronic Frailty Index). It is worth bearing in mind that frailty assessment tools were developed and evaluated to predict outcomes rather than guide clinical or surgical decision-making (Buta et al. 2015). Nonetheless, their integration into perioperative workflows can enhance risk stratification and support more person-centred care. The more commonly used tools are briefly described here.

The Clinical Frailty Scale (CFS) (Fig. 2.2) is a clinician-rated tool that evolved from the Canadian Study of Health and Aging (Rockwood 2005). The CFS summarises overall level of fitness, or frailty, of the older person on a scale ranging from

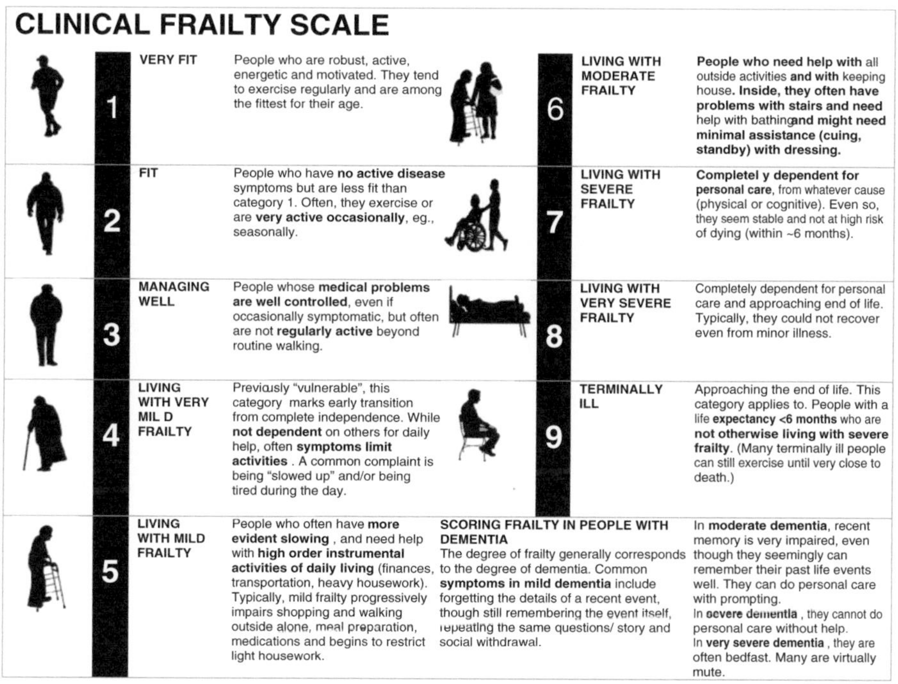

Fig. 2.2 The Clinical Frailty Scale. (Adapted from Rockwood and Theou 2020)

Table 2.2 Fried Frailty Criteria (Bambrick et al. 2021)

Criteria	Definition
Unintentional weight loss	**Meets criteria for weight loss if**: Self-reported loss of 10 lb (4.5 kg) in last year, or BMI <18.5 kg/m^2
Exhaustion	**Meets criteria for exhaustion if answer**: Self-reporting feeling lack of energy 'every day', or 'every week' in the last 4 weeks
Slowness	**Meets criteria for slow walking speed over 15 ft (4.57 m) if**: *Men* Height ≤173 cm, cut off ≥7 s Height >173 cm, cut off ≥6 s *Women* Height ≤159 cm, cut off ≥7 s Height >159 cm, cut off ≥6 s
Low physical activity level	**Meets criteria for low activity if**: Walk less than 30 min/day, or sit for most of the day
Weakness	**Meets criteria for grip strength weakness if**: *Men* ≤29 kg for BMI ≤24 ≤30 kg for BMI 24.1–26 ≤30 kg for BMI 26.1–28 ≤32 kg for BMI >28 *Women* ≤17 kg for BMI ≤23 ≤17.3 kg for BMI 23.1–26 ≤18 kg for BMI 26.1–29 ≤21 kg for BMI >29

BMI body mass index

1 (very fit) to 8 (living with severe frailty), and 9 (terminally ill). It is designed to be intuitive and easily used by non-geriatric medicine specialists (Theou et al. 2021). Its simplicity has made it the most widely used frailty tool in the surgical setting. The CFS is also useful in settings where rapid assessment is necessary due to time and resource constraints, such as during emergency care or critical illness. Hence, it has been incorporated into several perioperative guidelines, such as those from the Centre for Perioperative Care (CPOC) in the United Kingdom. This guideline recommends that all patients over 65 years of age, as well as those younger but are at risk, be assessed for frailty using the CFS preoperatively regardless of elective or emergency surgery. If a patient is identified as frail, they should further undergo a Comprehensive Geriatric Assessment (CGA) and optimisation prior to surgery. The UK National Emergency Laparatomy Audit (NELA) has also established standards for frailty assessment using CFS for patients aged 65 and over.

The Fried Frailty Criteria is another widely used tool for assessing frailty (Table 2.2). It comprised five key components that reflect physical capabilities and vulnerability in older adults.

An individual is classified as frail if they meet three or more of these criteria, pre-frail if they exhibit one or two and non-frail if none are present. This assessment requires scales for body weight, height measurement, a course to measure gait speed, stopwatch and a hand dynamometer. Such equipment may not always be routinely available. Also, this frailty assessment can take time to complete.

The FRAIL scale is a concise and easy-to-administer screening tool used to assess frailty in older adults, based on five key components (Van Kan et al. 2008). This includes Fatigue (self-reported tiredness), Resistance (difficulty walking up one flight of stairs), Ambulation (difficulty walking 100 m), Illnesses (the number of chronic conditions such as hypertension, diabetes or cardiovascular disease) and Loss of weight (self-reported unintentional weight loss). The presence of any of the five components is scored. A score of 0 indicates healthy status, 1–2 indicates pre-frail and 3–5 indicates frail.

Lastly, the Edmonton Frail Scale (EFS) is a comprehensive 10-item tool designed to assess frailty in older adults (Rolfson et al. 2006). These items include cognition (memory and orientation), functional status (ability to perform activities of daily living) and mood (signs of depression). The scale also assesses nutrition, polypharmacy and social support to provide a holistic view of an individual's frailty. By evaluating multiple aspects of health and well-being, the EFS helps clinicians stratify patients based on their risk of surgical complications, functional decline and other adverse outcomes. Subsequently, it can guide tailored treatment plans, identify patients in need of additional support and inform preoperative care to optimise outcomes in frail older patients.

Each tool identifies frailty differently. No frailty assessment tool has been considered 'the best' to be used in clinical practice. Regardless, what is most important is that formal frailty assessment is done. The 'best' tool to use is determined by respective clinical teams, based on the intended domains to be assessed, their familiarity and experience with the tool to be used.

2.5 Managing Frailty in the Context of Surgery

Frailty should be identified and addressed in both elective and emergency surgical contexts. In the elective setting, preoperative frailty assessment can support surgical risk stratification, inform clinical decision-making, optimise modifiable aspects of the frailty syndrome and aid prediction of postoperative outcomes. This can facilitate informed discussion with the person on the risks and benefits of surgery, and perhaps consider non-surgical alternatives, if appropriate. Thus, enabling shared decision-making that aligns with the person's goals and wishes. If the decision is not to proceed with surgery because the risks far outweigh the benefits, then treatment can promptly transition to alternative options.

For the person considering surgery, personalised preoperative management can be tailored to address the specific needs of frail patients. Frailty assessments can also influence the choice of surgery, as different approaches carry varying risk profiles. Additionally, frailty commonly co-exists with conditions such as multimorbidity, disability, cognitive impairment, malnutrition and sarcopenia which are modifiable and could be optimised. Addressing this can potentially translate to better surgical outcomes. This highlights the role for CGA and value of multidisciplinary prehabilitation (Skořepa et al. 2024). Prehabilitation has been shown to be an effective intervention to modify surgical risk and will be discussed in other sections of this book. Bearing in mind that frailty reflects a reduced ability to withstand a stressor event, and in this case surgery, identifying these risks in the preoperative period allows teams to proactively plan management in the postoperative stage. This includes early mobilisation, minimising functional decline, regular monitoring for delirium, nutritional support and careful management of comorbidities as targets for intervention in the recovery period. All these elements are central to the Enhanced Recovery After Surgery (ERAS) protocol. ERAS too has been shown to be beneficial for older adults undergoing surgery, many of whom are also frail.

In the emergency setting, frailty assessment is unlikely to make a difference in modifying the person's risk profile. However, it is valuable to guide clinicians determine the management plan. High-risk frail patients undergoing emergency surgery require close observation by experienced clinical teams in critical care areas, such as intensive care or high dependency unit. It also drives discussion around escalation and ceilings of care. Surgery may be futile in some of these situations, and consideration of other measures such as symptom control or palliative care may be more appropriate.

2.6 Frailty Pathway in Surgery

Frailty ultimately needs to be comprehensively managed across the entire surgical pathway. This pathway needs to be frailty-ready from the person's initial presentation, either when they present initially to primary care or as an emergency to the emergency department, all the way to their discharge and recovery following surgery (Fig. 2.3) (CPOC 2021). This 'frailty pathway' requires seamless transitions of care and information from primary care/emergency department, into the surgical setting and its transition back into the community. The identification of frailty, and those at risk of becoming frail, may have taken place for the first time as part of their surgical problem. Once the acute surgical period is over, the older person will need to have their frailty and other geriatric syndromes managed in appropriate clinical settings, for example, geriatric medicine clinics or primary care. This should be done alongside their longer-term recovery and rehabilitation. Information of the person's frailty status, care goals and treatment direction needs to be documented and made readily available to all relevant health providers.

Within the hospital setting is where the older adult will have the most clinical engagement. The cornerstone of a frailty-ready service here is the presence of a multidisciplinary team consisting of, but not limited to, surgeons, physicians with expertise in frailty, anaesthetists, therapists, dietitians and nurses. Such a team working collaboratively can help monitor and manage the issues related to frailty,

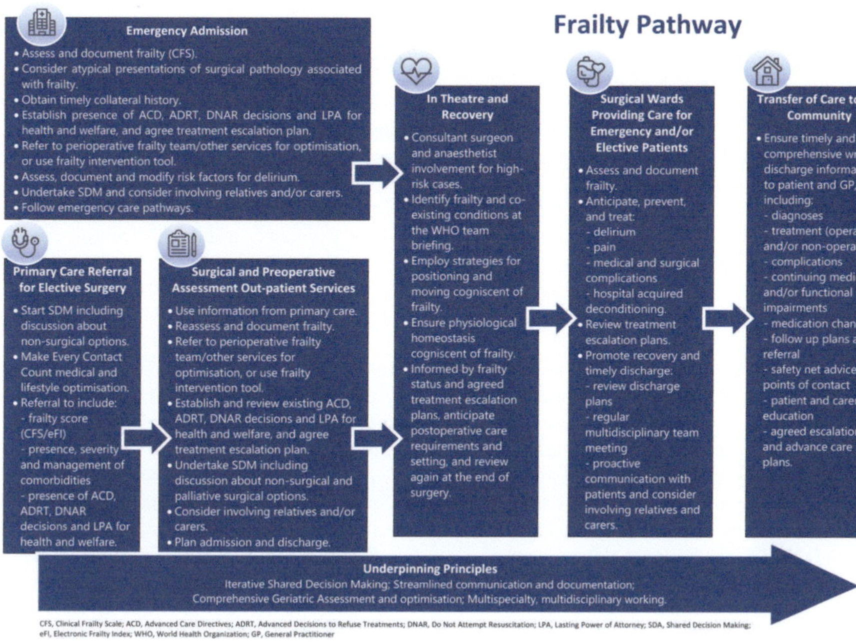

Fig. 2.3 Frailty pathway. (Adapted from the UK Guideline for Perioperative Care for People Living with Frailty Undergoing Elective and Emergency Surgery)

including cognitive dysfunction, nutritional deficits and physical deconditioning. The goal is to provide comprehensive care that addresses the medical, psychological and functional needs of the frail older person, ensuring better surgical outcomes. Training, education, audit, quality improvement and governance will need to be embedded within the service too. To ensure successful implementation and sustainability of this pathway, service providers and commissioners must work closely with healthcare professionals to ensure resources are available.

2.7 Conclusion

Frailty influences the outcome of older adults undergoing surgery. Its management requires the prompt identification of frailty which supports the decision-making process between the person and their clinical team. For those who proceed to have surgery, frailty guides the preoperative, intraoperative and postoperative management. This requires a workforce that is trained and well-equipped. Hospital commissioners and service providers must invest in this to ensure resources and mechanisms are in place to establish surgical services that are frailty-ready.

References

Afilalo J, Mottillo S, Eisenberg MJ, Alexander KP, Noiseux N, Perrault LP, Morin JF, Langlois Y, Ohayon SM, Monette J, Boivin JF, Shahian DM, Bergman H (2012) Addition of frailty and disability to cardiac surgery risk scores identifies elderly patients at high risk of mortality or major morbidity. Circ Cardiovasc Qual Outcomes 5(2):222–228. https://doi.org/10.1161/CIRCOUTCOMES.111.963157

Ahuja A, Baker T, Ramanan M (2024) Impact of frailty on outcomes after cardiac surgery. J Thorac Cardiovasc Surg. pii: S0022-5223(24)00511-7. Advance online publication. https://doi.org/10.1016/j.jtcvs.2024.05.025

Arya S, Long CA, Brahmbhatt R, Shafii S, Brewster LP, Veeraswamy R et al (2016) Preoperative frailty increases risk of nonhome discharge after elective vascular surgery in home-dwelling patients. Ann Vasc Surg 35:19–29

Bambrick P, Phelan N, Grant E, Byrne T, Harrison M, Mulcahy R, Cooke J (2021) Diet and Exercise for FRAILty (DEFRAIL): protocol for a study to examine the effect of a novel community-based group exercise and nutritional intervention, designed to reverse frailty in older adults. BMJ Open 11(6):e042408. https://doi.org/10.1136/bmjopen-2020-042408

Buta BJ, Walston JD, Godino JG, Park M, Kalyani RR, Xue Q, Bandeen-Roche K, Varadhan R (2015) Frailty assessment instruments: systematic characterization of the uses and contexts of highly-cited instruments. Ageing Res Rev 26:53–61. https://doi.org/10.1016/j.arr.2015.12.003

Chappidi MR, Kates M, Patel HD, Tosoian JJ, Kaye DR, Sopko NA, Lascano D, Liu JJ, McKiernan J, Bivalacqua TJ (2016) Frailty as a marker of adverse outcomes in patients with bladder cancer undergoing radical cystectomy. Urol Oncol 34(6):256.e1–256.e6. https://doi.org/10.1016/j.urolonc.2015.12.010

Chen CL, Chen CM, Wang CY, Ko PW, Chen CH, Hsieh CP, Chiu HC (2019) Frailty is associated with an increased risk of major adverse outcomes in elderly patients following surgical treatment of hip fracture. Sci Rep 9(1):19135. https://doi.org/10.1038/s41598-019-55459-2

Clegg A, Young J, Iliffe S, Rikkert MO, Rockwood K (2013) Frailty in elderly people. Lancet (London, England) 381(9868):752–762. https://doi.org/10.1016/S0140-6736(12)62167-9

Collard RM, Boter H, Schoevers RA, Olde Rikkert MG (2012) The prevalence of frailty in community-dwelling older persons: a systematic review. J Am Geriatr Soc 60(8):1487–1492. https://doi.org/10.1111/j.1532-5415.2012.04054.x

CPOC Publishes Guideline for People Living with Frailty in Collaboration with the BGS (2021) Centre for perioperative care. https://cpoc.org.uk/cpoc-publishes-guideline-people-living-frailty-collaboration-bgs

Deiner S, Westlake B, Dutton RP (2014) J Am Geriatr Soc 62(5):829–835. https://doi.org/10.1111/jgs.12794

Dent E, Hanlon P, Sim M, Jylhävä J, Liu Z, Vetrano DL, Stolz E, Pérez-Zepeda MU, Crabtree DR, Nicholson C, Job J, Ambagtsheer RC, Ward PR, Shi SM, Huynh Q, Hoogendijk EO (2023) Recent developments in frailty identification, management, risk factors and prevention: a narrative review of leading journals in geriatrics and gerontology. Ageing Res Rev 91:102082. https://doi.org/10.1016/j.arr.2023.102082

Doody P, Asamane EA, Aunger JA, Swales B, Lord JM, Greig CA, Whittaker AC (2022) The prevalence of frailty and pre-frailty among geriatric hospital inpatients and its association with economic prosperity and healthcare expenditure: a systematic review and meta-analysis of 467,779 geriatric hospital inpatients. Ageing Res Rev 80:101666. https://doi.org/10.1016/j.arr.2022.101666

Farhat JS, Velanovich V, Falvo AJ, Horst HM, Swartz A, Patton JH, Rubinfeld IS (2012) Are the frail destined to fail? Frailty index as predictor of surgical morbidity and mortality in the elderly. J Trauma Acute Care Surg 72(6):1526–1531. https://doi.org/10.1097/ta.0b013e3182542fab

Flexman AM, Charest-Morin R, Stobart L, Street J, Ryerson CJ (2016) Frailty and postoperative outcomes in patients undergoing surgery for degenerative spine disease. Spine J 16(11):1315–1323. https://doi.org/10.1016/j.spinee.2016.06.017

Fowler AJ, Abbott TEF, Prowle J, Pearse RM (2019) Age of patients undergoing surgery. Br J Surg 106(8):1012–1018. https://doi.org/10.1002/bjs.11148

Fried LP, Tangen C, Walston J et al (2001) Frailty in older adults: evidence for a phenotype. J Gerontol 56A:M1–M11

Gandossi CM, Zambon A, Ferrara MC, Tassistro E, Castoldi G, Colombo F, Mussi C, Martini E, Sergi G, Coin A, Zatti G, Trevisan C, Volpato S, Ungar A, Bellelli G, GIOG 2.0 Study Group, Società Italiana di Gerontologia e Geriatria (SIGG) (2023) Frailty and post-operative delirium influence on functional status in patients with hip fracture: the GIOG 2.0 study. Aging Clin Exp Res 35(11):2499–2506. https://doi.org/10.1007/s40520-023-02522-8

George EL, Hall DE, Youk A, Chen R, Kashikar A, Trickey AW, Varley PR, Shireman PK, Shinall MC Jr, Massarweh NN, Johanning J, Arya S (2021) Association between patient frailty and postoperative mortality across multiple noncardiac surgical specialties. JAMA Surg 156(1):e205152. https://doi.org/10.1001/jamasurg.2020.5152

Hubbard R, Story D (2015) Does frailty lie in the eyes of the beholder? Heart Lung Circ 24(6):525–526. https://doi.org/10.1016/j.hlc.2015.01.018

Johnson RL, Abdel MP, Frank RD, Chamberlain AM, Habermann EB, Mantilla CB (2019) Impact of frailty on outcomes after primary and revision total hip arthroplasty. J Arthroplast 34(1):56–64.e5. https://doi.org/10.1016/j.arth.2018.09.078

Joseph B, Pandit V, Zangbar B et al (2014) Superiority of frailty over age in predicting outcomes among geriatric trauma patients: a prospective analysis. JAMA Surg 149:766–772. https://doi.org/10.1001/jamasurg.2014.296

Khan M, Jehan F, Zeeshan M, Kulvatunyou N, Fain MJ, Saljuqi AT, O'Keeffe T, Joseph B (2019) Failure to rescue after emergency general surgery in geriatric patients: does frailty matter? J Surg Res 233:397–402. https://doi.org/10.1016/j.jss.2018.08.033

Kim DH, Rockwood K (2024) Frailty in older adults. N Engl J Med 391(6):538–548. https://doi.org/10.1056/nejmra2301292

Lee JA, Yanagawa B, An KR, Arora RC, Verma S, Friedrich JO, Canadian Cardiovascular Surgery Meta-Analysis Working Group (2021) Frailty and pre-frailty in cardiac surgery: a systematic review and meta-analysis of 66,448 patients. J Cardiothorac Surg 16(1):184. https://doi.org/10.1186/s13019-021-01541-8

Liu CY, Gong N, Liu W (2022) The association between preoperative frailty and postoperative delirium: a systematic review and meta-analysis. J Perianesth Nurs 37(1):53–62.e1. https://doi.org/10.1016/j.jopan.2020.12.006

Mandelbaum AD, Hadaya J, Ulloa JG, Patel R, McCallum JC, De Virgilio C, Benharash P (2021) Impact of frailty on clinical outcomes after carotid artery revascularization. Ann Vasc Surg 74:111–121. https://doi.org/10.1016/j.avsg.2020.12.039

Niemeläinen S, Huhtala H, Andersen J, Ehrlich A, Haukijärvi E, Koikkalainen S, Koskensalo S, Kössi J, Mattila A, Pinta T, Uotila-Nieminen M, Vihervaara H, Hyöty M, Jämsen E (2021) The Clinical Frailty Scale is a useful tool for predicting postoperative complications following elective colon cancer surgery at the age of 80 years and above: a prospective, multicentre observational study. Colorectal Dis 23(7):1824–1836. https://doi.org/10.1111/codi.15689

Ninomiya K, Takahira N, Ikeda T, Suzuki K, Sato R, Kazuo H (2023) Prevalence of frailty and associated factors among community-dwelling older adults after total hip arthroplasty. Hip Int 33(3):397–403. https://doi.org/10.1177/11207000211048180

Panayi AC, Orkaby AR, Sakthivel D, Endo Y, Varon D, Roh D, Orgill DP, Neppl RL, Javedan H, Bhasin S, Sinha I (2019) Impact of frailty on outcomes in surgical patients: a systematic review and meta-analysis. Am J Surg 218(2):393–400. https://doi.org/10.1016/j.amjsurg.2018.11.020

Parmar KL, Law J, Carter B, Hewitt J, Boyle JM, Casey P, Maitra I, Farrell IS, Pearce L, Moug SJ, ELF Study Group (2021) Frailty in older patients undergoing emergency laparotomy: results from the UK Observational Emergency Laparotomy and Frailty (ELF) Study. Ann Surg 273(4):709–718. https://doi.org/10.1097/SLA.0000000000003402

Partridge JS, Fuller M, Harari D, Taylor PR, Martin FC, Dhesi JK (2015) Frailty and poor functional status are common in arterial vascular surgical patients and affect postoperative outcomes. Int J Surg (London, England) 18:57–63. https://doi.org/10.1016/j.ijsu.2015.04.037

Rockwood K (2005) A global clinical measure of fitness and frailty in elderly people. Can Med Assoc J 173(5):489–495. https://doi.org/10.1503/cmaj.050051

Rockwood K, Mitnitski A (2007) Frailty in relation to the accumulation of deficits. J Gerontol A Biol Sci Med Sci 62:722–727. https://doi.org/10.1093/gerona/62.7.722

Rockwood K, Theou O (2020) Using the Clinical Frailty Scale in allocating scarce health care resources. Can Geriatr J 23:254–259. https://doi.org/10.5770/cgj.23.467

Rolfson DB, Majumdar SR, Tsuyuki RT, Tahir A, Rockwood K (2006) Validity and reliability of the Edmonton Frail Scale. Age Ageing 35(5):526–529. https://doi.org/10.1093/ageing/afl041

Skořepa P, Ford KL, Alsuwaylihi A, O'Connor D, Prado CM, Gomez D, Lobo DN (2024) The impact of prehabilitation on outcomes in frail and high-risk patients undergoing major abdominal surgery: a systematic review and meta-analysis. Clin Nutr 43(3):629–648. https://doi.org/10.1016/j.clnu.2024.01.020

Snitkjær C, Rehné Jensen L, Soylu LÍ, Hauge C, Kvist M, Jensen TK, Kokotovic D, Burcharth J (2024) Impact of clinical frailty on surgical and non-surgical complications after major emergency abdominal surgery. BJS Open 8(3):zrae039. https://doi.org/10.1093/bjsopen/zrae039

Sun X, Shen Y, Ji M, Feng S, Gao Y, Yang J, Shen J (2021) Frailty is an independent risk factor of one-year mortality after elective orthopedic surgery: a prospective cohort study. Aging 13(5):7190–7198. https://doi.org/10.18632/aging.202576

Theou O, Pérez-Zepeda MU, Van Der Valk AM, Searle SD, Howlett SE, Rockwood K (2021) A classification tree to assist with routine scoring of the Clinical Frailty Scale. Age Ageing 50(4):1406–1411. https://doi.org/10.1093/ageing/afab006

van de Ree CLP, Landers MJF, Kruithof N, de Munter L, Slaets JPJ, Gosens T, de Jongh MAC (2019) Effect of frailty on quality of life in elderly patients after hip fracture: a longitudinal study. BMJ Open 9(7):e025941. https://doi.org/10.1136/bmjopen-2018-025941

Van Kan GA, Rolland YM, Morley JE, Vellas B (2008) Frailty: toward a clinical definition. J Am Med Dir Assoc 9(2):71–72. https://doi.org/10.1016/j.jamda.2007.11.005

Varadaraj V, Chung S, Sheehan OC, Roth D, Schein OD, Bandeen-Roche K, Swenor BK (2021) Post-cataract surgery health outcomes in frail older patients. Invest Ophthalmol Vis Sci 62(8):63

Visser L, Banning LBD, El Moumni M, Zeebregts CJ, Pol RA (2019) The effect of frailty on outcome after vascular surgery. Eur J Vasc Endovasc Surg 58(5):762–769. https://doi.org/10.1016/j.ejvs.2019.04.031

Welsh SA, Pearson RC, Hussey K, Brittenden J, Orr DJ, Quinn T (2023) A systematic review of frailty assessment tools used in vascular surgery research. J Vasc Surg 78(6):1567–1579.e14. https://doi.org/10.1016/j.jvs.2023.06.010

Wu G, Cui C, Song Q (2024) Frailty and the incidence of surgical site infection after total hip or knee arthroplasty: a meta-analysis. Surgeon. pii: S1479-666X(24)00081-7. Advance online publication. https://doi.org/10.1016/j.surge.2024.07.008

Geriatric Assessment Models for the Frail Older Person

3

Matthew Zhixuan Chen

Take-Home Messages

- The prevalence of frailty is increasing in tandem with age.
- Frailty puts older surgical patients at risk of developing adverse outcomes.
- The decision to operate in frail older adults requires careful consideration and discussion based on overall risk–benefit assessment and individual goals and preferences.
- A tailored approach to preoperative, intraoperative and postoperative care that incorporates the comprehensive geriatric assessment (CGA) is required for frail older patients who may have unique vulnerabilities and complex health profiles, and can lead to improved outcomes.

3.1 Introduction

The world is ageing rapidly. From 1990 to 2019, the proportion of the world's population aged 65 years and above increased from 6% to 9%, and this figure is projected to nearly double to 16% by 2050 (UN, Department of Economic and Social Affairs, Population Division 2020). The prevalence of multimorbidity and frailty increases in tandem with age, with time spent in successive frailty states growing longer as

M. Z. Chen (✉)
Division of Geriatric Medicine, Department of Medicine, National University Hospital, Singapore, Singapore

Department of Medicine, Yong Loo Lin School of Medicine, National University of Singapore, Singapore, Singapore
e-mail: zhixuan_matthew_chen@nuhs.edu.sg

K.-Y. Tan et al. (eds.), *Mastering Geriatric Surgery*,
https://doi.org/10.1007/978-981-95-0665-1_3

frailty progresses (Chowdhury et al. 2023; Ofori-Asenso et al. 2019; Walsh et al. 2023). Unsurprisingly, the incidence of older adults who require surgery is growing as well, with highest rates of elective and non-elective procedures observed in the youngest-old and oldest-old, respectively (Becher et al. 2023; Deiner et al. 2014). What is more concerning is that more frail older adults have been undergoing major surgery, which has been attributed to an increase in non-elective surgeries being performed in this group (Becher et al. 2023).

While many conditions in later life are amenable to surgical intervention, the decision to operate in older adults requires careful consideration and discussion based on overall risk–benefit assessment and individual goals and preferences. A tailored approach to preoperative, intraoperative and postoperative care is required for frail older patients who may have unique vulnerabilities and complex health profiles. Comprehensive geriatric assessment (CGA) models provide an essential framework for evaluating and optimising the health of these patients, which can lead to improved surgical outcomes.

This chapter explores key geriatric assessment models and their application in the surgical care of frail older adults.

3.2 Understanding Frailty in Older Surgical Patients

Frailty is a dynamic clinical state where there is an increased vulnerability in developing adverse outcomes when exposed to a stressor such as surgery (Morley et al. 2013). These outcomes include functional decline, postoperative complications, prolonged Intensive Care Unit (ICU) stay, increased length of hospitalisation, hospital readmission, institutionalisation and mortality including in-hospital mortality (Cunha et al. 2019; Snitkjaer et al. 2025; Alsayari et al. 2025; Goh et al. 2024; Lin et al. 2016; Wen et al. 2023). While it is traditionally taught that all older patients are at increased risk of morbidity and mortality, there is now evidence showing that frailty is a better predictor than chronological age alone (Tian et al. 2023). This means that patients of the same age do not all have the same risk. Furthermore, 'eyeballing' which is subjective, inconsistent, has poor inter-rater reliability and can only pick up moderate frailty at best has been surpassed by more objective assessment tools (Dent et al. 2017; Hubbard and Story 2015; Yanagawa et al. 2018). Given that there can still be benefits such as symptom control and improved lifespan with surgery, it must be emphasised that frailty should not be viewed simplistically as a binary 'fit/not fit for surgery' indicator, and instead be used to inform shared decision-making and optimised during the perioperative period. Early identification of frail older patients may facilitate timely and targeted interventions such as rehabilitation, nutritional support, medication review and anaesthesia management to improve the likelihood of postoperative recovery. Understanding frailty and its concepts will help in the design of successful perioperative care models that can improve longer term health outcomes (Partridge et al. 2017; Eamer et al. 2018). The involvement of geriatricians with multidisciplinary collaboration is key to this success as their individual and collective training equips them with skillsets that are directly applicable to the needs of older people undergoing surgery (Rogerson et al. 2019).

There are two widely accepted conceptual models of frailty, namely the phenotypic model and the cumulative deficit model (Fried et al. 2001; Rockwood et al. 2007). While the phenotypic model defines frailty by the presence of at least three of the five physical criteria of weakness, slowness, low physical activity, fatigue and unintentional weight loss, the cumulative deficit model allows for a quantitative measure of frailty that reflects the accumulation of medical, functional and social deficits. Both approaches to frailty correlate moderately well with one another and have been validated in a wide variety of settings and populations.

Numerous validated tools are available for use in assessing frailty in older surgical patients and the more common ones are summarised in Table 3.1.

With the wide range of frailty assessment tools available for older surgical patients, decision on the most appropriate measure requires a balance between clinical needs, available resources and time constraints.

Clinical services that solely wish to look at preoperative risk assessment can select tools that correlate with surgical outcomes of interest. For those who want to provide a comprehensive evaluation of the older patient for the purpose of interventions, more detailed assessments such as the FI or CGA can be chosen to gain a broader understanding of the deficits, identify modifiable factors for prehabilitation and aid in shared decision-making. For patients with cognitive impairment, a tool such as the CFS may be more helpful as it relies on clinical observation and judgement rather than patient self-report.

For clinical services with limited time or resources, brief tools can be used either as a standalone or as a screening measure to determine whether to commit more resources in performing a more detailed assessment. It should be noted that certain

Table 3.1 Summary of validated tools commonly used in the assessment of frailty in older surgical patients

Tool	Description	Validated in
Frailty phenotype (or Cardiovascular Health Study frailty scale) (Fried et al. 2001)	Presence of at least three out of the five criteria: unintentional weight loss, weakness, exhaustion, slow gait speed and low physical activity Modified criteria available	• Elective and emergent cardiac surgery (Afilalo et al. 2012; Sundermann et al. 2011; Miguelena-Hycka et al. 2022; Lytwyn et al. 2017) • Elective transcatheter aortic valve replacement (Green et al. 2012, 2015; Afilalo et al. 2017) • Elective colorectal cancer surgery (Tan et al. 2012) • Elective major abdominal cancer surgery (Kinugasa et al. 2024) • Acute hip fracture surgery (Kistler et al. 2015)

(continued)

Table 3.1 (continued)

Tool	Description	Validated in
Frailty Index (FI) (Jones et al. 2004; Searle et al. 2008)	Quantifies frailty by counting health deficits such as comorbidities, symptoms and functional impairments. Variations of the original index available	• Elective and acute intermediate- and high-risk surgery (Lin et al. 2017) • Cardiac surgery (Johnson et al. 2024) • Vascular surgery (Braet et al. 2020) • Cancer surgery, including colorectal, gynaecologic and lung cancer surgery (Alsayari et al. 2025; Bhargavan et al. 2024; Tamburini et al. 2024; Chambers et al. 2021) • Head and neck surgery (Al Afif et al. 2024) • Elective spinal surgery (Camino-Willhuber et al. 2024; Manzetti et al. 2024) • Elective primary hip and knee replacement surgery (Ali et al. 2024) • Acute hip fracture surgery (Krishnan et al. 2014; Patel et al. 2014)
Clinical Frailty Scale (CFS) (Rockwood et al. 2005; Pulok et al. 2020)	A nine-point scale to assess the overall level of frailty based on clinical judgement, considering factors, including mobility, energy levels and physical function, with a score ranging from 1 (very fit) to 9 (terminally frail)	• Elective cardiac surgery (Sundermann et al. 2011) • Elective major vascular surgery (Ayyash et al. 2022) • Acute general surgery (Hewitt et al. 2015) • Emergency abdominal surgery (Goh et al. 2024; Fornaess et al. 2022) • Cancer surgery, including elective colon and urological cancer surgery (Bhargavan et al. 2024; Niemelainen et al. 2021; Sun et al. 2020)
Balducci Frailty Criteria (Balducci and Extermann 2000)	Considered to be part of a CGA, it defines frailty based on presence of factors such as functional dependence, three of more comorbidities, and/or at least one geriatric syndrome	• Elective cancer surgery (Kristjansson et al. 2010; Ronning et al. 2014) • Acute abdominal surgery (Kenig et al. 2015)

(continued)

Table 3.1 (continued)

Tool	Description	Validated in
Edmonton Frail Scale (EFS) (Rolfson et al. 2006)	Assesses frailty based on nine domains, including cognition, mood, nutrition and social support.	• Cardiac surgery (Lal et al. 2020; Sarkar et al. 2022; Castro et al. 2023) • Elective major abdominal surgery (He et al. 2020) • Elective colorectal cancer surgery (Richards et al. 2021) • Elective orthopaedic surgery (hip, knee, spine) (Roopsawang et al. 2020)
Vulnerable Elders-13 Survey (VES-13) (Saliba et al. 2001)	Assess frailty based on factors, including self-rated health, physical limitations, and ability to perform daily activities	• Acute abdominal surgery (Kenig et al. 2015) • Cardiac surgery (Kowalczuk-Wieteska et al. 2019) • Urological surgery (Tokura et al. 2023)
Groningen Frailty Indicator (GFI) (Bielderman et al. 2013)	A 15-item self-reported questionnaire that measures frailty across four key domains: physical, cognitive, social and psychological	• Acute abdominal surgery (Kenig et al. 2015) • Inpatient gastric and colorectal cancer surgery (Zhang et al. 2022) • Vascular surgery (Visser et al. 2019)
Multidimensional Frailty Score (MFS) (Kim et al. 2014)	A numerical assessment often calculated using a CGA that considers various factors across different domains, including physical function, cognitive ability, nutritional status, social well-being and medical history	• Elective intermediate- or high-risk general surgery (Kim et al. 2014) • Acute hip fracture surgery (Choi et al. 2017)

tools such as the Frailty Phenotype also require specialised equipment to measure hand grip strength as part of the assessment process. Tools that rely more on physical performance such as gait speed may be impractical in certain subgroup of patients such as those requiring emergency surgery.

While there is no one-size-fits-all tool currently available, the CGA remains the gold standard for frailty assessment and intervention in older adults, with majority of guidelines recommending the use of validated tools, including the frailty phenotype, CFS and EFS to routinely screen for frailty preoperatively (Tian et al. 2023; Dent et al. 2017, 2019; Partridge et al. 2012; Berian et al. 2018; Griffiths et al. 2014; Mohanty et al. 2016).

3.3 Comprehensive Geriatric Assessment

Traditional preoperative assessments focus primarily on risk assessment and assessment and management of individual organ systems/diseases and do not incorporate a CGA. This may lead to multiple referrals to different organ-specific specialities, suboptimal coordination of care, delays to treatment and neglect behavioural modification, environmental and rehabilitation needs that are critical to positive outcomes (Rogerson et al. 2019; Partridge et al. 2022). Postoperative care tends to be delivered by surgical teams, with only ad hoc support from medical or geriatric medicine teams on a consultation basis.

The CGA is a multidimensional and interdisciplinary diagnostic and therapeutic process to determine a frail older person's medical, functional, mental and social capabilities with the goal of ensuring that problems are identified, quantified and managed appropriately (Ellis et al. 2017). Its origins can be traced back to the 1930s, with Marjory Warren being one of the earliest advocates for setting up services dedicated for older adults (Warren 1943). It can be used to evaluate pre-existing comorbidities and diagnose previously unrecognised conditions, optimise perioperative risks through evidence-based multidisciplinary interventions, facilitate shared decision-making and plan for the perioperative period (Rogerson et al. 2019).

A 2018 Cochrane review on CGA for older people admitted to a surgical service looked at eight randomised trials, of which seven included patients with hip fracture and one included elective surgical oncology patients, and found that CGA led to significant mortality reduction, institutionalisation and probable reduction in healthcare delivery costs (Eamer et al. 2018). A subsequent randomised controlled trial looking at preoperative CGA led by geriatrician in patients aged 65 years and above undergoing elective vascular surgery demonstrated reduction in length of stay, delirium, cardiac and bowel/bladder complications, and institutionalisation (Partridge et al. 2017). A more recent systematic review in 2022 showed that perioperative CGA in older adults admitted to a surgical service (excluding orthopaedic ward) significantly reduced delirium and length of hospital stay by approximately 2 days when compared to usual/standard care (Veronese et al. 2022). The same study found that CGA when performed in older patients with hip fracture following trauma significantly reduced the risk of delirium, prevented functional decline, reduced mortality and disability in activities of daily living.

The components of the CGA in older surgical patients have been found to vary across different trials, with the most commonly included ones being functional status, cognitive function, nutritional status and medication review (Miller et al. 2022). The tools used to assess these areas varied across studies too. This observation can be explained from both a service delivery and clinical trials view, and reflects the reality in implementing such a complex intervention in a resource-conscious clinical environment. Table 3.2 shows the typical components in a CGA (Rogerson et al. 2019; Miller et al. 2022).

The composition of the assessment team depends on the services provided by the individual clinical service and is typically staffed by a core team comprising a physician (usually a geriatrician), nurse and social worker. An extended team of health

Table 3.2 Typical components of a CGA in older surgical patients

Component	Items to be assessed and optimised
Medical	• Diagnosis of previously unrecognised conditions • Screening for risk of geriatric syndromes such as falls, delirium, and incontinence • Evaluation and optimisation of – Comorbidities, including cardiac issues. – Anaemia – Pain control – Medications – Oral health – Nutrition – Vision/hearing
Mental health	• Evaluation and optimisation of – Cognition – Mood and anxiety
Functional capacity	• Evaluation and optimisation of – Basic activities of daily living (ADLs) – Instrumental activities of daily living (IADLs) – Gait and balance – Activity/exercise status
Social and financial support	• Evaluation and optimisation of – Informal support from family or friends – Social network such as daytime activities – Formal care provision – Lifestyle choices including smoking and exercise
Environment	• Evaluation and optimisation of – Home situation, facilities and safety – Accessibility to local resources
Goals of care	• Discuss current goals of care • Elicit advance care preferences

professionals such as physiotherapists, occupational therapists, speech therapists, dietitians, pharmacists and podiatrists can be called upon to provide inputs whenever appropriate.

The process of conducting a CGA usually begins with data gathering, which can be done through various sources, including patient self-report, patient and caregiver interview, or electronic health records. Using the information gathered, the multidisciplinary team engages in discussion and develops a pre-emptive treatment plan in partnership with the patient and/or caregiver. The treatment plan is then implemented, its response monitored and revised subsequently if required. Ensuring fidelity (i.e. how well the evidence-based intervention is replicated) is key to translating evidence into clinical services (Dhesi et al. 2019).

Figure 3.1 shows how a CGA and optimisation can be applied throughout the entire perioperative pathway.

While a large part of the existing literature is based on elective surgical settings, there is now growing evidence of the benefits of embedding CGA into emergency surgical settings, with data from the UK National Emergency Laparotomy Audit

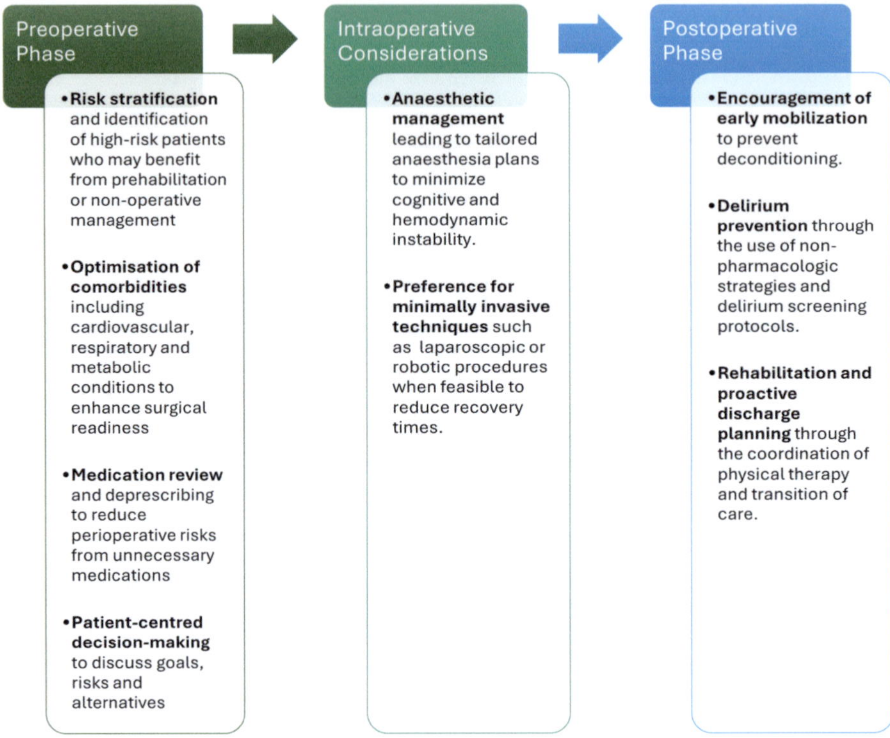

Fig. 3.1 Application of CGA to geriatric surgery

(NELA) demonstrating reduction in mortality rates and higher proportion of older people being discharged home as opposed to other care settings (Oliver et al. 2018; Aitken et al. 2020).

The Perioperative Care for Older People undergoing Surgery (POPS) is an example of a geriatrician-led multidisciplinary perioperative service that provides proactive input to all surgical subspecialities, including cardiac surgery, orthopaedics and trauma, vascular, gastrointestinal, gynaecology, urology, plastics, head and neck, and ophthalmology, and is being implemented across the English and Welsh National Health Services. Elective patients are referred to the service based on presence of multimorbidity (>2 comorbid conditions), geriatric syndromes, for example, frailty, functional limitation, difficult decision-making or complex surgery, while emergency surgical admissions requiring POPS input are identified by proactively screening admissions for multimorbidity, frailty (screened using the CFS), cognitive impairment, functional limitation and complexity of decision-making. It uses a preoperative CGA to optimise a patient's health and has been shown to improve quality of care and reduce postoperative complications, length of hospital stay, hospital readmissions and same-day cancellation of surgery (Waring et al. 2023; Jasper et al. 2019). Postoperative care is supported by the POPS team as well, though the collaborative model varies between surgical departments according to their respective working practices and patient population.

Similar models have been established elsewhere, for example, Singapore across different surgical specialities, including hip fracture, colorectal and vascular surgery, demonstrating that CGA-based models of care are translatable worldwide (Rogerson et al. 2019; Tan et al. 2011).

3.4 Challenges and Future Directions

Despite the clear benefits of geriatric assessment models for frail older adults, various barriers to implementation remain. There are still variations in models of care delivery for perioperative care, including the more established orthogeriatric services. In a 2020 survey of 23 orthogeriatric co-management programmes across the United States, nearly half adopted a shared care model, one in five used a consultation model, while the rest used a mix of shared care and consultation, with many reporting similar challenges in implementation (Rogers et al. 2020).

The limited availability of trained geriatric specialists is a global phenomenon which may lead to challenges in meeting the demands of the ageing population and scaling up of existing services (Gurwitz 2023). Efforts have been made previously to facilitate delivery of CGA by non-geriatricians in perioperative settings using a toolkit developed by Hospital Wide Comprehensive Geriatric Assessment (HOW-CGA) but this did not result in a change in clinical practice due to limited face validity, behavioural and cultural barriers (Dhesi et al. 2019). Constraints in time and resources in a busy perioperative practice may lead to suboptimal assessments, thereby impacting fidelity and tailoring of interventions. Engagement of stakeholders and involvement of the expertise at the appropriate part of the perioperative pathway should be addressed early to increase the chance of successful implementation of CGA-based perioperative care.

With the rapid advancement of technology in recent years, relevant digital tools can be leveraged upon for efficient CGA delivery and reduce the time and resources required for processes such as data gathering. Artificial intelligence is now more ready to be utilised and integrated to better predict surgical risks and outcomes, and augment the discovery of new pathways to deliver improved outcomes. Hybrid models incorporating both CGA and prehabilitation-based models of care can be examined to look at longer term outcomes, including patient-reported outcome measures, process measures and cost-effectiveness (Partridge et al. 2022). Geriatric medical education, including cross speciality training of healthcare professionals, should continue to develop to address geriatric competencies in all members of the workforce involved in the care of older adults and create a collaborative environment for service delivery, quality improvement and research. Implementation science methodology should be adopted to ensure that perioperative CGA pathways are scaled up timely, with outcomes measured through studies using big data (Sbai et al. 2020).

3.5 Conclusion

Geriatric assessment models play a crucial role in the care of frail older adults undergoing surgery. Perioperative models of CGA are supported by a growing evidence base and incorporated into numerous guidelines and recommendations. By providing a structured approach to evaluating and optimising health, these models help to mitigate risks, enhance recovery and improve surgical outcomes. As the population ages, continued research and innovation in this field will be essential to meeting the needs of this vulnerable population, with a focus on policy development at the local, national and international level to effect mindset and systemic change.

References

Afilalo J, Mottillo S, Eisenberg MJ, Alexander KP, Noiseux N, Perrault LP et al (2012) Addition of frailty and disability to cardiac surgery risk scores identifies elderly patients at high risk of mortality or major morbidity. Circ Cardiovasc Qual Outcomes 5(2):222–228. https://doi.org/10.1161/CIRCOUTCOMES.111.963157

Afilalo J, Lauck S, Kim DH, Lefevre T, Piazza N, Lachapelle K et al (2017) Frailty in older adults undergoing aortic valve replacement: the FRAILTY-AVR study. J Am Coll Cardiol 70(6):689–700. https://doi.org/10.1016/j.jacc.2017.06.024

Aitken RM, Partridge JSL, Oliver CM, Murray D, Hare S, Lockwood S et al (2020) Older patients undergoing emergency laparotomy: observations from the National Emergency Laparotomy Audit (NELA) years 1-4. Age Ageing 49(4):656–663. https://doi.org/10.1093/ageing/afaa075

Al Afif A, Rosen P, Gardella J, Norwood TG, Abbas A, Moore LS et al (2024) Predicting outcomes in head and neck surgery with modified frailty index and surgical apgar scores. Oral Oncol 159:107045. https://doi.org/10.1016/j.oraloncology.2024.107045

Ali M, Safri MK, Abdullah M, Nisar F, Lakdawala HA, Abbas M et al (2024) Modified frailty index as a predictor of adverse outcomes in elective primary hip and knee replacement surgery patients at a tertiary care hospital in Pakistan: a cross-sectional study. Cureus 16(3):e55783. https://doi.org/10.7759/cureus.55783

Alsayari R, McKechnie T, Kazi T, Heimann L, Sachdeva A, Lee Y et al (2025) Modified frailty index for patients undergoing surgery for colorectal cancer: analysis of the national inpatient sample from 2015 to 2019. Am Surg 91(1):76–85. https://doi.org/10.1177/00031348241269398

Ayyash R, Knight J, Kothmann E, Eid M, Ayyash K, Colling K et al (2022) Utility and reliability of the Clinical Frailty Scale in patients scheduled for major vascular surgery: a prospective, observational, multicentre observer-blinded study. Perioper Med (Lond) 11(1):6. https://doi.org/10.1186/s13741-022-00240-9

Balducci L, Extermann M (2000) Management of cancer in the older person: a practical approach. Oncologist 5(3):224–237. https://doi.org/10.1634/theoncologist.5-3-224

Becher RD, Vander Wyk B, Leo-Summers L, Desai MM, Gill TM (2023) The incidence and cumulative risk of major surgery in older persons in the United States. Ann Surg 277(1):87–92. https://doi.org/10.1097/SLA.0000000000005077

Berian JR, Rosenthal RA, Baker TL, Coleman J, Finlayson E, Katlic MR et al (2018) Hospital standards to promote optimal surgical care of the older adult: a report from the coalition for quality in geriatric surgery. Ann Surg 267(2):280–290. https://doi.org/10.1097/SLA.0000000000002185

Bhargavan R, Philip FA, Km JK, Augustine P, Thomas S (2024) Comparison of modified frailty index, clinical frailty scale, ECOG score, and ASA PS score in predicting postoperative outcomes in cancer surgery: a prospective study. Indian J Surg Oncol 15(4):938–945. https://doi.org/10.1007/s13193-024-01995-x

Bielderman A, van der Schans CP, van Lieshout MR, de Greef MH, Boersma F, Krijnen WP et al (2013) Multidimensional structure of the Groningen Frailty Indicator in community-dwelling older people. BMC Geriatr 13:86. https://doi.org/10.1186/1471-2318-13-86

Braet DJ, Taaffe JP, Dombrovskiy VY, Bath J, Kruse RL, Vogel TR (2020) Modified frailty index as an indicator for outcomes, discharge status, and readmission after lower extremity bypass surgery for critical limb ischemia. J Vasc Nurs 38(4):171–175. https://doi.org/10.1016/j.jvn.2020.08.002

Camino-Willhuber G, Choi J, Holc F, Oyadomari S, Guiroy A, Bow H et al (2024) Utility of the modified 5-items frailty index to predict complications and mortality after elective cervical, thoracic and lumbar posterior spine fusion surgery: multicentric analysis from ACS-NSQIP database. Global Spine J 14(3):839–845. https://doi.org/10.1177/21925682221124101

Castro ML, Alves M, Martins A, Luisa Papoila A, Botelho MA, Fragata J (2023) Reproducibility and validity of the Portuguese Edmonton Frail Scale version in cardiac surgery patients. Rev Port Cardiol 42(4):295–304. https://doi.org/10.1016/j.repc.2022.03.009

Chambers LM, Chalif J, Yao M, Chichura A, Morton M, Gruner M et al (2021) Modified frailty index predicts postoperative complications in women with gynecologic cancer undergoing cytoreductive surgery and hyperthermic intraperitoneal chemotherapy. Gynecol Oncol 162(2):368–374. https://doi.org/10.1016/j.ygyno.2021.05.013

Choi JY, Cho KJ, Kim SW, Yoon SJ, Kang MG, Kim KI et al (2017) Prediction of mortality and postoperative complications using the hip-multidimensional frailty score in elderly patients with hip fracture. Sci Rep 7:42966. https://doi.org/10.1038/srep42966

Chowdhury SR, Chandra Das D, Sunna TC, Beyene J, Hossain A (2023) Global and regional prevalence of multimorbidity in the adult population in community settings: a systematic review and meta-analysis. EClinicalMedicine 57:101860. https://doi.org/10.1016/j.eclinm.2023.101860

Cunha AIL, Veronese N, de Melo BS, Ricci NA (2019) Frailty as a predictor of adverse outcomes in hospitalized older adults: a systematic review and meta-analysis. Ageing Res Rev 56:100960. https://doi.org/10.1016/j.arr.2019.100960

Deiner S, Westlake B, Dutton RP (2014) Patterns of surgical care and complications in elderly adults. J Am Geriatr Soc 62(5):829–835. https://doi.org/10.1111/jgs.12794

Dent E, Lien C, Lim WS, Wong WC, Wong CH, Ng TP et al (2017) The Asia-Pacific clinical practice guidelines for the management of frailty. J Am Med Dir Assoc 18(7):564–575. https://doi.org/10.1016/j.jamda.2017.04.018

Dent E, Morley JE, Cruz-Jentoft AJ, Woodhouse L, Rodriguez-Manas L, Fried LP et al (2019) Physical frailty: ICFSR international clinical practice guidelines for identification and management. J Nutr Health Aging 23(9):771–787. https://doi.org/10.1007/s12603-019-1273-z

Dhesi J, Moonesinghe SR, Partridge J (2019) Comprehensive geriatric assessment in the perioperative setting; where next? Age Ageing 48(5):624–627. https://doi.org/10.1093/ageing/afz069

Eamer G, Taheri A, Chen SS, Daviduck Q, Chambers T, Shi X et al (2018) Comprehensive geriatric assessment for older people admitted to a surgical service. Cochrane Database Syst Rev 1(1):CD012485. https://doi.org/10.1002/14651858.CD012485.pub2

Ellis G, Gardner M, Tsiachristas A, Langhorne P, Burke O, Harwood RH et al (2017) Comprehensive geriatric assessment for older adults admitted to hospital. Cochrane Database Syst Rev 9(9):CD006211. https://doi.org/10.1002/14651858.CD006211.pub3

Fornaess KM, Nome PL, Aakre EK, Hegvik TA, Jammer I (2022) Clinical frailty scale: inter-rater reliability of retrospective scoring in emergency abdominal surgery. Acta Anaesthesiol Scand 66(1):25–29. https://doi.org/10.1111/aas.13974

Fried LP, Tangen CM, Walston J, Newman AB, Hirsch C, Gottdiener J et al (2001) Frailty in older adults: evidence for a phenotype. J Gerontol A Biol Sci Med Sci 56(3):M146–M156

Goh SSN, Zhao J, Drakeford PA, Chen Q, Lim WW, Li AL et al (2024) Assessing the impact of frailty in elderly patients undergoing emergency laparotomies in Singapore. Ann Acad Med Singap 53(6):352–360. https://doi.org/10.47102/annals-acadmedsg.2023155

Green P, Woglom AE, Genereux P, Daneault B, Paradis JM, Schnell S et al (2012) The impact of frailty status on survival after transcatheter aortic valve replacement in older adults with severe

aortic stenosis: a single-center experience. JACC Cardiovasc Interv 5(9):974–981. https://doi.org/10.1016/j.jcin.2012.06.011
Green P, Arnold SV, Cohen DJ, Kirtane AJ, Kodali SK, Brown DL et al (2015) Relation of frailty to outcomes after transcatheter aortic valve replacement (from the PARTNER trial). Am J Cardiol 116(2):264–269. https://doi.org/10.1016/j.amjcard.2015.03.061
Griffiths R, Beech F, Brown A, Dhesi J, Foo I, Goodall J et al (2014) Peri-operative care of the elderly 2014: Association of Anaesthetists of Great Britain and Ireland. Anaesthesia 69(Suppl 1):81–98. https://doi.org/10.1111/anae.12524
Gurwitz JH (2023) The paradoxical decline of geriatric medicine as a profession. JAMA 330(8):693–694. https://doi.org/10.1001/jama.2023.11110
He Y, Li LW, Hao Y, Sim EY, Ng KL, Lee R et al (2020) Assessment of predictive validity and feasibility of Edmonton Frail Scale in identifying postoperative complications among elderly patients: a prospective observational study. Sci Rep 10(1):14682. https://doi.org/10.1038/s41598-020-71140-5
Hewitt J, Moug SJ, Middleton M, Chakrabarti M, Stechman MJ, McCarthy K et al (2015) Prevalence of frailty and its association with mortality in general surgery. Am J Surg 209(2):254–259. https://doi.org/10.1016/j.amjsurg.2014.05.022
Hubbard RE, Story DA (2015) Does frailty lie in the eyes of the beholder? Heart Lung Circ 24(6):525–526. https://doi.org/10.1016/j.hlc.2015.01.018
Jasper EV, Dhesi JK, Partridge JS, Sevdalis N (2019) Scaling up perioperative medicine for older people undergoing surgery (POPS) services; use of a logic model approach. Clin Med (Lond) 19(6):478–484. https://doi.org/10.7861/clinmed.2019-0223
Johnson A, Hore E, Milne B, Muscedere J, Peng Y, McIsaac DI et al (2024) A frailty index to predict mortality, resource utilization and costs in patients undergoing coronary artery bypass graft surgery in Ontario. CJC Open 6(2 Part A):72–81. https://doi.org/10.1016/j.cjco.2023.10.010
Jones DM, Song X, Rockwood K (2004) Operationalizing a frailty index from a standardized comprehensive geriatric assessment. J Am Geriatr Soc 52(11):1929–1933. https://doi.org/10.1111/j.1532-5415.2004.52521.x
Kenig J, Zychiewicz B, Olszewska U, Barczynski M, Nowak W (2015) Six screening instruments for frailty in older patients qualified for emergency abdominal surgery. Arch Gerontol Geriatr 61(3):437–442. https://doi.org/10.1016/j.archger.2015.06.018
Kim SW, Han HS, Jung HW, Kim KI, Hwang DW, Kang SB et al (2014) Multidimensional frailty score for the prediction of postoperative mortality risk. JAMA Surg 149(7):633–640. https://doi.org/10.1001/jamasurg.2014.241
Kinugasa Y, Ida M, Kawaguchi M (2024) Fried Frailty Phenotype Questionnaire scores and postoperative patient-reported outcomes of patients undergoing major abdominal cancer surgery: a secondary analysis. Geriatr Gerontol Int 24(5):464–469. https://doi.org/10.1111/ggi.14872
Kistler EA, Nicholas JA, Kates SL, Friedman SM (2015) Frailty and short-term outcomes in patients with hip fracture. Geriatr Orthop Surg Rehabil 6(3):209–214. https://doi.org/10.1177/2151458515591170
Kowalczuk-Wieteska A, Parys M, Majchrzyk I, Zembala M, Zembala M (2019) Can the Vulnerable Elders-13 Survey (VES-13) scale replace the EuroSCORE scale in predicting complications in patients over 60 years of age undergoing cardiac surgery? Postepy Kardiol Interwencyjnej 15(2):211–217. https://doi.org/10.5114/aic.2019.86014
Krishnan M, Beck S, Havelock W, Eeles E, Hubbard RE, Johansen A (2014) Predicting outcome after hip fracture: using a frailty index to integrate comprehensive geriatric assessment results. Age Ageing 43(1):122–126. https://doi.org/10.1093/ageing/aft084
Kristjansson SR, Nesbakken A, Jordhoy MS, Skovlund E, Audisio RA, Johannessen HO et al (2010) Comprehensive geriatric assessment can predict complications in elderly patients after elective surgery for colorectal cancer: a prospective observational cohort study. Crit Rev Oncol Hematol 76(3):208–217. https://doi.org/10.1016/j.critrevonc.2009.11.002
Lal S, Gray A, Kim E, Bunton RW, Davis P, Galvin IF et al (2020) Frailty in elderly patients undergoing cardiac surgery increases hospital stay and 12-month readmission rate. Heart Lung Circ 29(8):1187–1194. https://doi.org/10.1016/j.hlc.2019.10.007

Lin HS, Watts JN, Peel NM, Hubbard RE (2016) Frailty and post-operative outcomes in older surgical patients: a systematic review. BMC Geriatr 16(1):157. https://doi.org/10.1186/s12877-016-0329-8

Lin H, Peel NM, Scott IA, Vardesh DL, Sivalingam P, McBride RL et al (2017) Perioperative assessment of older surgical patients using a frailty index-feasibility and association with adverse post-operative outcomes. Anaesth Intensive Care 45(6):676–682. https://doi.org/10.1177/0310057X1704500605

Lytwyn J, Stammers AN, Kehler DS, Jung P, Alexander B, Hiebert BM et al (2017) The impact of frailty on functional survival in patients 1 year after cardiac surgery. J Thorac Cardiovasc Surg 154(6):1990–1999. https://doi.org/10.1016/j.jtcvs.2017.06.040

Manzetti M, Ruffilli A, Viroli G, Traversari M, Ialuna M, Salamanna F et al (2024) Frailty influence on postoperative surgical site infections after surgery for degenerative spine disease and adult spine deformity. Can a frailty index be a valuable summary risk indicator? A systematic review and metanalysis of the current literature. Global Spine J:21925682241235605. https://doi.org/10.1177/21925682241235605

Miguelena-Hycka J, Lopez-Menendez J, Prada PC, Garcia MM, Vigil-Escalera C, Harmand MG et al (2022) Changes in frailty status after cardiac surgery. A prospective cohort study. Arch Gerontol Geriatr 98:104568. https://doi.org/10.1016/j.archger.2021.104568

Miller RL, Barnes JD, Mouton R, Braude P, Hinchliffe R (2022) Comprehensive geriatric assessment (CGA) in perioperative care: a systematic review of a complex intervention. BMJ Open 12(10):e062729. https://doi.org/10.1136/bmjopen-2022-062729

Mohanty S, Rosenthal RA, Russell MM, Neuman MD, Ko CY, Esnaola NF (2016) Optimal perioperative management of the geriatric patient: a best practices guideline from the American College of Surgeons NSQIP and the American Geriatrics Society. J Am Coll Surg 222(5):930–947. https://doi.org/10.1016/j.jamcollsurg.2015.12.026

Morley JE, Vellas B, van Kan GA, Anker SD, Bauer JM, Bernabei R et al (2013) Frailty consensus: a call to action. J Am Med Dir Assoc 14(6):392–397. https://doi.org/10.1016/j.jamda.2013.03.022

Niemelainen S, Huhtala H, Andersen J, Ehrlich A, Haukijarvi E, Koikkalainen S et al (2021) The clinical frailty scale is a useful tool for predicting postoperative complications following elective colon cancer surgery at the age of 80 years and above: a prospective, multicentre observational study. Colorectal Dis 23(7):1824–1836. https://doi.org/10.1111/codi.15689

Ofori-Asenso R, Chin KL, Mazidi M, Zomer E, Ilomaki J, Zullo AR et al (2019) Global incidence of frailty and prefrailty among community-dwelling older adults: a systematic review and meta-analysis. JAMA Netw Open 2(8):e198398. https://doi.org/10.1001/jamanetworkopen.2019.8398

Oliver CM, Bassett MG, Poulton TE, Anderson ID, Murray DM, Grocott MP et al (2018) Organisational factors and mortality after an emergency laparotomy: multilevel analysis of 39 903 National Emergency Laparotomy Audit patients. Br J Anaesth 121(6):1346–1356. https://doi.org/10.1016/j.bja.2018.07.040

Partridge JS, Harari D, Dhesi JK (2012) Frailty in the older surgical patient: a review. Age Ageing 41(2):142–147. https://doi.org/10.1093/ageing/afr182

Partridge JS, Harari D, Martin FC, Peacock JL, Bell R, Mohammed A et al (2017) Randomized clinical trial of comprehensive geriatric assessment and optimization in vascular surgery. Br J Surg 104(6):679–687. https://doi.org/10.1002/bjs.10459

Partridge JSL, Moonesinghe SR, Lees N, Dhesi JK (2022) Perioperative care for older people. Age Ageing 51(8). https://doi.org/10.1093/ageing/afac194

Patel KV, Brennan KL, Brennan ML, Jupiter DC, Shar A, Davis ML (2014) Association of a modified frailty index with mortality after femoral neck fracture in patients aged 60 years and older. Clin Orthop Relat Res 472(3):1010–1017. https://doi.org/10.1007/s11999-013-3334-7

Pulok MH, Theou O, van der Valk AM, Rockwood K (2020) The role of illness acuity on the association between frailty and mortality in emergency department patients referred to internal medicine. Age Ageing 49(6):1071–1079. https://doi.org/10.1093/ageing/afaa089

Richards SJG, Cherry TJ, Frizelle FA, Eglinton TW (2021) Pre-operative frailty is predictive of adverse post-operative outcomes in colorectal cancer patients. ANZ J Surg 91(3):379–386. https://doi.org/10.1111/ans.16319

Rockwood K, Song X, MacKnight C, Bergman H, Hogan DB, McDowell I et al (2005) A global clinical measure of fitness and frailty in elderly people. CMAJ 173(5):489–495. https://doi.org/10.1503/cmaj.050051

Rockwood K, Andrew M, Mitnitski A (2007) A comparison of two approaches to measuring frailty in elderly people. J Gerontol A Biol Sci Med Sci 62(7):738–743

Rogers SE, Ko JS, McNicoll L, Mendelson DA (2020) The diverse implementation of geriatrics-orthopedics comanagement programs in the United States. J Am Geriatr Soc 68(8):1714–1719. https://doi.org/10.1111/jgs.16677

Rogerson A, Partridge JS, Dhesi JK (2019) Perioperative medicine for older people. Ann Acad Med Singap 48(11):376–381

Rolfson DB, Majumdar SR, Tsuyuki RT, Tahir A, Rockwood K (2006) Validity and reliability of the Edmonton Frail Scale. Age Ageing 35(5):526–529. https://doi.org/10.1093/ageing/afl041

Ronning B, Wyller TB, Jordhoy MS, Nesbakken A, Bakka A, Seljeflot I et al (2014) Frailty indicators and functional status in older patients after colorectal cancer surgery. J Geriatr Oncol 5(1):26–32. https://doi.org/10.1016/j.jgo.2013.08.001

Roopsawang I, Thompson H, Zaslavsky O, Belza B (2020) Predicting hospital outcomes with the reported Edmonton Frail Scale-Thai version in orthopaedic older patients. J Clin Nurs 29(23–24):4708–4719. https://doi.org/10.1111/jocn.15512

Saliba D, Elliott M, Rubenstein LZ, Solomon DH, Young RT, Kamberg CJ et al (2001) The Vulnerable Elders Survey: a tool for identifying vulnerable older people in the community. J Am Geriatr Soc 49(12):1691–1699. https://doi.org/10.1046/j.1532-5415.2001.49281.x

Sarkar S, MacLeod J, Hassan A, Brunt KR, Palmer K, Legare JF (2022) Enhanced telehealth home-monitoring intervention for vulnerable and frail patients after cardiac surgery (THE-FACS Pilot Intervention Study). BMC Geriatr 22(1):836. https://doi.org/10.1186/s12877-022-03531-4

Sbai M, Martin F, Partridge J, Dhesi J (2020) Comprehensive geriatric assessment (CGA) in the perioperative setting: the current state of play. J R Coll Physicians Edinb 50(4):356–358. https://doi.org/10.4997/JRCPE.2020.401

Searle SD, Mitnitski A, Gahbauer EA, Gill TM, Rockwood K (2008) A standard procedure for creating a frailty index. BMC Geriatr 8:24. https://doi.org/10.1186/1471-2318-8-24

Snitkjaer C, Jensen TK, Kokotovic D, Burcharth J (2025) The cumulative risk and severity of postoperative complications in patients with frailty undergoing major emergency abdominal surgery—a prospective cohort study. World J Surg 49(1):55–65. https://doi.org/10.1002/wjs.12407

Sun CY, Huang CC, Tsai YS, Chang YT, Ou CH, Su WC et al (2020) Clinical frailty scale in predicting postoperative outcomes in older patients undergoing curative surgery for urologic malignancies: a prospective observational cohort study. Urology 144:38–45. https://doi.org/10.1016/j.urology.2020.06.069

Sundermann S, Dademasch A, Praetorius J, Kempfert J, Dewey T, Falk V et al (2011) Comprehensive assessment of frailty for elderly high-risk patients undergoing cardiac surgery. Eur J Cardiothorac Surg 39(1):33–37. https://doi.org/10.1016/j.ejcts.2010.04.013

Tamburini N, Dolcetti F, Fabbri N, Azzolina D, Greco S, Maniscalco P et al (2024) Impact of modified frailty index on readmissions following surgery for NSCLC. Thorac Cardiovasc Surg. https://doi.org/10.1055/a-2287-2341

Tan KY, Tan P, Tan L (2011) A collaborative transdisciplinary "geriatric surgery service" ensures consistent successful outcomes in elderly colorectal surgery patients. World J Surg 35(7):1608–1614. https://doi.org/10.1007/s00268-011-1112-9

Tan KY, Kawamura YJ, Tokomitsu A, Tang T (2012) Assessment for frailty is useful for predicting morbidity in elderly patients undergoing colorectal cancer resection whose comorbidities are already optimized. Am J Surg 204(2):139–143. https://doi.org/10.1016/j.amjsurg.2011.08.012

Tian B, Stahel PF, Picetti E, Campanelli G, Di Saverio S, Moore E et al (2023) Assessing and managing frailty in emergency laparotomy: a WSES position paper. World J Emerg Surg 18(1):38. https://doi.org/10.1186/s13017-023-00506-7

Tokura Y, Kawai T, Takei K, Ujiie T, Kanatani A, Yamada Y et al (2023) Geriatric 8 and Vulnerable Elders Survey-13 predict length of hospital stay and postoperative complications in Japanese patients undergoing urological surgery. J Geriatr Oncol 14(6):101558. https://doi.org/10.1016/j.jgo.2023.101558

UN, Department of Economic and Social Affairs, Population Division (2020) World population ageing 2019 (ST/ESA/SER.A/444)

Veronese N, Custodero C, Demurtas J, Smith L, Barbagallo M, Maggi S et al (2022) Comprehensive geriatric assessment in older people: an umbrella review of health outcomes. Age Ageing 51(5). https://doi.org/10.1093/ageing/afac104

Visser L, Banning LBD, El Moumni M, Zeebregts CJ, Pol RA (2019) The effect of frailty on outcome after vascular surgery. Eur J Vasc Endovasc Surg 58(5):762–769. https://doi.org/10.1016/j.ejvs.2019.04.031

Walsh B, Fogg C, Harris S, Roderick P, de Lusignan S, England T et al (2023) Frailty transitions and prevalence in an ageing population: longitudinal analysis of primary care data from an open cohort of adults aged 50 and over in England, 2006-2017. Age Ageing 52(5). https://doi.org/10.1093/ageing/afad058

Waring J, Martin GP, Hartley P, Partridge JSL, Dhesi JK (2023) Implementing a perioperative care of older people undergoing surgery (POPS) service: findings from a multi-site qualitative implementation study. Age Ageing 52(8). https://doi.org/10.1093/ageing/afad149

Warren MW (1943) Care of chronic sick. Br Med J 2(4329):822–823. https://doi.org/10.1136/bmj.2.4329.822

Wen H, Liu T, Li J (2023) Association between frailty and clinical post-operative outcomes in patients following hip arthroplasty: a systematic review and meta-analysis. Int Orthop 47(3):667–675. https://doi.org/10.1007/s00264-022-05657-x

Yanagawa B, Graham MM, Afilalo J, Hassan A, Arora RC (2018) Frailty as a risk predictor in cardiac surgery: beyond the eyeball test. J Thorac Cardiovasc Surg 156(1):172–6 e2. https://doi.org/10.1016/j.jtcvs.2018.01.103

Zhang Q, Zhang M, Hu S, Meng L, Xi J, Xu A et al (2022) Prevalence and risk factors of preoperative frailty in Chinese elderly inpatients with gastric and colorectal cancer undergoing surgery: a single-center cross-sectional study using the Groningen Frailty Indicator. Support Care Cancer 30(1):677–686. https://doi.org/10.1007/s00520-021-06483-4

Sarcopenia and Its Impact on Surgical Outcomes

4

Jing-Ting Wu and Frederick H. Koh

Take-Home Messages

- Sarcopenia significantly affects surgical outcomes, leading to increased complications, prolonged hospital stays, and higher mortality rates.
- Early identification and targeted interventions are crucial for optimizing surgical outcomes in these patients.
- A comprehensive approach that includes preoperative, perioperative, and postoperative strategies is essential for managing sarcopenic patients in surgical settings.

4.1 The Emerging Concept of Sarcopenia

Sarcopenia is characterized by the progressive and widespread loss of skeletal muscle mass and function, resulting in physical disability, reduced quality of life, and increased mortality. Over the past decade, several organizations, including the International Working Group on Sarcopenia (IWGS) (Fielding et al. 2011), the Foundation for the National Institutes of Health (FNIH) (Studenski et al. 2014), the Asian Working Group for Sarcopenia (AWGS) (Chen et al. 2020), and the European Working Group on Sarcopenia in Older People (EWGSOP) (Cruz-Jentoft et al. 2019), have established global standards for defining sarcopenia. According to their consensus, sarcopenia is defined by three key criteria: (1) loss of skeletal muscle mass along with (2) loss of muscle strength and/or (3) reduced physical

J.-T. Wu · F. H. Koh (✉)
SingHealth Duke-NUS Muscle Health Programme and Department of General Surgery, Sengkang General Hospital, SingHealth, Singapore, Singapore
e-mail: frederick.koh.h.x@singhealth.com.sg

K.-Y. Tan et al. (eds.), *Mastering Geriatric Surgery*,
https://doi.org/10.1007/978-981-95-0665-1_4

performance. The presence of all three criteria satisfies the diagnosis of severe sarcopenia.

4.1.1 "Sarcopenia" Instead of "Frailty"

Traditionally, frailty has been the dominant paradigm for evaluating vulnerability in older adults, emerging evidence suggests that sarcopenia is more precise and relevant tool in certain contexts, including surgical risk assessment. Sarcopenia is focused specifically on muscle mass and function, which are critical determinants of mobility, independence, and physical resilience. It can be measured using clear, objective methods like bioelectrical impedance analysis (BIA) (Koh et al. 2024), dual-energy X-ray absorptiometry (DEXA), or grip strength testing. In contrast, frailty is a broader, multidimensional concept encompassing physical, cognitive, and psychological factors that often rely on subjective evaluations or multifactorial indices, and can vary based on clinician judgment or the specific tools used. While frailty is useful, it often lacks the granularity to identify specific physical deficits like muscle weakness, which can have direct surgical implications.

4.1.2 Pathophysiology of Sarcopenia

Pathophysiologically, sarcopenia involves a complex interplay between protein metabolism, hormonal changes, inflammation, and neuromuscular factors. It is a multifactorial syndrome, where both intrinsic and extrinsic factors such as lifestyle contribute to the overall decline in muscle function as one ages (Fig. 4.1).

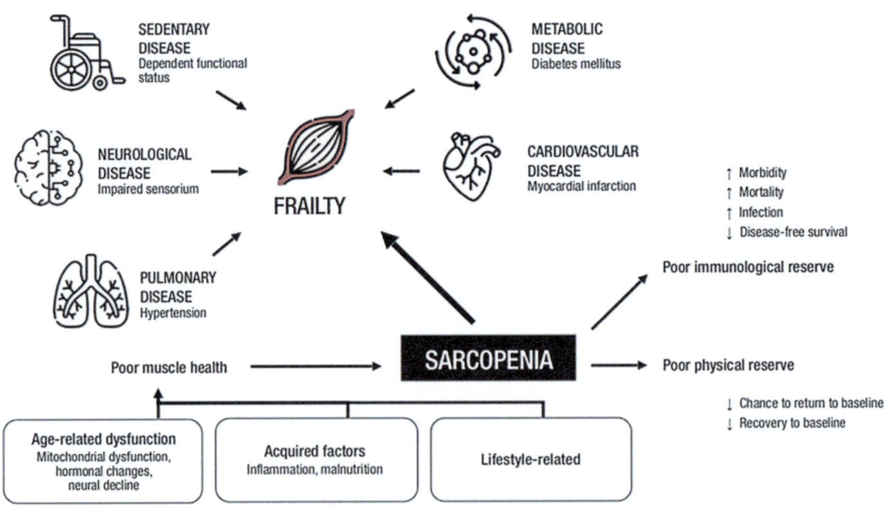

Fig. 4.1 Pathophysiology of sarcopenia

4.1.2.1 Muscle Protein Turnover

Sarcopenia results from an imbalance between protein synthesis and degradation. In healthy individuals, muscle protein turnover is a dynamic process. Proteins within muscle cells are constantly being synthesized and degraded. This balance is disrupted in sarcopenia, where there is a shift toward increased protein breakdown and decreased protein synthesis, leading to muscle wasting. Factors such as oxidative stress, mitochondrial dysfunction, and impaired autophagy play a role in this process (Li et al. 2022). The reduced capacity for muscle repair and regeneration exacerbates the loss of muscle mass and function.

4.1.2.2 Hormonal Changes

Age-related hormonal changes significantly impact both men and women, contributing to the development and progression of sarcopenic obesity. Insulin resistance, a common feature in the elder person, impairs muscle protein synthesis. In men, the decline in testosterone levels with age is a key factor. Testosterone, an anabolic hormone, promotes protein synthesis in skeletal muscle cells. As men age, their testosterone levels drop, and obesity further exacerbates this by converting testosterone to estradiol in adipose tissue through the aromatization process, leading to hypogonadism and subsequent sarcopenia (Shin et al. 2018).

In postmenopausal women, hormonal changes also drive body composition alterations that include increased adipose tissue and decreased muscle mass. The reduction in estradiol and the rise in FSH levels are primary contributors to these changes. Additionally, the decline in growth hormone (GH) levels with age and obesity affects muscle mass, further participating in the pathogenesis of sarcopenia. The complex interplay between various hormonal pathways underscores the need for a comprehensive approach to manage sarcopenia (Batsis and Villareal 2018).

4.1.2.3 Inflammatory Processes

Chronic low-grade inflammation associated with aging, indicated by higher levels of proinflammatory cytokines like IL-1β, IL-6, and TNFα, and lower levels of anti-inflammatory cytokines, aggravates changes in the muscle tissue microenvironment and hinders muscle regeneration. This persistent low-grade inflammation, known as inflammaging, disrupts immune regulation and significantly contributes to the onset of sarcopenia (Kalinkovich et al. 2022). These cytokines promote muscle protein breakdown and inhibit muscle repair and regeneration. The inflammatory milieu in sarcopenia is thought to be driven by a combination of factors, including increased fat mass, cellular senescence, and immune system aging. Anti-inflammatory treatments and lifestyle modifications that reduce systemic inflammation are important considerations in the management of sarcopenia.

4.1.2.4 Neuromuscular Factors

Motor neuron loss and muscle denervation play critical roles in sarcopenia. Age-related loss of motor neurons leads to reduced muscle fiber recruitment and subsequent muscle atrophy. The decline in neuromuscular function also affects the quality of muscle contractions, contributing to reduced strength and endurance (Figueiredo et al. 2006). Strategies to enhance neuromuscular health, such as targeted exercise programs and neuromuscular electrical stimulation, are being investigated as potential interventions to combat sarcopenia.

4.1.2.5 Lifestyle Factors and Chronic Medical Conditions

Physical inactivity and poor nutrition significantly contribute to the development of sarcopenia. Sedentary behavior leads to muscle disuse, while inadequate protein and caloric intake fail to support muscle maintenance and repair.

4.2 Prevalence of Sarcopenia in the World and Singapore

Sarcopenia primarily affects the older person, with prevalence rates increasing with age. Globally, to quote the data from the International Sarcopenia Initiative, the prevalence of sarcopenia is estimated to be 1–29% among community-dwelling individuals, 14–33% in long-term care facilities, and 10% in acute care hospitals (Shafiee et al. 2017).

Understanding the epidemiology of sarcopenia is crucial for developing targeted interventions and preventive strategies. In Singapore, sarcopenia is notably prevalent among the older person. Almost 90% of community-dwelling Singaporean aged ≥60 years have poor muscle health, highlighting an urgent need for targeted interventions to promote muscle health (Gupta et al. 2024).

Sarcopenia is prevalent in surgical patients, particularly in those undergoing major surgeries such as abdominal, orthopedic, and thoracic procedures (Wu et al. 2024). With the advent of better surgical techniques and increased life expectancy, there has been a steady growth of surgical procedures performed in geriatric patients (Lee et al. 2022). The high prevalence underscores the importance of routine screening for sarcopenia in surgical patients, particularly those at higher risk. Early identification allows for timely interventions that can improve surgical outcomes and reduce postoperative complications (Koh et al. 2021).

Age is the primary risk factor for sarcopenia. However, comorbid conditions such as cancer, cardiovascular disease, and diabetes also significantly increase the risk. Malnutrition and physical inactivity further exacerbate sarcopenia in these patients (Shen et al. 2019). Understanding the risk factors for sarcopenia in surgical patients is crucial for developing targeted strategies to mitigate its impact.

4.3 Impact of Sarcopenia on Surgical Outcomes

4.3.1 Intraoperative Challenges

Sarcopenic patients present unique intraoperative challenges. Reduced muscle mass and strength can complicate positioning and access during surgery. Sarcopenic patients are more susceptible to pressure ulcers, especially during long surgeries where immobility and poor circulation can damage skin and tissue. This results from reduced muscle padding around bony prominences (Galivanche et al. 2020). Surgeons may need to modify techniques to accommodate these patients.

Anesthesia management may also be affected, as sarcopenic patients often have altered pharmacokinetics and increased sensitivity to anesthetic agents (Shi et al. 2021). The body's ability to metabolize these drugs is affected by reduced muscle mass, leading to prolonged effects or heightened sensitivity to anesthesia. In sarcopenic patients undergoing abdominal surgery, reduced muscle mass can result in prolonged sedation or recovery times after general anesthesia. This increases the risk of complications such as delayed extubation and postoperative delirium. The loss of muscle mass associated with sarcopenia affects not only skeletal muscles but also the respiratory muscles, such as the diaphragm and intercostal muscles (Bone et al. 2017). This can reduce the patient's ability to manage ventilation during and after surgery, leading to difficulties in breathing and an increased risk of postoperative respiratory complications. Intraoperative monitoring and adjustments are crucial to ensure patient safety and optimal surgical outcomes.

Sarcopenia can lead to muscle atrophy, making surgeries that require muscle manipulation, like hernia repairs, more difficult. Weakened and atrophied muscles can be fragile, harder to manipulate, and may not hold sutures or surgical anchors as well as healthy muscles, although whether it helps predict surgical outcomes remains to be determined (Clark et al. 2020).

4.3.2 Postoperative Outcomes

4.3.2.1 Surgical Outcomes

Sarcopenia is a recognized independent predictor of poor surgical outcomes, linked with higher postoperative mortality across various conditions, including colorectal surgery, gastric cancer (Huang et al. 2016), hepatocellular carcinoma (Voron et al. 2015), pancreatic cancer (Peng et al. 2012), biliary cancer (Chakedis et al. 2018), and even vascular and cardiac surgery (Antoniou et al. 2019; Okamura et al. 2019). A meta-analysis by Trejo-Avila et al., which reviewed 44 observational studies encompassing 18,891 colorectal cancer patients, identified a significant association between sarcopenia and an increased risk of overall postoperative complications, including infections and cardiopulmonary issues (Trejo-Avila et al. 2021). Additionally, sarcopenia was correlated with general postoperative infections like pneumonia and urinary tract infections. These patients often experience longer hospital stays and higher mortality rates. Functional recovery is also compromised, leading to delayed return to baseline activities.

Sarcopenia is increasingly recognized as a strong predictor of adverse outcomes even in emergency general surgery (Trotter et al. 2018) and abdominal trauma (Ming et al. 2022). Muscle mass and function are critical indicators of a patient's ability to tolerate surgical stress and recover effectively, and sarcopenic individuals often have diminished physiological reserves to cope with the trauma of surgery. As a result, identifying sarcopenia preoperatively, even in emergency contexts, can provide valuable prognostic information, allowing surgical teams to better anticipate complications and adjust perioperative care to improve outcomes.

One proposed mechanism for these outcomes is that sarcopenia leads to a heightened postoperative inflammatory response (Reisinger et al. 2016), evidenced by elevated plasma levels of inflammatory markers such as calprotectin and an increased neutrophil-to-lymphocyte ratio. However, most studies on anastomotic leakage did not find a significant difference in its occurrence based on sarcopenia status, with one notable exception identifying psoas density as an independent predictor (Herrod et al. 2019). The variability in outcomes across studies is largely due to differing definitions and measurement methods for sarcopenia, underscoring the need for standardized diagnostic criteria.

4.3.2.2 Oncological Outcomes

Sarcopenia has been linked to incomplete neoadjuvant therapy (Abe et al. 2022) and reduced tolerance to postoperative chemotherapy, which in turn adversely affects prognosis and overall survival. The decrease in muscle mass makes patients more susceptible to chemotherapy's toxic effects, likely due to altered drug pharmacokinetics, thereby reducing the efficacy of treatment (Antoun et al. 2013).

Several meta-analyses have revealed that sarcopenic patients exhibit significantly shorter overall survival, disease-free survival, and cancer-specific survival (Trejo-Avila et al. 2021; Xie et al. 2021) compared to non-sarcopenic patients. These findings underscore the critical importance of early detection and prevention of sarcopenia in individuals undergoing oncological surgery.

The underlying mechanisms contributing to poorer oncological outcomes in sarcopenic patients remain poorly understood. One proposed explanation involves an immunological impact associated with compromised muscle health. In colorectal cancer, skeletal muscle has been linked to tumor-infiltrating lymphocytes (TILs), where an increase in TILs (such as CD3+, CD8+, CD4+, and FOXP3+ T cells) not only enhances the immune response against tumor growth but also serves as a predictor for better chemotherapy responses (Reisinger et al. 2016). This immunological mechanism has been observed in other cancers, including gastric, gynecological, and hepatobiliary malignancies.

4.3.2.3 Quality of Life

The presence of sarcopenia significantly diminishes the quality of life for surgical patients. The reduction in muscle mass and strength leads to increased physical frailty, impaired mobility, and a greater dependency on caregivers for daily activities.

4.3.2.4 Healthcare Costs

Sarcopenia contributes to increased healthcare costs due to prolonged hospitalizations (Koh et al. 2024), higher complication rates, and the need for extensive -operative rehabilitation and care, including readmission rates (Xia et al. 2020). The economic burden of managing sarcopenic patients is substantial, underscoring the importance of early intervention and effective management strategies.

4.4 Management Strategies: Prehabilitation

Multimodal "prehabilitation'," which aligns with the principles of Enhanced Recovery After Surgery (ERAS), emphasizes the cumulative benefits of small improvements in various aspects of patient care. The preoperative period presents a vital opportunity to improve a patient's health, establishing a "buffer" to mitigate the expected decrease in physiological reserve after surgery. Prehabilitation focuses on boosting a patient's functional capacity through targeted preoperative strategies to enhance postoperative recovery and outcomes (Wu et al. 2024; Koh et al. 2021). Understanding that physical condition, psychological health, and nutrition are crucial to surgical success, prehabilitation programs are increasingly adopting a holistic approach. These programs combine exercise, nutritional guidance, and psychological support to address essential health factors, ultimately optimizing surgical outcomes (Fig. 4.2).

4.4.1 Physical Activity Modification

The primary goal of exercise prehabilitation is to boost physiological reserve and fitness, which are key modifiable risk factors that can decrease surgical complications. Two essential components of exercise prehabilitation are aerobic/endurance and resistance/strength exercises. High-risk populations, such as frail or sarcopenic patients, may benefit significantly from these programs. Aerobic training, which focuses on improving cardiovascular fitness through prolonged low-intensity activity, primarily engages slow-twitch muscle fibers. This type of exercise promotes mitochondrial biogenesis, ATP production, and increases muscle mass and strength

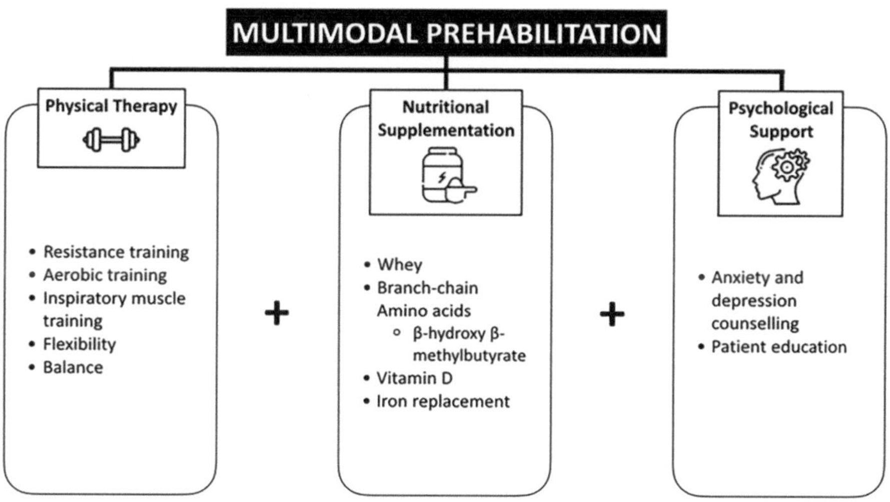

Fig. 4.2 Components of a multimodal prehabilitation

in older adults (Chen et al. 2017). Aerobic exercise activates energy-sensing networks, which initiate mitochondrial biogenesis (Radak et al. 2020). Additionally, aerobic exercise reduces catabolic gene expression (Yan et al. 2012), increases muscle protein synthesis, and enhances autophagy in skeletal muscle, vital for muscle integrity.

Resistance exercise, on the other hand, targets muscle hypertrophy and strength by engaging fast-twitch muscle fibers through short bursts of high-intensity activity against external loads. Resistance training (RT) is crucial for preventing muscle atrophy as it stimulates protein synthesis and muscle hypertrophy, leading to increased muscle mass, strength, and functional performance, particularly in sarcopenic patients (Lichtenberg et al. 2019). RT activates the mTOR pathway, which plays a central role in protein synthesis and muscle growth (Goodman et al. 2011), while promoting protein synthesis. RT also increases testosterone levels, the main anabolic hormone maintaining muscle mass and function. Additionally, RT suppresses catabolic networks that drive muscle degradation, notably by reducing myostatin levels—a potent inhibitor of muscle regeneration and growth—thereby supporting muscle preservation and growth (Negaresh et al. 2019).

4.4.2 Nutritional Assessment and Conditioning

Preoperative evaluation of sarcopenia is crucial for risk stratification and optimization. Identifying sarcopenic patients allows for targeted interventions to improve surgical outcomes. Comprehensive preoperative assessments, including functional status and nutritional evaluations, are essential for developing individualized care plans.

Nutritional status is a critical predictor of postoperative complications, with markers like preoperative serum albumin levels being linked to outcomes such as morbidity, mortality, and length of hospital stay (van der Kroft et al. 2015). Nutritional conditioning before surgery aims to correct deficiencies and increase functional reserve, reducing the risk of adverse outcomes. However, nutritional interventions should be tailored to each individual's needs, rather than adopting a "one-size-fits-all" approach—illustrated by a case where carbohydrate loading, instead of improving clinical outcomes, actually exacerbated tumor proliferation in estrogen receptor-positive cancers in breast cancer patients (Lende et al. 2019).

No standardized nutritional regimen exists for sarcopenic patients, and interventions often focus on protein supplementation to promote anabolism. Sarcopenia involves dysregulation of muscle protein synthesis and breakdown, and supplements like branched-chain amino acids (BCAAs) (TCTR 2019) and whey protein, which are rich in essential amino acids like leucine (Kobayashi 2018), can enhance protein synthesis and reduce muscle degradation. Additionally, whey protein offers antioxidant and anti-inflammatory properties that may counteract the oxidative stress associated with both sarcopenia and surgical stress (Gilmartin et al. 2020).

Given the role of muscle in glucose metabolism, sarcopenia is closely linked to insulin resistance, a condition exacerbated by surgical stress and associated with increased postoperative complications (Perrone et al. 2011). Perioperative carbohydrate loading has shown promise in reducing insulin resistance and preserving muscle mass, though more research is needed to confirm its benefits in sarcopenic patients.

Other nutrients, such as vitamin D, omega-3 fatty acids, and vitamin B12, may complement protein supplementation by improving muscle strength, balance, and mitochondrial function. Vitamin D, in particular, is crucial for muscle contraction and function, especially in older adults, where deficiency is common. Omega-3 fatty acids and vitamin B12 have also been shown to enhance muscle health, while emerging supplements like epicatechin and urolithin A offer additional potential benefits for muscle growth and function.

4.4.3 Psychological Support and Counseling

The often-overlooked yet essential component of prehabilitation begins with psychological rehab. Psychological distress is closely linked to adverse surgical outcomes, as anxiety and depression can heighten pain sensitivity (Tsimopoulou et al. 2015) and hinder adherence to prehabilitation programs, diminishing their effectiveness. These emotional states can exacerbate pain and stress, leading to increased glucocorticoid levels that impede wound healing (Gouin and Kiecolt-Glaser 2011), particularly harmful for high-risk patients with limited functional reserves. Research indicates that preoperative anxiety can negatively impact patient satisfaction, and that cognitive and psychological well-being significantly affect mortality rates in geriatric surgical patients (Tang et al. 2020). Additionally, psychosocial factors like anxiety can result in longer hospital stays, higher readmission rates, and decreased muscle mass and function in older adults (Dent and Hoogendijk 2014).

To address these challenges, screening for anxiety and depression using tools like the GAD-7 and PHQ-9 is crucial. Those identified as high-risk can benefit from psychological interventions such as referrals to mental health professionals, cognitive behavioral therapy, and relaxation techniques. Incorporating technology, such as virtual reality and smartphone apps, can enhance psychological support (Vailati Riboni et al. 2020). Despite the clear link between psychological factors and surgical outcomes, these aspects are frequently neglected in patient risk assessments. Recognizing and addressing these factors can significantly improve patient care and manage surgical stress more effectively.

4.5 Grounded by Science and Spreading the Word

The scientific basis for the management of sarcopenia is robust, with extensive evidence supporting the benefits of prehabilitation and early intervention. Numerous studies highlight the physiological mechanisms by which sarcopenia affects surgical outcomes and the benefits of addressing these through targeted interventions. The Surgical Prehabiltiation for Comprehensive Enhance Recovery (SUPREME)

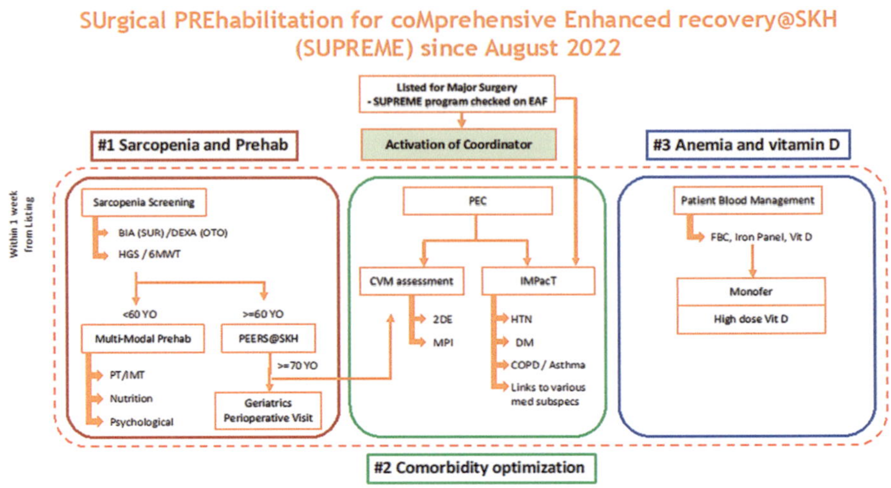

Fig. 4.3 SUPREME workflow with three key components: sarcopenia screening, comorbidity optimization, iron and vitamin D supplementation

program was introduced in 2020, first in the colorectal surgical service in the author's institution, to systemize a systematic screening process for patients undergoing major surgery. SUPREME screens for three main components—sarcopenia, early comorbidity optimization, and supplementation of iron as well as vitamin D (Fig. 4.3).

Preliminary results at 6 months have shown that a systematic multimodal prehabilitation program that not only address sarcopenia, but also includes tackling of vitamin D insufficiency, iron deficiency, and uncontrolled comorbidities, was able to allow sarcopenic patients to obtain similar morbidity rates, mean duration of stay, postoperative functional outcomes, and quality of life up to 6 months postoperatively compared to their non-sarcopenic counterparts. Through multivariate analysis, it was also demonstrated that with prehabilitation performed for all patients identified to be high-risk, sarcopenia was no longer an independent variable to predict for worse outcomes. This study lays the groundwork for advancing coordinated efforts to create customized multimodal prehabilitation programs specifically for sarcopenic patients.

Current treatments for sarcopenia largely focus on lifestyle modifications and nutritional supplementation, but these approaches have limited effectiveness for individuals who are immobile or cannot tolerate preoperative enteral nutrition. Emerging therapeutics are being explored through the identification of targetable cellular regions. Multiomics profiling studies aim to provide a detailed understanding of the molecular changes and signaling pathways involved in sarcopenia (Liu et al. 2022), potentially leading to new clinical applications. Regenerative medicine and stem cell therapies, which offer mitochondrial restoration and immune modulation, hold promise for treating sarcopenia at a molecular level (Cai et al. 2022). Pharmacological treatments, such as myostatin inhibitors and selective androgen receptor modulators (SARMs), are being investigated to improve muscle growth and function by targeting key muscle metabolism pathways. Advanced rehabilitation techniques, including neuromuscular electrical stimulation, also show potential for enhancing muscle function.

Further research is necessary to confirm the safety and effectiveness of these new therapies. Additionally, new assessment methods, such as point-of-care ultrasound devices for measuring intramuscular adipose tissue (Sun et al. 2024), could enable regular monitoring of sarcopenia and track the efficacy of prehabilitation programs. Ultimately, a multimodal, multidisciplinary approach tailored to each individual's clinical, lifestyle, genetic, and molecular profile may offer the best strategy to address this growing health issue in the aging population.

In Singapore, the development of a Delphi consensus statement has already laid the groundwork for guiding the perioperative management of sarcopenia. This consensus, detailed in a study by Koh et al. (2024), provides evidence-based recommendations tailored to the local healthcare context for optimizing the care of sarcopenic patients undergoing major surgeries (Table 4.1). This initiative marks a significant step forward in standardizing and improving the management of sarcopenia in the perioperative setting within Singapore.

Implementing such a multifaceted system requires careful coordination of care across various disciplines, which can be a determining factor in the success or failure of prehabilitation programs. The complexity of these interventions means that the effectiveness of a program often depends on how well different components—such as nutritional support, exercise regimens, and psychological rehabilitation—are integrated and tailored to individual patient needs. Inconsistent outcomes across

Table 4.1 A modified Delphi consensus for perioperative management of sarcopenia in patients undergoing major surgeries in Singapore (Koh et al. 2024)

Statement	Quality of evidence
Statement 1: Patients going for major surgery do not need to be screened for sarcopenia but should be assessed for the diagnosis of sarcopenia	High
Statement 2: There are benefits and limitations to different imaging modalities for the assessment of lean muscle mass	Low-moderate
Statement 3: Sarcopenic patients undergoing major abdominal and gastrointestinal surgery should at least receive bimodal prehabilitation that includes resistance training and nutritional therapy	Moderate-high
Statement 4: Treating to target: Nutrition and resistance training should be personalized using a treat-to-target approach	Low-moderate
Statement 5: Prehabilitation can reduce healthcare costs	Low-moderate
Statement 6: 3 other pillars to consider for prehabilitation include financial, psychological and social support	Low-moderate
Statement 7: Rehabilitation improves outcomes in patients undergoing major surgery especially in patients with adjuvant therapy	Moderate-high
Statement 8: Optimizing a patient's Quality-of-Life should be a goal of rehabilitation	Low-moderate

different programs may reflect variations in how effectively these elements are coordinated. Ensuring that each component is delivered in a cohesive and patient-centered manner is crucial for maximizing the benefits of prehabilitation and improving surgical outcomes for sarcopenic patients.

4.6 Conclusion

Sarcopenia poses significant challenges in the surgical setting, impacting postoperative outcomes, oncological prognosis, quality of life, and healthcare costs. Through effective multimodal prehabilitation strategies and initiatives, there is a potential to mitigate these negative effects and improve surgical outcomes. Grounded by increasing scientific and clinical evidences, these approaches offer a pathway to better management and care for sarcopenic patients, particularly in aging populations like Singapore.

References

Abe S, Nozawa H, Kawai K, Sasaki K, Murono K, Emoto S et al (2022) Poor nutrition and sarcopenia are related to systemic inflammatory response in patients with rectal cancer undergoing preoperative chemoradiotherapy. Int J Colorectal Dis 37. https://doi.org/10.1007/s00384-021-04039-w

Antoniou GA, Rojoa D, Antoniou SA, Alfahad A, Torella F, Juszczak MT (2019) Effect of low skeletal muscle mass on post-operative survival of patients with abdominal aortic aneurysm: a prognostic factor review and meta-analysis of time-to-event data. Eur J Vasc Endovasc Surg 58. https://doi.org/10.1016/j.ejvs.2019.03.020

Antoun S, Borget I, Lanoy E (2013) Impact of sarcopenia on the prognosis and treatment toxicities in patients diagnosed with cancer. Curr Opin Support Palliat Care 7. https://doi.org/10.1097/SPC.0000000000000011

Batsis JA, Villareal DT (2018) Sarcopenic obesity in older adults: aetiology, epidemiology and treatment strategies. Nat Rev Endocrinol 14. https://doi.org/10.1038/s41574-018-0062-9

Bone AE, Hepgul N, Kon S, Maddocks M (2017) Sarcopenia and frailty in chronic respiratory disease. Chron Respir Dis 14. https://doi.org/10.1177/1479972316679664

Cai Z, Liu D, Yang Y, Xie W, He M, Yu D et al (2022) The role and therapeutic potential of stem cells in skeletal muscle in sarcopenia. Stem Cell Res Ther 13. https://doi.org/10.1186/s13287-022-02706-5

Chakedis J, Spolverato G, Beal EW, Woelfel I, Bagante F, Merath K et al (2018) Pre-operative sarcopenia identifies patients at risk for poor survival after resection of biliary tract cancers. J Gastrointest Surg 22. https://doi.org/10.1007/s11605-018-3802-1

Chen HT, Chung YC, Chen YJ, Ho SY, Wu HJ (2017) Effects of different types of exercise on body composition, muscle strength, and IGF-1 in the elderly with sarcopenic obesity. J Am Geriatr Soc 65. https://doi.org/10.1111/jgs.14722

Chen LK, Woo J, Assantachai P, Auyeung TW, Chou MY, Iijima K et al (2020) Asian Working Group for Sarcopenia: 2019 consensus update on sarcopenia diagnosis and treatment. J Am Med Dir Assoc 21. https://doi.org/10.1016/j.jamda.2019.12.012

Clark ST, Malietzis G, Grove TN, Jenkins JT, Windsor ACJ, Kontovounisios C et al (2020) The emerging role of sarcopenia as a prognostic indicator in patients undergoing abdominal wall hernia repairs: a systematic review of the literature. Hernia 24. https://doi.org/10.1007/s10029-020-02179-6

Cruz-Jentoft AJ, Bahat G, Bauer J, Boirie Y, Bruyère O, Cederholm T et al (2019) Sarcopenia: revised European consensus on definition and diagnosis. Age Ageing 48. https://doi.org/10.1093/ageing/afy169

Dent E, Hoogendijk EO (2014) Psychosocial factors modify the association of frailty with adverse outcomes: a prospective study of hospitalised older people. BMC Geriatr 14. https://doi.org/10.1186/1471-2318-14-108

Fielding R, Vellas B, Evans W (2011) Sarcopenia: an undiagnosed condition in older adults. Current consensus definition: prevalence, etiology, and consequences. International Working Group on Sarcopenia. J Am Med Dir Assoc 12:249–256. https://doi.org/10.1016/j.jamda.2011.01.003. Sarcopenia

Figueiredo PA, Mota MP, Appell HJ, Duarte J (2006) Ceasing of muscle function with aging: is it the consequence of intrinsic muscle degeneration or a secondary effect of neuronal impairments? Eur Rev Aging Phys Act 3. https://doi.org/10.1007/s11556-006-0011-9

Galivanche AR, Kebaish KJ, Adrados M, Ottesen TD, Varthi AG, Rubin LE et al (2020) Postoperative pressure ulcers after geriatric hip fracture surgery are predicted by defined preoperative comorbidities and postoperative complications. J Am Acad Orthop Surg 28. https://doi.org/10.5435/JAAOS-D-19-00104

Gilmartin S, O'Brien N, Giblin L (2020) Whey for sarcopenia; can whey peptides, hydrolysates or proteins play a beneficial role? Foods 9. https://doi.org/10.3390/foods9060750

Goodman CA, Frey JW, Mabrey DM, Jacobs BL, Lincoln HC, You JS et al (2011) The role of skeletal muscle mTOR in the regulation of mechanical load-induced growth. J Physiol 589. https://doi.org/10.1113/jphysiol.2011.218255

Gouin JP, Kiecolt-Glaser JK (2011) The impact of psychological stress on wound healing: methods and mechanisms. Immunol Allergy Clin N Am 31. https://doi.org/10.1016/j.iac.2010.09.010

Gupta P, Vu TA, Man REK, Fenwick EK, Tay L, Yee Sien N et al (2024) The prevalence patterns and risk factor profiles of poor muscle health and its associated components in multiethnic older Asians: the PIONEER study. J Cachexia Sarcopenia Muscle 15:1376–1387. https://doi.org/10.1002/jcsm.13483

Herrod PJJ, Boyd-Carson H, Doleman B, Trotter J, Schlichtemeier S, Sathanapally G et al (2019) Quick and simple; psoas density measurement is an independent predictor of anastomotic leak and other complications after colorectal resection. Tech Coloproctol 23. https://doi.org/10.1007/s10151-019-1928-0

Huang DD, Chen XX, Chen XY, Wang SL, Shen X, Chen XL et al (2016) Sarcopenia predicts 1-year mortality in elderly patients undergoing curative gastrectomy for gastric cancer: a prospective study. J Cancer Res Clin Oncol 142. https://doi.org/10.1007/s00432-016-2230-4

Kalinkovich A, Becker M, Livshits G (2022) New horizons in the treatment of age-associated obesity, sarcopenia and osteoporosis. Drugs Aging. https://doi.org/10.1007/s40266-022-00960-z

Kobayashi H (2018) Amino acid nutrition in the prevention and treatment of sarcopenia. Yakugaku Zasshi 138. https://doi.org/10.1248/yakushi.18-00091-4

Koh FH, Chua JM, Tan JL, Foo F-J, Tan WJ, Sivarajah SS et al (2021) Paradigm shift in gastrointestinal surgery—combating sarcopenia with prehabilitation: multimodal review of clinical and scientific data. World. J Gastrointest Surg 13. https://doi.org/10.4240/wjgs.v13.i8.734

Koh FH, Chew LM, Wong N, Kow AW, Yap D, Ng S et al (2024) Perioperative management of sarcopenia in patients undergoing major surgeries in Singapore: a modified Delphi consensus. Int J Surg. https://doi.org/10.1097/js9.0000000000001515

Lee YZ, Dharmawan A, Zhang X, Chua DYC, Low JK (2022) The changing landscape of general surgery in the elderly—trends over a decade in a tertiary centre in Singapore. ANZ J Surg 92:2018–2024. https://doi.org/10.1111/ans.17674

Lende TH, Austdal M, Varhaugvik AE, Skaland I, Gudlaugsson E, Kvaløy JT et al (2019) Influence of pre-operative oral carbohydrate loading vs. standard fasting on tumor proliferation and clinical outcome in breast cancer patients—a randomized trial. BMC Cancer 19. https://doi.org/10.1186/s12885-019-6275-z

Li CW, Yu K, Shyh-Chang N, Jiang Z, Liu T, Ma S et al (2022) Pathogenesis of sarcopenia and the relationship with fat mass: descriptive review. J Cachexia Sarcopenia Muscle 13. https://doi.org/10.1002/jcsm.12901

Lichtenberg T, Von Stengel S, Sieber C, Kemmler W (2019) The favorable effects of a high-intensity resistance training on sarcopenia in older community-dwelling men with osteosarcopenia: the randomized controlled frost study. Clin Interv Aging 14. https://doi.org/10.2147/CIA.S225618

Liu JC, Dong SS, Shen H, Yang DY, Chen BB, Ma XY et al (2022) Multi-omics research in sarcopenia: current progress and future prospects. Ageing Res Rev 76. https://doi.org/10.1016/j.arr.2022.101576

Ming YJ, Howley P, Holmes M, Gani J, Pockney P (2022) Sarcopenia 'made simple' and outcomes from emergency laparotomy. ANZ J Surg 92:3198–3203. https://doi.org/10.1111/ans.17759

Negaresh R, Ranjbar R, Baker J, Habibi A, Mokhtarzade M, Gharibvand M et al (2019) Skeletal muscle hypertrophy, insulin-like growth factor 1, myostatin and follistatin in healthy and sarcopenic elderly men: the effect of whole-body resistance training. Int J Prev Med 10. https://doi.org/10.4103/ijpvm.IJPVM_310_17

Okamura H, Kimura N, Tanno K, Mieno M, Matsumoto H, Yamaguchi A et al (2019) The impact of preoperative sarcopenia, defined based on psoas muscle area, on long-term outcomes of heart valve surgery. J Thorac Cardiovasc Surg 157. https://doi.org/10.1016/j.jtcvs.2018.06.098

Peng P, Hyder O, Firoozmand A, Kneuertz P, Schulick RD, Huang D et al (2012) Impact of sarcopenia on outcomes following resection of pancreatic adenocarcinoma. J Gastrointest Surg 16. https://doi.org/10.1007/s11605-012-1923-5

Perrone F, Da-Silva-Filho AC, Adôrno IF, Anabuki NT, Leal FS, Colombo T et al (2011) Effects of preoperative feeding with a whey protein plus carbohydrate drink on the acute phase response and insulin resistance. A randomized trial. Nutr J 10. https://doi.org/10.1186/1475-2891-10-66

Radak Z, Suzuki K, Posa A, Petrovszky Z, Koltai E, Boldogh I (2020) The systemic role of SIRT1 in exercise mediated adaptation. Redox Biol 35. https://doi.org/10.1016/j.redox.2020.101467

Reisinger KW, Derikx JPM, van Vugt JLA, Von Meyenfeldt MF, Hulsewé KW, Olde Damink SWM et al (2016) Sarcopenia is associated with an increased inflammatory response to surgery in colorectal cancer. Clin Nutr 35. https://doi.org/10.1016/j.clnu.2015.07.005

Shafiee G, Keshtkar A, Soltani A, Ahadi Z, Larijani B, Heshmat R (2017) Prevalence of sarcopenia in the world: a systematic review and meta- analysis of general population studies. J Diabetes Metab Disord 16. https://doi.org/10.1186/s40200-017-0302-x

Shen Y, Chen J, Chen X, Hou LS, Lin X, Yang M (2019) Prevalence and associated factors of sarcopenia in nursing home residents: a systematic review and meta-analysis. J Am Med Dir Assoc 20. https://doi.org/10.1016/j.jamda.2018.09.012

Shi Y, Zhou L, Yan E, Yang L, Yang C, Liu C (2021) Sarcopenia and perioperative management of elderly surgical patients. Front Biosci Landmark 26. https://doi.org/10.52586/4995

Shin MJ, Jeon YK, Kim IJ (2018) Testosterone and Sarcopenia. World J Mens Health 36. https://doi.org/10.5534/wjmh.180001

Studenski SA, Peters KW, Alley DE, Cawthon PM, Mclean RR, Harris TB et al (2014) The FNIH Sarcopenia Project: rationale, study and final estimates. J Gerontol Med Sci 69:547–558. https://doi.org/10.1093/gerona/glu010

Sun C, Zhao T, Yang W, Guo G, Wang H, Li C et al (2024) Reduced muscle strength is closely linked to computed tomography-defined myosteatosis among inpatients with cirrhosis. Postgrad Med J 100. https://doi.org/10.1093/postmj/qgad097

Tang VL, Jing B, Boscardin J, Ngo S, Silvestrini M, Finlayson E et al (2020) Association of functional, cognitive, and psychological measures with 1-year mortality in patients undergoing major surgery. JAMA Surg 155. https://doi.org/10.1001/jamasurg.2020.0091

TCTR (2019) The role of branch chain amino acid granules in treatment of sarcopenia in cirrhotic patient. https://Trialsearch.Who.Int/Trial2Aspx?TrialID=TCTR20190904006

Trejo-Avila M, Bozada-Gutiérrez K, Valenzuela-Salazar C, Herrera-Esquivel J, Moreno-Portillo M (2021) Sarcopenia predicts worse postoperative outcomes and decreased survival rates in patients with colorectal cancer: a systematic review and meta-analysis. Int J Colorectal Dis 36. https://doi.org/10.1007/s00384-021-03839-4

Trotter J, Johnston J, Ng A, Gatt M, MacFie J, McNaught CE (2018) Is sarcopenia a useful predictor of outcome in patients after emergency laparotomy? A study using the NELA database. Ann R Coll Surg Engl 100. https://doi.org/10.1308/rcsann.2017.0230

Tsimopoulou I, Pasquali S, Howard R, Desai A, Gourevitch D, Tolosa I et al (2015) Psychological prehabilitation before cancer surgery: a systematic review. Ann Surg Oncol 22. https://doi.org/10.1245/s10434-015-4550-z

Vailati Riboni F, Comazzi B, Bercovitz K, Castelnuovo G, Molinari E, Pagnini F (2020) Technologically-enhanced psychological interventions for older adults: a scoping review. BMC Geriatr 20. https://doi.org/10.1186/s12877-020-01594-9

van der Kroft G, Janssen-Heijnen MLG, van Berlo CLH, Konsten JLM (2015) Evaluation of nutritional status as an independent predictor of post-operative complications and morbidity after gastro-intestinal surgery. Clin Nutr ESPEN 10. https://doi.org/10.1016/j.clnesp.2015.05.005

Voron T, Tselikas L, Pietrasz D, Pigneur F, Laurent A, Compagnon P et al (2015) Sarcopenia impacts on short- and long-term results of hepatectomy for hepatocellular carcinoma. Ann Surg 261. https://doi.org/10.1097/SLA.0000000000000743

Wu J, Chi H, Kok S, Chua JMW, Huang XX, Zhang S et al (2024) Multimodal prerehabilitation for elderly patients with sarcopenia in colorectal surgery. Ann Coloproctol 40:3–12. https://doi.org/10.3393/ac.2022.01207.0172

Xia L, Zhao R, Wan Q, Wu Y, Zhou Y, Wang Y et al (2020) Sarcopenia and adverse health-related outcomes: an umbrella review of meta-analyses of observational studies. Cancer Med 9:7964–7978. https://doi.org/10.1002/cam4.3428

Xie H, Wei L, Liu M, Yuan G, Tang S, Gan J (2021) Preoperative computed tomography-assessed sarcopenia as a predictor of complications and long-term prognosis in patients with colorectal cancer: a systematic review and meta-analysis. Langenbeck's. Arch Surg 406. https://doi.org/10.1007/s00423-021-02274-x

Yan Z, Lira VA, Greene NP (2012) Exercise training-induced regulation of mitochondrial quality. Exerc Sport Sci Rev 40. https://doi.org/10.1097/JES.0b013e3182575599

The Importance of Functional Recovery After Surgery

5

Jayachandran Balachandran

Take-Home Messages

- Functional independence is a high-priority patient-centered outcome.
- Identifying risk factors preoperatively and mitigating them can enhance functional recovery.

5.1 Introduction

With the aging of the population, an increased demand for surgical services can be anticipated. Older adults undergoing surgical procedures are at increased risk for postoperative morbidity and mortality (Bentrem et al. 2009) and may prioritize quality over quantity-of-life years (Fried et al. 2002). Patient-centered care requires that clinicians pay attention to outcomes that matter most to patients. Loss of the ability to live independently is a high-priority patient-centered outcome. Loss of independence (LOI) is defined as one of three changes: a decline in function according to activities of daily living (ADLs), a decline in mobility requiring new mobility aid, or an increase in care needs, such as the need for new home-care services or discharge to a nonhome destination (Berian et al. 2016).

J. Balachandran (✉)
National University Hospital, Singapore, Singapore
e-mail: balachandran_J@nuhs.edu.sg

K.-Y. Tan et al. (eds.), *Mastering Geriatric Surgery*,
https://doi.org/10.1007/978-981-95-0665-1_5

5.2 Functional Recovery After Surgery

Functional recovery is important in older persons as it is associated with decreased postoperative complication and improved quality of life post-surgery. Loss of independence, as defined by a decrease in function or mobility or increase in care needs after surgery, was strongly associated with readmission, postoperative complication across a wide spectrum of surgeries and death (Berian et al. 2016). Maintenance of baseline levels of function and independence and reduction in premature disability after a surgical procedure are critical from a physical, psychological, social, and economic standpoint (Kwon et al. 2012). A survey result showed that 70% of older persons would not choose a treatment that causes severe functional disability, even if survival was assured as emphasis is on the quality of life (Fried et al. 2011). Patients defined recovery as returning to previous habits and routines, resolving symptoms and mental strains caused by surgery, regaining independence in daily tasks, and enjoying life (Rajabiyazdi et al. 2021). Many geriatric patients consider functional decline as a fate worse than death (Becher et al. 2020). The onset and worsening of postoperative disability defined as the need for personal assistance to perform daily activities such as bathing, dressing, and transferring marks a serious decline in functional health (Stabenau et al. 2018). Increased disability confers a greater risk of institutionalization and death and reduction in quality of life.

Major surgery is a leading cause of disability and loss of independence. Surgery is a major stressor to functional status and must be considered in the context of a general decline in functional status associated with “healthy aging.” A healthy 65-year-old is expected to have 9.5 years of functional independence, whereas an 85-year-old is expected to have an average of 3.3 years of independent function (Katz et al. 1983). Thus, major surgery in older persons increases the risk of functional decline with increasing age. Functional dependence is also associated with other adverse outcomes, such as nursing home placement and greater use of formal and informal home services, all of which place substantial burden on informal caregivers and healthcare resources (Kemper 1992).

Functional recovery after surgery depends on the disability status preoperatively. In one of the studies, disability was assessed using four basic activities (bathing, dressing, walking, and transferring), five instrumental activities (shopping, housework, meal preparation, taking medications, and managing finances), and three mobility activities (walk 1/4 mile, climb flight of stairs, and lift/carry ten pounds). For these 12 activities, disability was operationalized as the need for personal assistance or inability to do the task. Older persons with no disability before surgery transitioned to a trajectory of rapid improvement about half of the time. For those with moderate or severe disability before surgery, however, transition to a favorable postsurgery trajectory was uncommon (Stabenau et al. 2018).

5.3 Functional Decline

One of the most feared complications of major surgery is the loss of independence (Gill et al. 2022). Major surgery in older persons puts them at risk of functional decline and disability (Becher et al. 2020). A significant proportion of older patients undergoing major surgery experienced functional decline at 1 month (45.3%), 3 months (30.1%), and 1 year (28.3%) (Kwon et al. 2012). Patients experience significant functional decline in activities of daily living (ADL) after 1 week postoperatively, with 50% of patients reporting dependency for dressing and bathing and 30% requiring assistance for eating and grooming (Lawrence et al. 2004). About 39% adults aged 80 years and older were unable to return directly home after non-cardiac surgery (Polanczyk et al. 2001). Although patients may be fully recovered in their ability to care for themselves and their affairs within 3 months, they may not be back to preöperative strength and conditioning levels for more than 6 months (Lawrence et al. 2004). More patients reported decline than improvement in at least one EQ-5D functional domain 30 days after surgery but not 1 year after surgery (Ladha et al. 2021).

A study that systematically mapped the natural history of long-term recovery of functional independence and identified predictors of recovery in patients 60 years or older after major, elective open abdominal operations found that the temporal order of recovery was cognitive status (by 3 weeks, after a mild decline); timed up and go (6 weeks); ADL, the SF-Physical Component Scale, and Functional Reach (6 weeks to 3 months); and IADL (3–6 months). Slowest to recover was grip strength, for which mean function had not returned to baseline after 6 months. Better preoperative physical performance status and serious postoperative complications consistently predicted recovery. In addition, worse depressive status may be linked to recovery. So, potentially modifiable variables influence recovery, and sequential acute events (operation and postoperative complications) are especially powerful in slowing recovery and perhaps permanently increasing dependence (Lawrence et al. 2004).

5.3.1 Factors Associated with Functional Decline

There are multiple risk factors associated with functional decline for older adults. In one of the studies, they found that ASA class, smoking, LOS, cancer, and male sex were associated with a significant functional decline at some point after surgery (Kwon et al. 2012). In another study, poor preoperative physical performance (measured by gait speed, functional reach, and handgrip strength), depression, and serious postoperative complications were associated with poor ADL recovery after abdominal surgery (Lawrence et al. 2004). Frailty, sensory impairment, nonelective surgery, and smoking are some of the risk factors associated with functional decline. Frailty leaves older patients at risk for poor health outcomes, complications, and prolonged length of stay both during hospitalization and after surgery, including readmission and death (Li et al. 2018; Makary et al. 2010). Sensory impairment such as hearing loss is predictive of postoperative delirium, which in turn can lead to functional disability (Vidán et al. 2009). Nonelective surgery puts patients at risk of severe physiological insult, further reducing physiological reserve and priming older patients for disability and dependency. Nonfrailty and elective surgery were associated with recovery to presurgical function, whereas hearing impairment and greater increases in postsurgical disability were associated with protracted disability and dependency (Becher et al. 2020). Older patients undergoing orthopedic surgery have shown that preoperative functional status is an important predictor of postoperative function. Patients undergoing nonorthopedic surgery, higher preoperative activity level, defined as "those who left their homes as a result of their own efforts at least twice a week," were associated with fewer complications (Seymour and Pringle 1983). Functional decline was associated with worse preoperative fitness and moderate or severe postoperative complications (Ladha et al. 2021).

5.4 Strategies to Enhance Functional Recovery

5.4.1 Preoperative Assessment

Frailty is associated with poor outcomes across most surgical specialties and is also potentially modifiable in the preoperative phase of care. Preoperative assessment helps optimize each patient preoperatively. Preoperative assessment should include a standard evaluation of health and an assessment for frailty, functional status, physical capacity, and cognitive ability, hearing impairment, depression, and social support. The GOSAFE study suggests that preoperative assessment of older adult's fitness for elective surgery should require evaluation of cognition, functional status, and mental health (Montroni et al. 2022). Figure 5.1 highlights a potential decision-making tool for identifying those patients who may benefit most from a preoperative exercise training program (Tew et al. 2018).

5.4.2 Prehabilitation

Improving fitness before surgery through exercise training seems a logical step in achieving this and is termed "prehabilitation." Theoretically, by increasing the functional capacity before operation, the prehabilitated patient retains a higher level of functional ability perioperatively when compared with the non-prehabilitated patient and more rapidly recovers to a minimal level of functional independence after operation (Fig. 5.2) (Banugo and Amoako 2017).

Prehabilitation may involve physical conditioning, nutritional assessment, and supplementation, as well as psychological/emotional conditioning, including the teaching of anxiety-coping techniques. A study comparing "trimodal" prehabilitation (exercise, nutrition, and coping strategies for anxiety) with postoperative

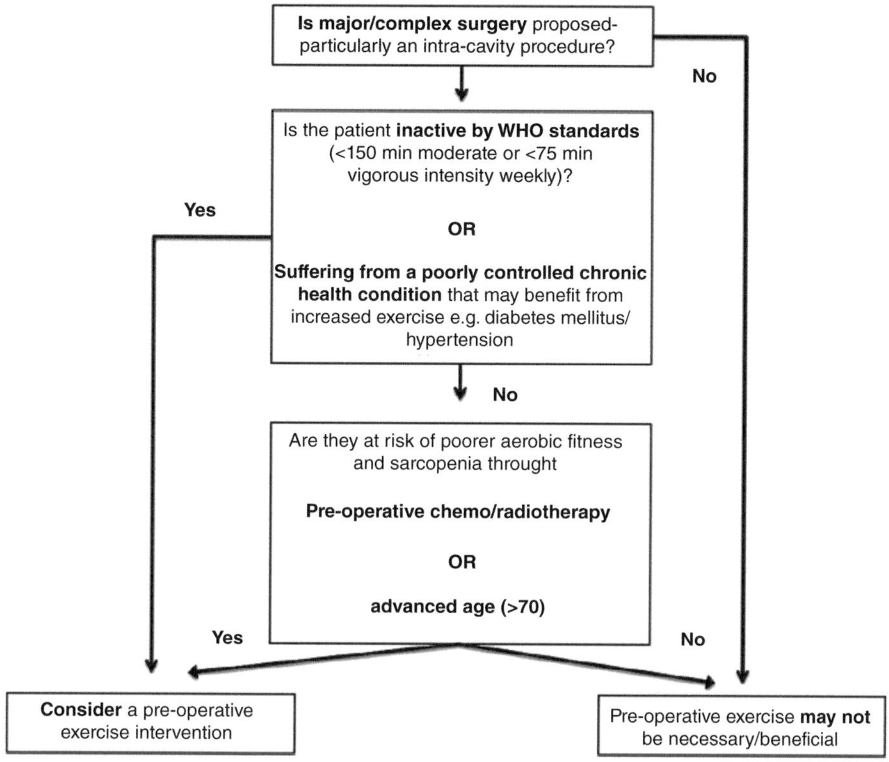

Fig. 5.1 Flow chart to assist clinicians in identifying patients who may benefit from preoperative exercise training (Tew et al. 2018)

rehabilitation (identical to the prehabilitation regimen, but only performed after surgery) showed significantly improved physical functioning in prehabilitation group compared to rehabilitation group as assessed using the 6 MWT (Minnella et al. 2017). In another study, it is demonstrated that prehabilitation is most effective in generating both pre- and postoperative improvements in physical functioning among patients with lower baseline fitness and walking capacity (Minnella et al. 2016). Similarly physical prehabilitation has demonstrated beneficial effects on postoperative recovery in high-risk patients with age >70 years and ASA score III/IV undergoing major abdominal surgery (Barberan-Garcia et al. 2018). Exercise-focused prehabilitation is also feasible in rectal cancer patients undergoing neoadjuvant chemoradiation therapy using the preoperative period to improve functional outcomes (Moug et al. 2019). Since preservation of functional capacity and physical independence are essential postoperative outcomes for senior adults, it is important to incorporate prehabilitation in the geriatric surgical pathway (Ghignone et al. 2020).

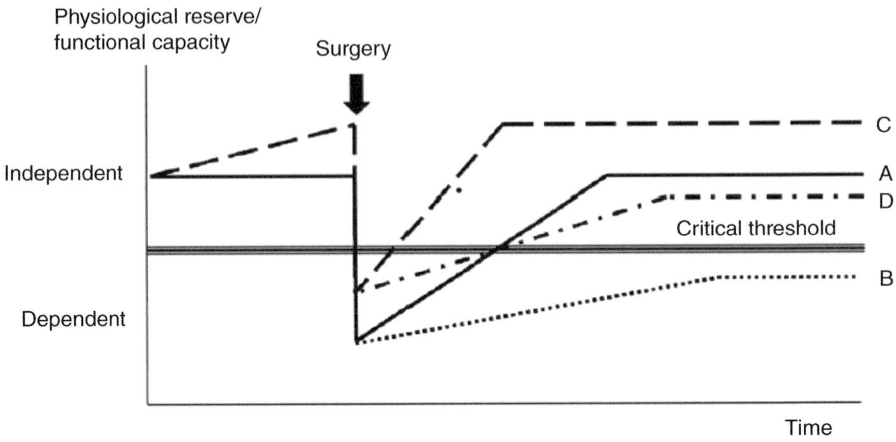

Fig. 5.2 The prehabilitation concept. Following major surgical intervention, all patients experience an acute drop in physiological reserve/functional capacity followed by a recovery and rehabilitation phase (A). A low physiological reserve/functional capacity may increase the risk of perioperative complications and lead to a slower, sometimes incomplete recovery (B). A prehabilitated patient may possess greater physiological reserve/functional capacity at the time of surgery, facilitating a more rapid and complete recovery (C). Crucially, in the event of a complicated recovery, prehabilitated patients may be better placed to retain their functional independence and quality of life in the longer term (D) (Tew et al. 2018)

5.4.3 Prehabilitation Program (Physical Conditioning)

Physical conditioning component of preop usually consists of inspiratory muscle training, aerobic and resistance training. The prehab program is usually conducted for 2–4 weeks.

Inspiratory muscle training is usually done with inspiratory threshold-loading device with the load typically in the range of 10–60% on maximal inspiratory pressure. The frequency of inspiratory muscle training ranged from three sessions per week, with sessions lasting 15 min (range 10–30 min). Perceived exertion was used to guide the progression of training, aiming to maintain a moderate/somewhat hard or hard intensity during each session (Tew et al. 2018).

Aerobic training is done on level ground or cycle ergometer or treadmill or recumbent cross-trainer. The training can be continuous or interval or circuit based. The aerobic training intensity is guided using heart rate response, rate of perceived exertion, or both. The duration of aerobic training is commonly 30–45 min per session; frequency of 3–7 times per week (Tew et al. 2018).

Resistance training is usually done with elastic resistance bands or functional exercise or dumbbells or fixed resistance machines. Intensity for resistance training is based on patient's repetition maximum. Volume of resistance training is either two sets of 10–12 repetitions for each exercise or 8–15 repetitions maximum. The frequency of resistance training ranged from 2 to 4 sessions per week (Tew et al. 2018).

5.4.4 Nutritional Status Improvement

Oral nutritional supplements should be recommended to all malnourished cancer and high-risk patients undergoing major abdominal surgery, in particular to sarcopenic senior adults. This includes patients who meet one or more of the following criteria: weight loss >10–15% within 6 months, BMI <18.5 kg/m^2, NRS >5, and preoperative serum albumin <30 g/L (Weimann et al. 2017).

5.4.5 Delirium Prevention

The best treatment for delirium is prevention. It is also important to detect delirium early when it happens. Simple strategies can be put in place after surgery: pain control, optimization of physical environment (sleep hygiene, presence of family at bedside), easy access of vision and hearing aids, early removal of catheters, and minimization of psychoactive medications could sensibly reduce the risk of delirium. Further postoperative early mobilization, frequent physical activity, and daily cognitive reorientation can reduce delirium (Mohanty et al. 2016).

5.4.6 Enhanced Recovery After Surgery (ERAS)

The ERAS protocols are designed to minimize the physiological stress associated with surgery. The key elements of an enhanced recovery pathway are preoperative education, minimal invasive surgery, intraoperative fluid management, early removal of lines and drains, active pain control, early feeding, and mobilization and multidisciplinary management. The beneficial effects of ERAS pathways in reducing postoperative cardiovascular and respiratory complications in the general population are well-established (Ljungqvist and Hubner 2018; Gonzalez-Ayora et al. 2016). This benefit of reducing postoperative pulmonary complication enhances functional outcomes and QOL for older patients following surgery. ERAS protocols are feasible and equally effective in the geriatric surgical population compared to the general population (Hallam et al. 2018). The success of ERAS pathways requires the participation of all stakeholders involved in the care pathway, including the patient, the surgery team, anesthesia, nursing, physical and occupational therapy, the patient's primary care physician or geriatrician, and oncologist. Minimally invasive surgery (MIS) has already been widely demonstrated to be beneficial in terms of lower mortality and morbidity for older adult patients (Antoniou et al. 2015) and should nowadays be considered the standard surgical approach. MIS and ERAS protocols should always be offered together to enhance their synergic effects.

References

Antoniou SA, Antoniou GA, Koch OO, Pointner R, Granderath FA (2015) Laparoscopic colorectal surgery confers lower mortality in the elderly: a systematic review and meta-analysis of 66,483 patients. Surg Endosc 29:322–333

Banugo P, Amoako D (2017) Prehabilitation. BJA Educ 17(12):401–405

Barberan-Garcia A, Ubré M, Roca J, Lacy AM, Burgos F, Risco R et al (2018) Personalised prehabilitation in high-risk patients undergoing elective major abdominal surgery: a randomized blinded controlled trial. Ann Surg 267:50

Becher RD, Murphy TE, Gahbauer EA, Leo-Summers L, Stabenau HF, Gill TM (2020) Factors associated with functional recovery among older survivors of major surgery. Ann Surg 272(1):92–98

Bentrem DJ, Cohen ME, Hynes DM, Ko CY, Bilimoria KY (2009) Identification of specific quality improvement opportunities for the elderly undergoing gastrointestinal surgery. Arch Surg 144(11):1013–1020

Berian JR, Mohanty S, Ko CY, Rosenthal RA, Robinson TN (2016) Association of loss of independence with readmission and death after discharge in older patients after surgical procedures. JAMA Surg 151(9):e161689

Fried TR, Bradley EH, Towle VR, Allore H (2002) Understanding the treatment preferences of seriously ill patients. N Engl J Med 346(14):1061–1066

Fried TR, Tinetti M, Agostini J, Iannone L, Towle V (2011) Health outcome prioritization to elicit preferences of older persons with multiple health conditions. Patient Educ Couns 83(2):278–282

Ghignone F, Hernandez P, Mahmoud NN, Ugolini G (2020) Functional recovery in senior adults undergoing surgery for colorectal cancer: assessment tools and strategies to preserve functional status. Eur J Surg Oncol 46(3):387–393

Gill TM, Murphy TE, Gahbauer EA, Leo-Summers L, Becher RD (2022) Geriatric vulnerability and the burden of disability after major surgery. J Am Geriatr Soc 70(5):1471–1480

Gonzalez-Ayora S, Pastor C, Guadalajara H, Ramirez JM, Royo P, Redondo E et al (2016) Enhanced recovery care after colorectal surgery in elderly patients. Compliance and outcomes of a multicenter study from the Spanish working group on ERAS. Int J Colorectal Dis 31:1625–1631

Hallam S, Rickard F, Reeves N, Messenger D, Shabbir J (2018) Compliance with enhanced recovery protocols in elderly patients undergoing colorectal resection. Ann R Coll Surg Engl 100(7):570–579

Katz S, Branch LG, Branson MH, Papsidero JA, Beck JC, Greer DS (1983) Active life expectancy. N Engl J Med 309(20):1218–1224

Kemper P (1992) The use of formal and informal home care by the disabled elderly. Health Serv Res 27(4):421

Kwon S, Symons R, Yukawa M, Dasher N, Legner V, Flum DR (2012) Evaluating the association of preoperative functional status and postoperative functional decline in older patients undergoing major surgery. Am Surg 78(12):1336–1344

Ladha KS, Cuthbertson BH, Abbott TEF, Pearse RM, Wijeysundera DN (2021) Functional decline after major elective non-cardiac surgery: a multicentre prospective cohort study. Anaesthesia 76(12):1593–1599

Lawrence VA, Hazuda HP, Cornell JE, Pederson T, Bradshaw PT, Mulrow CD, Page CP (2004) Functional independence after major abdominal surgery in the elderly. J Am Coll Surg 199(5):762–772

Li Y, Pederson JL, Churchill TA, Wagg AS, Holroyd-Leduc JM, Alagiakrishnan K et al (2018) Impact of frailty on outcomes after discharge in older surgical patients: a prospective cohort study. CMAJ 190(7):E184–E190

Ljungqvist O, Hubner M (2018) Enhanced recovery after surgery—ERAS—principles, practice and feasibility in the elderly. Aging Clin Exp Res 30:249–252

Makary MA, Segev DL, Pronovost PJ, Syin D, Bandeen-Roche K, Patel P et al (2010) Frailty as a predictor of surgical outcomes in older patients. J Am Coll Surg 210(6):901–908

Minnella EM, Awasthi R, Gillis C, Fiore JF Jr, Liberman AS, Charlebois P et al (2016) Patients with poor baseline walking capacity are most likely to improve their functional status with multimodal prehabilitation. Surgery 160(4):1070–1079
Minnella EM, Bousquet-Dion G, Awasthi R, Scheede-Bergdahl C, Carli F (2017) Multimodal prehabilitation improves functional capacity before and after colorectal surgery for cancer: a five-year research experience. Acta Oncol 56(2):295–300
Mohanty S, Rosenthal RA, Russell MM, Neuman MD, Ko CY, Esnaola NF (2016) Optimal perioperative management of the geriatric patient: a best practices guideline from the American College of Surgeons NSQIP and the American Geriatrics Society. J Am Coll Surg 222(5):930–947
Montroni I, Ugolini G, Saur NM, Rostoft S, Spinelli A, Van Leeuwen BL et al (2022) Quality of life in older adults after major cancer surgery: the GOSAFE international study. JNCI J Natl Cancer Inst 114(7):969–978
Moug SJ, Mutrie N, Barry SJE, Mackay G, Steele RJC, Boachie C et al (2019) Prehabilitation is feasible in patients with rectal cancer undergoing neoadjuvant chemoradiotherapy and may minimize physical deterioration: results from the REx trial. Colorectal Dis 21(5):548–562
Polanczyk CA, Marcantonio E, Goldman L, Rohde LE, Orav J, Mangione CM, Lee TH (2001) Impact of age on perioperative complications and length of stay in patients undergoing noncardiac surgery. Ann Intern Med 134(8):637–643
Rajabiyazdi F, Alam R, Pal A, Montanez J, Law S, Pecorelli N et al (2021) Understanding the meaning of recovery to patients undergoing abdominal surgery. JAMA Surg 156(8):758–765
Seymour DG, Pringle R (1983) Post-operative complications in the elderly surgical patient. Gerontology 29(4):262–270
Stabenau HF, Becher RD, Gahbauer EA, Leo-Summers L, Allore HG, Gill TM (2018) Functional trajectories before and after major surgery in older adults. Ann Surg 268(6):911–917
Tew GA, Ayyash R, Durrand J, Danjoux G (2018) Clinical guideline and recommendations on pre-operative exercise training in patients awaiting major non-cardiac surgery. Anaesthesia 73(6):750–768
Vidán MT, Sánchez E, Alonso M, Montero B, Ortiz J, Serra JA (2009) An intervention integrated into daily clinical practice reduces the incidence of delirium during hospitalization in elderly patients. J Am Geriatr Soc 57(11):2029–2036
Weimann A, Braga M, Carli F, Higashiguchi T, Hübner M, Klek S et al (2017) ESPEN guideline: clinical nutrition in surgery. Clin Nutr 36(3):623–650

Perioperative Medication Considerations for the Older Person

6

Thuy Bui, Tori Burfield, and Caitlin Mulqueen

Take-Home Messages

- Physiological changes and polypharmacy in the older person can significantly influence medication management during the perioperative period.
- The optimal approach to perioperative medication management for many medicines across various surgical procedures remains largely guided by limited evidence and consensus-based recommendations.
- Effective perioperative medication management requires comprehensive evaluation of patient, medication, and surgical factors by a multidisciplinary team to determine the overall risk–benefit of continuing or withholding medications.

6.1 Impact of Physiological Changes in the Older Person Requiring Surgery

As individuals age, several physiological changes occur that can significantly impact medication management during the perioperative period. Altered pharmacokinetic, pharmacodynamic and homeostatic responses, in addition to comorbidities, increase the risk of adverse drug reactions and complications (Hughes 1998). While

T. Bui (✉) · C. Mulqueen
Pharmacy Department, Alfred Health, Melbourne, VIC, Australia
e-mail: T.Bui@alfred.org.au; C.Mulqueen@alfred.org.au

T. Burfield
Pharmacy Department, Princess Alexandra Hospital, Woolloongabba, QLD, Australia
e-mail: Victoria.Burfield@health.qld.gov.au

K.-Y. Tan et al. (eds.), *Mastering Geriatric Surgery*,
https://doi.org/10.1007/978-981-95-0665-1_6

Table 6.1 Pharmacokinetic changes in the ageing person and clinical consequences (Hughes 1998; Drenth-van Maanen et al. 2020)

Pharmacokinetic consideration	Changes with ageing	Clinical consequence
Absorption	• Gastrointestinal tract changes, e.g. ↓ intestinal blood flow, gastric acid production and gut motility, delayed gastric emptying	• Mostly not of clinical significance
Distribution	• ↓ Lean muscle mass • ↓ Total body water • ↑ Body fat • ↓ Serum albumin levels	• Affects the volume of distribution of hydrophilic and lipophilic medications, leading to altered medication concentrations and varying therapeutic effect • ↑ Effect of highly protein-bound medications like warfarin or phenytoin
Metabolism	• ↓ Hepatic function and blood flow	• ↓ Metabolism and ↑ accumulation/toxicity of medications
Excretion	• ↓ Renal function	• ↓ Clearance and ↑ accumulation/toxicity of medications

pharmacokinetic changes are well understood (see Table 6.1), pharmacodynamic changes, such as heightened sensitivity to central nervous system depressants like opioids or benzodiazepines, are less clear (Hughes 1998). Furthermore, many older persons have various comorbidities, such as diabetes, hypertension or cognitive decline, often requiring polypharmacy, which raises the risk of drug interactions. These factors highlight the need for careful and individualised medication management in the perioperative period to minimise adverse events and optimise surgical outcomes.

6.2 Polypharmacy in the Older Person and Surgery

Polypharmacy, defined as the use of five or more medications (Masnoon et al. 2017), is a common concern in older persons, particularly those undergoing surgery. As the population ages, so does the prevalence of polypharmacy, with studies showing that 45% of older persons aged >65 years take five or more medications (Kim et al. 2024). This prevalence increases in individuals with multiple comorbidities requiring surgical intervention (Kim et al. 2024). The complexity of managing medications in these individuals increases significantly due to the presence of chronic conditions such as hypertension, diabetes, heart disease and osteoarthritis, which often require long-term medication use. Common classes of medications in older persons requiring surgery include antihypertensives, anticoagulants, analgesics, antidiabetics and statins (Gao et al. 2018; Hales et al. 2019).

Pre-existing medications can pose significant risks during the perioperative period. Anticoagulants increase bleeding risk, while diabetes medications may require adjustment while fasting for surgery to prevent hypoglycaemia. Non-steroidal anti-inflammatory drugs (NSAIDs), often used for pain, increase the risk of bleeding and kidney complications (Forsyth et al. 2018; Bongiovanni et al. 2021; Bell et al. 2018), and medications affecting cognition, such as benzodiazepines and anticholinergics, can interact with anaesthetics, raising the risk of delirium and prolonged recovery (Duprey et al. 2022). Polypharmacy combined with medications newly administered in the perioperative period heightens the risk of adverse interactions. A careful preoperative medication review and development of an individualised plan, which includes discontinuing or adjusting medications prior to surgery, is essential to minimise complications. Comprehensive medication management, including clear communication between healthcare providers and the patient and close monitoring during the perioperative period, is vital to optimise surgical outcomes in older persons.

6.3 Perioperative Medication Review

6.3.1 Preoperative Considerations for Elective Surgery

Prior to elective surgery, a patient should ideally be reviewed by a multidisciplinary team which may include anaesthetists, surgeons, nurses, pharmacists, other allied health clinicians such as physiotherapists and dietitians or other medical doctors such as perioperative medicine physicians, endocrinologists or geriatricians (Kwan et al. 2007; Hale et al. 2013; Bui et al. 2022; Sim et al. 2023). This review may take place in a preadmission (or pre-anaesthetic) clinic (PAC), or it could be completed over the phone prior to surgery. A vital component of this pre-surgery assessment is obtaining a best possible medication history (BPMH), which ensures an accurate medication list is available to all relevant clinicians. Evidence has demonstrated that a multidisciplinary approach in PAC, particularly with involvement of a pharmacist, leads to fewer errors in patient medication lists (Kwan et al. 2007; Dooley et al. 2008; Marotti et al. 2011; George et al. 2011).

After obtaining a BPMH, the multidisciplinary team collaborates to recommend necessary medication modifications prior to surgery. These recommendations are based on a comprehensive evaluation of patient-specific factors, surgical considerations including anaesthetic requirements and medication-related factors (see Fig. 6.1). Once a perioperative medication plan has been developed, a designated team member, such as the PAC pharmacist or nurse, communicates the plan to the patient and works with them to ensure adherence, considering individual needs, such as cognitive status or family involvement, particularly for older persons. Many older persons rely on dose administration aids to manage their medications at home, which presents a challenge when medications are required to be identified and withheld preoperatively. In this instance, the designated PAC team member liaises with their community pharmacy colleagues to ensure dose administration aids are adjusted accordingly in preparation for surgery.

Surgical Factors

- Intent of surgery (e.g. curative, palliative)
- Nature and location of surgery, including impact on available routes of medicine administration and medicine absorption (e.g. open versus laparoscopic surgery)
- Classification of surgery (e.g. major versus minor surgery)
- The urgency of surgery (e.g. emergency versus elective surgery)
- Timing of surgery (e.g. imminent versus weeks to months to prepare, morning versus afternoon case) and duration
- Type of anaesthesia (e.g. general anaesthesia versus regional anaesthesia versus local anaesthesia plus sedation)
- Enhanced recovery after surgery (ERAS®) program availability

Medicine Factors

- Indication
- Pharmacokinetics and pharmacodynamics
- Side effects
- Interactions (e.g. drug-drug, drug-disease and drug-nutrient interactions)
- Drug formulation

Patient Factors

- Age extremes (e.g. neonates, children and older people)
- Comorbidities
- Renal and/or hepatic impairment and level of impairment
- Respiratory compromise/risk of post operative pulmonary complications
- Pregnancy or breastfeeding
- Weight extremes (e.g. obesity and cachexia)
- Frailty and function
- Cognition (e.g. literacy, health literacy, ability to understand and execute medicine plans in the perioperative period)
- Pharmacogenomic factors
- Cultural and religious background
- Communicaton barriers (e.g. language, literacy and health literacy, hearing and vision impairment)

Fig. 6.1 Preoperative medication planning is a risk–benefit relationship between patient factors, medicine factors and surgical factors (Bui et al. 2022; reproduced with permission from Advanced Pharmacy Australia)

6.3.2 Preoperative Optimisation

Many PACs are evolving into preoperative optimisation clinics, particularly for older persons, with goals of reducing surgical complications and enhancing recovery outcomes (NICE 2020). These clinics offer immediate access to a range of healthcare professionals, including geriatricians, endocrinologists, specialist nurses, anaesthetists, pharmacists, physiotherapists and other allied health clinicians such as physiotherapists and dietitians (Sim et al. 2023). The multidisciplinary team not only provides recommendations for preoperative medication management but also works to optimise a patient's overall health status and manage their pre-existing comorbidities preoperatively. This could include optimisation of blood pressure management, diagnosis and management of preoperative anaemia or optimisation of glycaemic control. Preoperative optimisation clinics also present an excellent opportunity for comprehensive geriatric assessments, including frailty assessments, and deprescribing opportunities using established deprescribing models such as the Beers Criteria or Screening Tool of Older Persons Potentially Inappropriate Prescriptions (STOPPS) (Forget et al. 2020; Zietlow et al. 2022; Quek et al. 2023).

6.3.3 Postoperative Medication Considerations

Postoperative medication management is equally as important and should be considered early in the perioperative period for older persons. This involves ensuring safe and timely administration of both regular and new postoperative medications (Bui et al. 2022). A study in Australia demonstrated improved prescribing of a patient's regular medications and postoperative venous thromboembolism prophylaxis with collaborative prescribing between the pharmacist and the medical team in PAC (Hale et al. 2013).

The PAC pharmacist, as part of the multidisciplinary team, can also provide recommendations for postoperative medication considerations. For example, patients who will be unable to take medications orally postoperatively may require alternative administration routes and medication formulations for their regular medications to be continued postoperatively. Identifying these patients early prevents delays to medication administration postoperatively, ensuring better management of comorbid conditions during the postoperative period.

6.3.4 Perioperative Medication Considerations in Emergency Surgery

Perioperative medication management in emergency surgery is also critical, particularly for older persons. The multidisciplinary team, including those in the emergency department, surgical units, operating suites and critical care units, must collaborate to minimise medication-related harm. For older persons requiring emergency surgery, having an up-to-date BPMH is essential for all clinicians involved, including surgeons, anaesthetists and geriatricians. This medication history facilitates informed decision-making in time-critical situations. Rates of cognitive impairment in older persons undergoing emergency surgery can be as high as 70%, making it challenging to obtain a BPMH (Moug et al. 2016). Therefore, the involvement of a pharmacist in the multidisciplinary team is invaluable as they can provide pharmacokinetic and pharmacodynamic advice to guide medication management in emergency situations, particularly when there is insufficient time to withhold medications prior to surgery.

6.4 Drug Class Subsections

For any medication, a risk analysis should be completed to determine if it is safe for the patient to continue that medication in the perioperative period. The likelihood of the patient's condition worsening with temporary withdrawal of treatment needs to be weighed against potential interactions with the surgery itself or the anaesthetic if the treatment is continued. Evidence for perioperative medication management is continually evolving as new medications come to market, and more experience and research on, becomes available for different medications. The general principles of perioperative medication management apply; if there is no significant interaction between medications, the surgery and the anaesthetic, then medications should be continued to maintain control of the underlying comorbidity. Perioperative medication management for older persons is further complicated by higher rates of cognitive impairment, which can increase the risk of medication misadventure. The following sections will discuss key considerations for different medication classes commonly requiring review in the perioperative period (see Table 6.2 for a summary including useful guidelines and resources). These considerations are best practice where there is adequate time to withhold medications prior to surgery. In some time-critical situations, it may not be practical to follow these considerations, and a risk–benefit decision should be made. In general, perioperative medication management aims to ensure patient safety before, during and after surgery.

Table 6.2 Summary of perioperative management of common medications and useful resources

Medication classes	General recommendations	Useful guidelines or resources
Diabetes	• Optimise preoperative control to prevent postoperative complications • Medication changes while fasting except sodium glucose co-transporter 2 inhibitors which require a longer withholding period	• ADS-ANZCA Perioperative Diabetes Guidelines and Hyperglycaemia Guidelines (ADS-ANZCA 2022) • American Diabetes Association Standards of Care (American Diabetes Association 2024) • Centre for Perioperative Care Guideline for Perioperative Care for People with Diabetes Mellitus Undergoing Elective and Emergency Surgery (Centre for Perioperative Care 2021) • UKCPA Handbook of Perioperative Medicines, https://periop-handbook.ukclinicalpharmacy.org/
Osteoporosis	• Optimise bone health following minimal trauma fracture • Continue except withhold oral bisphosphonates on the day of surgery	• Preoperative Management of Endocrine, Hormonal, and Urologic Medications: Society for Perioperative Assessment and Quality Improvement (SPAQI) Consensus Statement (Pfeifer et al. 2021) • The Royal Australian College of General Practitioners (RACGP) Osteoporosis risk assessment, diagnosis and management guideline (RACGP-OA 2017) • UKCPA Handbook of Perioperative Medicines, https://periop-handbook.ukclinicalpharmacy.org/
Adrenal	• Continue • Consider stress dosing intra-operatively and postoperatively in those at risk of adrenal crisis	• Preoperative Management of Endocrine, Hormonal, and Urologic Medications: Society for Perioperative Assessment and Quality Improvement (SPAQI) Consensus Statement (Pfeifer et al. 2021) • UKCPA Handbook of Perioperative Medicines, https://periop-handbook.ukclinicalpharmacy.org/
Other endocrine conditions	• Continue • Consider risk of postoperative venous thromboembolism with hormone replacement therapy	

(continued)

Table 6.2 (continued)

Medication classes	General recommendations	Useful guidelines or resources
Alzheimer's disease	• Continue and monitor for potential interactions with anaesthetic agents	• Preoperative Management of Medications for Neurologic Diseases: Society of Perioperative Assessment and Quality Improvement (SPAQI) Consensus Statement (Oprea et al. 2022a) • UKCPA Handbook of Perioperative Medicines, https://periop-handbook.ukclinicalpharmacy.org/
Parkinson's disease	• Continue unless advised otherwise by specialist	
Antiplatelets	• Dependent on antiplatelet, indication and surgical considerations • If patient on dual antiplatelet therapy, consider aspirin monotherapy in perioperative period	• AHA/ACC/ACS/ASNC/HRS/SCA/SCCT/SCMR/SVM Guideline for perioperative cardiovascular management of noncardiac surgery: a report of the American College of Cardiology/American Heart Association Joint Committee on Clinical Practice Guidelines (Thompson et al. 2024) • ESC Guidelines on cardiovascular assessment and management of patients undergoing non-cardiac surgery (Halvorsen et al. 2022) • Clinical Excellence Commission Guidelines on perioperative management of anticoagulant and antiplatelet agents (Clinical Excellence Commission 2018) • American College of Chest Physicians Clinical Practice Guideline on the Perioperative Management of Antithrombotic Therapy (Douketis et al. 2022) • UKCPA Handbook of Perioperative Medicines, https://periop-handbook.ukclinicalpharmacy.org/
Oral anticoagulants	• Dependent on anticoagulant, kidney function, indication, thrombotic risk and surgical or anaesthetic considerations	
Renin–angiotensin system inhibitors	• Individualised approach to patient and surgical considerations	• AHA/ACC/ACS/ASNC/HRS/SCA/SCCT/SCMR/SVM Guideline for perioperative cardiovascular management of noncardiac surgery: a report of the American College of Cardiology/American Heart Association Joint Committee on Clinical Practice Guidelines (Thompson et al. 2024) • Preoperative management of cardiovascular medications: a Society for Perioperative Assessment and Quality Improvement (SPAQI) consensus statement (Sahai et al. 2022) • UKCPA Handbook of Perioperative Medicines, https://periop-handbook.ukclinicalpharmacy.org/
Beta-blockers	• Continue • Avoid initiation immediately before surgery	

(continued)

Table 6.2 (continued)

Medication classes	General recommendations	Useful guidelines or resources
Diuretics	• Patient preference	• Preoperative management of cardiovascular medications: a Society for Perioperative Assessment and Quality Improvement (SPAQ) consensus statement (Sahai et al. 2022) • UKCPA Handbook of Perioperative Medicines, https://periop-handbook.ukclinicalpharmacy.org/
Psychotropics	• Continue	• The Maudsley Prescribing Guidelines in Psychiatry (Taylor et al. 2021) • UKCPA Handbook of Perioperative Medicines, https://periop-handbook.ukclinicalpharmacy.org/
Rheumatological	• Dependent on medication, risk of infection versus flare-up of disease, surgical considerations	• Australian recommendations on perioperative use of disease-modifying anti-rheumatic drugs in people with inflammatory arthritis undergoing elective surgery (Buchbinder et al. 2023) • American College of Rheumatology/American Association of Hip and Knee Surgeons Guideline for the Perioperative Management of Antirheumatic Medication in Patients with Rheumatic Disease Undergoing Elective Total Hip or Knee Arthroplasty (Goodman et al. 2022) • Preoperative Management of Medications for Rheumatologic and HIV Diseases: Society of Perioperative Assessment and Quality Improvement (SPAQI) Consensus Statement (Russell et al. 2022) • UKCPA Handbook of Perioperative Medicines, https://periop-handbook.ukclinicalpharmacy.org/
Herbal medicines	• Withhold for a minimum of 1 week prior to surgery	• Complementary/Natural Medicines Database, https://naturalmedicines.therapeuticresearch.com • UKCPA Handbook of Perioperative Medicines, https://periop-handbook.ukclinicalpharmacy.org/

6.4.1 Endocrinology Medications

There are many endocrine conditions that the older person may be prescribed medications to manage. In the perioperative setting, not all of these conditions require changes to medications. This section will focus on selected conditions where medication changes may be required.

6.4.1.1 Diabetes

Diabetes affects a significant proportion of the population, with 26% of adults aged 65 years or older in the United States being diagnosed with diabetes (Lee and Halter 2017; American Diabetes Association 2024). While there is a larger proportion of older persons diagnosed with type 2 diabetes, the incidence of older persons having type 1 diabetes has increased due to advancements in diabetes management and increased life expectancy (Pratley et al. 2020; Xu et al. 2018). Perioperative diabetes management is a complicated balance of avoiding hypoglycaemia while patients are fasting but also maintaining sufficient insulin levels to prevent hyperglycaemia. Hyperglycaemia in the perioperative period has been associated with adverse outcomes, including surgical site infections and cardiac complications, leading to increased morbidity, length of hospital stays and mortality (ADS-ANZCA 2022). New therapies for diabetes have been developed to not only improve glycaemic control but also prevent cardiac and renal complications. However, these newer therapies have been found to present different challenges in the perioperative setting [e.g. sodium-glucose transporter 2 inhibitor (SGLT2i)-induced euglycaemic ketoacidosis in the perioperative period].

The general principles that guide perioperative diabetes decision-making are to withhold oral hypoglycaemics on the day of surgery to prevent hypoglycaemia while the patient is fasting. International guidelines differ, with some countries only withholding oral hypoglycaemics that predispose the patient to a hypoglycaemic event while fasting. Other countries choose to withhold all oral hypoglycaemic agents to simplify the perioperative medication advice for patients (UKCPA 2021; ADS-ANZCA 2022; American Diabetes Association 2024). Some classes of oral hypoglycaemics may require longer withhold periods due to their pharmacokinetics and side effect profile [e.g. SGLT2i and glucagon-like-peptide 1 agonists (GLP1)]. For patients who are prescribed insulin, it is more complicated as they still require basal insulin, even when fasting. An accurate medication history that includes injectable therapies is essential to ensure optimal perioperative advice is provided to the patient as insulin is available in several different long-, short- and mixed-acting formulations. It is important to assess the patient's baseline diabetes control (e.g. HbA1c), fasting blood sugar levels (BSLs) and recent hypoglycaemic episodes. This information will guide whether a more conservative perioperative insulin management plan is required. Many international guidelines exist to guide perioperative diabetes management of specific insulin types, non-insulin injectables and oral hypoglycaemics (Pfeifer et al. 2021; American Diabetes Association 2024; ADS-ANZCA 2022; Centre for Perioperative Care 2021; Jinjing et al. 2021).

Postoperatively, patients with diabetes should return to their usual diabetes medications as soon as they are eating and drinking adequately. Special attention should be given to converting patients from intravenous insulin and glucose infusions back to their usual subcutaneous insulin regimen. The pharmacokinetics of subcutaneous insulin therapy needs to be considered as intravenous insulin has a very short elimination half-life. Therefore, it is often recommended there be overlap between the intravenous insulin and subcutaneous insulin, with subcutaneous insulin restarted in relation to meals. BSLs should be closely monitored postoperatively as several factors may contribute to variations in the patient's usual BSLs (e.g. surgical stress response, infection, postoperative nausea and vomiting or changes to regular diet). Oral hypoglycaemic agents can typically be restarted once patients are eating and drinking adequately again; however, special consideration should be given to patients with additional surgery plans (SGLT2i), nausea and vomiting (GLP1) or administration of iodinated contrast or acute kidney injury (metformin).

6.4.1.2 Osteoporosis

In Australia, the prevalence of osteoporosis and osteopenia in older persons is 17%, and highest for women over 75 years old (AIHW 2024). Older persons with a history of osteoporosis should be asked about medications prescribed for their osteoporosis. Some patients may omit these medications from their current medications list as they may be taken once a week or administered by injection every 6 months. In the perioperative period, oral bisphosphonates should be withheld on the day of surgery to prevent oesophageal adverse effects from lying supine during surgery and reduced oesophageal sphincter pressure from anaesthetics (Pfeifer et al. 2021; UKCPA 2019a). Other medications for osteoporosis, including supplements such as vitamin D (colecalciferol) and calcium, can be continued in the perioperative period.

The perioperative period may also be an opportunity to recommend therapy for untreated osteoporosis for older persons presenting for emergency surgery following a minimal trauma fracture. Australian guidelines recommend initiating treatment following a minimal trauma fracture of the hip or spine in older persons (>50 years old) without confirmation of low bone mineral density (BMD). For fractures at other sites, BMD should be assessed to guide treatment (RACGP-OA 2017).

6.4.1.3 Adrenal

Older persons are at increased risk of comorbid conditions which may require treatment with long-term corticosteroids. Doses of 5–10 mg or greater of prednisolone for a duration of more than 3–4 weeks are more likely to cause hypothalamo-pituitary-adrenal axis suppression (UKCPA 2019c; Woodcock et al. 2020; Pfeifer et al. 2021). Due to the increased stress response experienced during surgery, these patients may be at risk of adrenal crisis. It is often recommended that patients continue their usual corticosteroid dose in the lead up to surgery and anaesthetic guidelines propose intraoperative stress dosing of steroids (e.g. with intravenous hydrocortisone). It is important these patients are identified prior to surgery and discussed with the anaesthetist so that they can decide whether stress dosing is required on the day of surgery (Pfeifer et al. 2021). Postoperative stress dosing of steroids may also be required in some cases, under the guidance of an endocrinologist.

6.4.1.4 Other Endocrine Conditions

For other endocrine conditions such as hormone replacement therapy (HRT) and thyroid replacement therapy, medication modification or cessation preoperatively is not typically recommended. It is important to maintain adequate control of these conditions before and after surgery. Oral hormone replacement therapies may increase the risk of venous thromboembolism. Most HRT use in older women, however, is administered topically, which reduces systemic absorption and, therefore, adverse effects (Järvstråt et al. 2015; MIMS Australia 2024). Additional consideration should be given to postoperative venous thromboembolism prophylaxis for older persons taking oral forms of HRT. Thyroid function should also be considered if clinically appropriate, for example, in the setting of postoperative atrial fibrillation.

6.4.2 Neurological Medications

Increasing age is one of the biggest risk factors for the development of neurological conditions. The prevalence of conditions such as dementia, stroke and Parkinson's has increased two- to threefold in the last 30 years (Oprea et al. 2022a; Dumurgier and Tzourio 2020; Feigin et al. 2021). Often it is recommended to continue medications used to treat neurological conditions in the perioperative period to maintain control of the underlying disease. However, there are some specific situations and medications clinicians need to consider when planning for surgery for these patients. This section will focus on Alzheimer's disease and Parkinson's disease. For older persons with a history of stroke, the perioperative medication management is similar to patients with a history of cardiovascular disease (e.g. anticoagulants, statins; see 'Cardiovascular medications' section for more information).

6.4.2.1 Alzheimer's Disease and Other Dementias

Older persons who have Alzheimer's disease (AD) or other types of dementia often require assistance from family members or carers to manage their medications due to the nature of their disease. It is important to involve the patient's family or caregivers in the perioperative medication planning. This may also include liaising with primary care providers such as community pharmacies or aged care facilities to ensure medication changes are enacted prior to surgery. This section will discuss perioperative considerations for acetylcholinesterase inhibitors used to treat AD. Patients with dementia may also require antipsychotic medications; see 'Antipsychotic medications' section for further information.

Reversible acetylcholinesterase inhibitors such as rivastigmine and donepezil are often used to treat AD. These medications do not modify disease progression, but in the short term, they do improve cognition, alertness and function. These medications may interact with neuromuscular blockade during surgery. They may prolong the neuromuscular block of suxamethonium (succinylcholine) or reduce the effectiveness of non-depolarising muscle relaxants (Oprea et al. 2022a; UKCPA 2019b). Despite these interactions, it is often recommended that these medications continue throughout the perioperative period (Oprea et al. 2022a). There is concern that stopping these medications for greater than 2–3 days could lead to an irreversible decline in a patient's cognition. Anaesthetists should be advised if a patient is taking one of these medications and adjust the anaesthetic plan accordingly if neuromuscular blockade is required (UKCPA 2019b). If a patient is using a rivastigmine patch, they should be advised that it can be worn during surgery; however, they should place the patch in a location that is distant to the operative site if possible. Otherwise, the patch may need to be removed and replaced once clinically appropriate postoperatively.

6.4.2.2 Parkinson's Disease

The prevalence of Parkinson's disease (PD) has risen over the past 30 years due to our ageing population (Ben-Schlomo et al. 2024). The perioperative management of older persons with PD is challenging due to both the medications used to treat PD and the risk of PD symptom exacerbation during the perioperative period. Dopaminergic and anticholinergic medications are common treatments for PD. These medications may be associated with adverse effects such as delirium, orthostatic hypotension or dopaminergic adverse effects. While there are no direct interactions with anaesthetic medications, it is important to promptly identify the cause of these symptoms in the perioperative period if experienced by a patient (Oprea et al. 2022a; Ben-Schlomo et al. 2024).

The pharmacokinetics of PD medications results in frequent dosing intervals throughout the day. On the day of surgery, it can be difficult to maintain a patient's regular dosing schedule (Oprea et al. 2022a). It is vital that a BPMH is completed prior to surgery. Patients should be advised to take regular doses prior to surgery, as per their usual dosing regimen. On the day of surgery, consideration should be given to intraoperative dosing to maintain a patient's usual dosing regimen if possible. Expert opinion suggests that two or three doses of PD medications can be missed without impacting symptoms (Therapeutic Guidelines 2018). Individual patient experience and symptom control, however, should be factored into the decision-making. There are some surgeries that result in a delay to oral intake. It is important to identify these patients early and consideration given to transitioning their oral therapy to the transdermal route. Dosing calculators are available to guide the conversion of a patient's total daily levodopa equivalent dose to a transdermal formulation (Therapeutic Guidelines 2018).

While it is usually recommended to continue these medications throughout the perioperative period, for PD-related surgery (e.g. deep brain stimulator insertion), it may be advised to withhold PD medications prior to surgery (Oprea et al. 2022a).

6.4.3 Cardiovascular Medications

6.4.3.1 Antiplatelets

Antiplatelets, including aspirin and $P2Y_{12}$ inhibitors, are taken for a range of indications, most commonly coronary heart disease, cerebrovascular disease and peripheral arterial disease. A national survey conducted in the United States found that more than half of patients aged 70 years and over were taking an antiplatelet (Gu et al. 2015). Antiplatelets require an individualised perioperative management plan. This plan should be formulated after confirmation of a patient's indication for taking antiplatelet therapy, involvement of a patient's surgeon and specialist managing the antiplatelet(s) and after consideration of a patient's thromboembolic risk and bleeding risk of the procedure (Clinical Excellence Commission 2018; Thompson et al. 2024). Specific consideration should also be given to patients taking antiplatelet therapy following percutaneous coronary intervention (PCI), including the type of PCI and surgery timing in relation to the PCI timing. If the antiplatelet is to be interrupted perioperatively, the timing of both interruption and resumption should be guided by the agent's pharmacokinetic and pharmacodynamic properties, including whether the agent reversibly or irreversibly inhibits platelet function (Douketis et al. 2022; Halvorsen et al. 2022). Furthermore, if patients are taking both aspirin and a $P2Y_{12}$ inhibitor concurrently [dual antiplatelet therapy (DAPT)], consideration should be given to continuing aspirin as single antiplatelet therapy in the perioperative period while the $P2Y_{12}$ inhibitor is withheld.

6.4.3.2 Oral Anticoagulants

Oral anticoagulants (OAC), including vitamin K antagonists (VKA) and direct oral anticoagulants (DOAC), are commonly taken for venous thromboembolism (VTE), atrial fibrillation (AF) and valvular heart disease. An estimated 1 in 4 patients taking an anticoagulant will require surgery within 2 years, presenting both bleeding and thrombotic risks perioperatively, particularly in older persons (Halvorsen et al. 2022). Similar to antiplatelets, anticoagulants require an individualised perioperative management plan formulated by a patient's surgeon and specialist managing the anticoagulant. In formulating this plan, specific surgical factors (including urgency of surgery, bleeding risk and type of anaesthesia), patient factors (including age, thromboembolic risk, history of bleeding complications and renal function) and medicine factors (including indication, pharmacokinetics and pharmacodynamics) should be considered (Halvorsen et al. 2022; Thompson et al. 2024). Several resources are available to assist with surgical bleeding risk and thromboembolic risk assessment and medicine factor considerations (Douketis et al. 2022; Halvorsen et al. 2022; Spyropoulos et al. 2019; Thompson et al. 2024). If a VKA is to be interrupted perioperatively and a patient has a high thromboembolic risk, consideration should also be given to the need for preoperative bridging anticoagulation with a parenteral heparin. Preoperative bridging anticoagulation while a DOAC is interrupted is generally not required (Thompson et al. 2024).

6.4.3.3 Renin–Angiotensin System (RAS) Inhibitors

Renin–angiotensin system (RAS) inhibitors, comprising angiotensin-converting-enzyme inhibitors (ACE-I) and angiotensin II receptor blockers (ARB), are commonly prescribed for hypertension, heart failure and chronic kidney disease. Continuing these medicines perioperatively with anaesthesia, fluid shifts and blood loss has been associated with increased risk of intraoperative hypotension, which may contribute to complications such as acute kidney injury (Legrand et al. 2024). Due to a lack of evidence, there is uncertainty surrounding their optimal management in the perioperative period. They are frequently withheld preoperatively to prevent intraoperative hypotension and, in turn, reduce the risk of myocardial injury and death, particularly in older persons (Ackland et al. 2024). Recent evidence supports a reduction in intraoperative hypotension when RAS inhibitors are withheld preoperatively. Rates of postoperative complications or death, however, were similar for withholding and continuing RAS inhibitors preoperatively (Legrand et al. 2024). While awaiting further evidence, an individualised approach for the perioperative management of RAS inhibitors is recommended (Sahai et al. 2022). RAS inhibitors are generally continued in surgeries with minimal risk of intraoperative hypotension such as intracranial procedures or day surgery.

6.4.3.4 Beta-Blockers

Beta-blockers are prescribed for a range of cardiovascular conditions, and their use in the perioperative period has been extensively studied (Sahai et al. 2022). For those on established beta-blocker therapy, beta-blockers should be continued throughout the perioperative period as acutely discontinuing treatment has been associated with harm (Sahai et al. 2022; Thompson et al. 2024). For those newly commenced on beta-blockers, a period of at least 7 days is recommended between commencement and surgery (Thompson et al. 2024). This is to ensure there is sufficient time to assess tolerability and titrate the dose as well as to reduce mortality risk. Finally, in the absence of an immediate need for beta-blocker treatment, beta-blockers should not be commenced on the day of surgery due to an increase in postoperative mortality risk (Thompson et al. 2024).

6.4.3.5 Diuretics

Loop diuretics, thiazide diuretics and aldosterone antagonists are the most prescribed diuretic classes. Evidence to support their management in the perioperative period is lacking. There are a range of concerns relating to their continuation, including hypovolemia and subsequent hypotension, electrolyte disturbances and postoperative acute kidney injury. It is unclear, however, if withholding diuretics on the morning of surgery will alleviate these concerns. To formulate a perioperative plan, a patient's individual history and fluid status must be considered. The practicality of a patient managing a strong urge to urinate immediately prior to, and during, a procedure should also be considered, particularly for older persons (Sahai et al. 2022).

6.4.3.6 Other Cardiovascular Medications

Evidence relating to the optimal perioperative management of statins and other antihypertensives, including calcium channel blockers and alpha-2 receptor agonists, is lacking. These agents, however, are generally continued perioperatively (Thompson et al. 2024).

6.4.4 Psychotropics Medications

6.4.4.1 Benzodiazepines

Benzodiazepines are one of the most prescribed medication classes for older persons. They are predominantly prescribed for the management of anxiety and insomnia symptoms (Kudoh et al. 2004). Continuation of chronic benzodiazepines preoperatively increases the risk of CNS depression, which is further increased when given concomitantly with other CNS depressants such as perioperative analgesics. Preoperative benzodiazepine use also increases the risk of delirium, especially in older persons. On the other hand, interruption to chronic benzodiazepine use preoperatively may exacerbate anxiety and insomnia symptoms or cause withdrawal symptoms. Therefore, benzodiazepines are generally recommended to be continued preoperatively (Oprea et al. 2022b; Taylor et al. 2021). It should be noted that a single preoperative benzodiazepine dose to treat anxiety has not been shown to increase the risk of delirium (Mahanna-Gabrielli et al. 2023).

6.4.4.2 Antipsychotics

Antipsychotics are largely used for the treatment of schizophrenia and bipolar disease (Harbell et al. 2021). They can also be used for the management of dementia-associated agitation, aggression and psychosis (Therapeutic Guidelines 2021). Most antipsychotics can increase the risk of CNS depression, QT interval prolongation, hypotension as a result of alpha-1 blockade, intraoperative hypothermia and reduced seizure threshold. This risk is enhanced when administered with other medications also associated with these side effects (Oprea et al. 2022b, Taylor et al. 2021). Furthermore, antipsychotics are predominantly metabolised by the cytochrome P450 system, resulting in various drug–drug interactions that require consideration in the perioperative period (Harbell et al. 2021). Interrupting antipsychotic use preoperatively, however, may increase the risk of psychotic symptom relapse and postoperative confusion and agitation. Preoperative use of antipsychotics is likely safe with side effect and drug–drug interaction consideration, and they are generally recommended to be continued (Oprea et al. 2022b, Taylor et al. 2021).

6.4.4.3 Antidepressants

A national survey conducted in the United States found that 19% of patients aged 60 years and over were taking an antidepressant (Brody and Gu 2020). Use of antidepressants in the perioperative period is not without risks, and consideration should be given to the anaesthetic agents to be used. Interruption preoperatively, however, may lead to a relapse of symptoms or withdrawal symptoms (see Table 6.3) (Harbell et al. 2021; Oprea et al. 2022b; Taylor et al. 2021).

6.4.5 Rheumatological Medications

Rheumatological diseases are common in older persons, secondary to the effects of ageing on the musculoskeletal and immune systems. Rheumatoid arthritis (RA) affects approximately 1% of individuals aged over 65 years (GBD 2023), while conditions like lupus, polymyalgia rheumatica (PMR) and giant cell arteritis (GCA) are less frequent (Poudel and Yu 2020). These diseases and their treatments, including disease-modifying antirheumatic drugs (DMARDs), increase the risk of surgical complications such as infections, delayed wound healing and cardiovascular events. Perioperative management of DMARDs must balance the risk of

Table 6.3 Considerations and recommendations for antidepressants in the perioperative period (Harbell et al. 2021, Oprea et al. 2022b, Taylor et al. 2021)

Antidepressant class	Perioperative risks	Preoperative recommendation
Selective serotonin reuptake inhibitors (SSRIs), serotonin-norepinephrine reuptake inhibitors (SNRIs)	Serotonin syndrome Bleeding (due to antiplatelet effect) QT interval prolongation	Continue
Tricyclic antidepressants (TCAs)	CNS depression Hypotension (due to alpha-1 blockade) Serotonin syndrome QT interval prolongation Seizure threshold lowering Bleeding (amitriptyline, clomipramine) Anticholinergic	Continue
Monoamine oxidase inhibitors (MAOIs)	Hypertensive crisis (with indirect acting sympathomimetic agents) Serotonin syndrome	Continue with careful consideration of anaesthetic agents used

complications from continuing treatment with the potential for disease flare-ups if treatment is withheld. RA flare-ups occur in 10–20% of patients undergoing surgery, but RA patients have a 50% increased risk of prosthetic joint infection compared to those with osteoarthritis, complicating their recovery (Goodman et al. 2022). Active RA and ageing further elevate infection risk, with older persons having 2–3 times the risk of serious infections requiring hospitalisation or an emergency department visit (Widdifield et al. 2013).

Managing RA flare-ups and preventing joint damage or disability are crucial for a patient's postoperative recovery. A comprehensive preoperative evaluation, including a review of medications and disease status, is essential, with collaboration between the surgical and rheumatology specialists (see Fig. 6.2). Addressing patient concerns about past infections and flare-ups is key when developing an individualised perioperative medication management plan. If therapy interruption is chosen, it is generally recommended to resume therapy 1–2 weeks after surgery or once sutures are removed, provided wound healing is adequate and no signs of infection are present (Goodman et al. 2022; Russell et al. 2022; Buchbinder et al. 2023).

6.4.5.1 NSAIDs and Corticosteroids

NSAIDs may increase the risk of bleeding or kidney dysfunction after surgery (Russell et al. 2022). Guidelines recommend withholding NSAIDs 7 days preoperatively or based on their half-life (see Chap. 8, Table 8.4) (Russell et al. 2022). For example, ibuprofen, with a short half-life, can be withheld for 1 day prior to surgery, while celecoxib, a selective COX-2 inhibitor with no antiplatelet effect, may be continued prior to surgery. The impact of withholding NSAIDs on pain and function should be assessed, as alternative short-acting NSAIDs or other analgesia may be

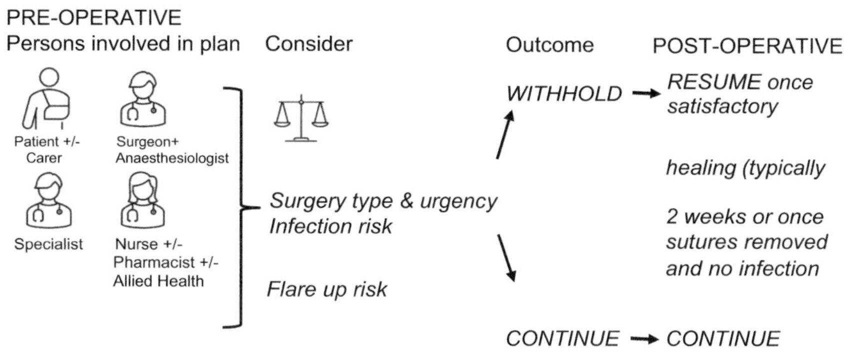

Fig. 6.2 Approach to perioperative management of medications for rheumatological disease

necessary. For corticosteroids, the current daily dose should be continued perioperatively rather than administering supraphysiological doses on the day of surgery. Limited evidence suggests that higher doses (>15 mg/day) may increase the risk of hyperglycaemia, infection and impaired wound healing (Goodman et al. 2022; Russell et al. 2022).

6.4.5.2 Conventional DMARDs

Evidence for the optimal perioperative medication management of conventional DMARDs such as methotrexate, leflunomide, hydroxychloroquine, sulfasalazine and apremilast is limited, with most studies focusing on methotrexate and leflunomide in RA patients undergoing elective orthopaedic surgery (Buchbinder et al. 2023; Goodman et al. 2022). Data supporting recommendations is mainly indirect or of low-to-moderate quality, often based on consensus (Buchbinder et al. 2023, Goodman et al. 2022). Discontinuation of conventional DMARDs perioperatively may increase the risk of flare without significantly reducing postoperative infections (Buchbinder et al. 2023, Goodman et al. 2022). Guidelines generally recommend continuing conventional DMARDs perioperatively (Goodman et al. 2022, Russell et al. 2022, Buchbinder et al. 2023), although they may be withheld in patients with a history of serious or recurrent infections (Goodman et al. 2022, Russell et al. 2022, Buchbinder et al. 2023).

6.4.5.3 Biologic DMARDs

Biologic agents such as tumour necrosis factor (TNF) inhibitors and interleukin inhibitors suppress the immune system, often requiring a "drug holiday" before elective surgery. Typically, these agents should be withheld for one dosing cycle, with surgery scheduled towards the end of the dosing interval (Goodman et al. 2022, Russell et al. 2022, Buchbinder et al. 2023). This recommendation is based on low-quality evidence showing no difference in postoperative outcomes between short and longer interruptions (Goodman et al. 2022). In patients with difficult-to-control disease, continuing therapy may be more appropriate, whereas a longer interruption period may be considered for those with severe or recurrent infections or a shorter interruption period considered when the benefit of surgery outweighs the infection risk (Goodman et al. 2022, Russell et al. 2022, Buchbinder et al. 2023).

6.4.5.4 Targeted Synthetic DMARDs

Traditionally, the recommendation has been to withhold janus kinase (JAK) inhibitors (e.g. tofacitinib, baricitinib, upadacitinib) for 7 days preoperatively due to concerns with prolonged immunological activity beyond the short serum half-life of the medications (Goodman et al. 2022; Buchbinder et al. 2023). However, recent trial data suggests that interruption of tofacitinib therapy can lead to rapid disease progression (Kaine et al. 2020). Therefore, a recently updated guideline recommends withholding JAK inhibitors for only 3 days prior to surgery, based on their pharmacokinetics (Goodman et al. 2022). The interruption period may be longer in those with a history of severe or recurrent infections.

6.4.5.5 Other Immunosuppressant Medications

Mycophenolate, azathioprine, cyclosporine, tacrolimus or voclosporin are other immunosuppressant medications indicated for systemic lupus erythematosus (SLE) and several other non-rheumatological conditions such as skin disorders and prevention of organ transplant rejection. For SLE, it is recommended to continue these medications in severe cases and consider withholding them for 1 week prior to surgery in patients with non-severe SLE (Goodman et al. 2022, Russell et al. 2022).

6.4.6 Herbal Medicines

The World Health Organization defines herbal medicines as 'herbs, herbal materials, herbal preparations and finished herbal products, that contain as active ingredients parts of plants, or other plant materials, or combinations' (World Health Organisation 2024). Examples of herbal medicines include echinacea, garlic, gingko, ginseng and St. John's wort (Lazo et al. 2024). The prevalence of herbal medicine use varies widely in the literature. A study conducted in the United States found 1 in 4 patients waiting for surgery were using herbal medicine. Furthermore, surgeons and anaesthetists were usually not informed of the herbal medicine use and only half of the patients withheld these medicines before surgery (Leung et al. 2001). Herbal medicine use is also most prevalent in older persons, with approximately 1 in 4 patients taking herbal medicines, aged 65 years and over (Harnett et al. 2023).

Literature on the implications of herbal medicine use in the perioperative period is limited. It is expected, however, that these medicines may have several effects on major organ systems in this period (see Table 6.4) (Lazo et al. 2024).

Given the possible implications of herbal medicine use during the perioperative period, it is important that a patient's herbal medicine use is identified during preoperative assessment with a BPMH. Perioperative interruption to herbal medicine therapy for 1–2 weeks prior to surgery is often advisable where possible (Lazo et al.

Table 6.4 Examples of common herbal medicines and possible adverse effects in the perioperative period (Lazo et al. 2024)

	Associated common herbal medicines	Possible adverse effects in the perioperative period
Central nervous system	Ashwagandha, black cohosh, turmeric, valerian	Increased sedation
	Valerian	Increased anaesthetic requirement
Cardiovascular system	Green tea, licorice	Tachycardia, hypertension
	Ashwagandha	Hypotension
	Black cohosh	Bradycardia
Respiratory function	Lion's mane	Acute respiratory distress syndrome
Endocrine function	Garlic, ginger, ginseng, lion's mane	Hypoglycaemia
Hepatic function	Ashwagandha, black cohosh, echinacea, green tea, valerian	Liver damage and/or dysfunction
Renal function	Licorice	Acute tubular necrosis, acute renal failure
	Licorice	Hypokalaemia
Gastrointestinal function	Black cohosh, garlic, ginger, ginseng, milk thistle, saw palmetto, St. John's wort	Nausea, vomiting, diarrhoea
	Echinacea	Constipation
	Ginger	Abdominal pain
Haemostasis	Garlic, gingko, ginseng, green tea, lion's mane, saw palmetto, St. John's wort	Antiplatelet effect
	Garlic, ginger, gingko, ginseng, green tea, licorice, milk thistle, saw palmetto, St. John's wort, turmeric	Anticoagulant effect
	Black cohosh, green tea	Procoagulant effect
Drug metabolism	Echinacea, licorice, peppermint, saw palmetto, turmeric, valerian	Inhibit cytochrome P450 enzyme system
	Echinacea, St. John's wort	Induce cytochrome P450 enzyme system

2024). If this is not possible or in the case of emergency surgery, herbal medicine use is generally not a reason to cancel or postpone surgery.

6.5 Considerations for Common Medications Initiated After Surgery

When managing postoperative care in older persons, several key considerations must be taken into account for medications aimed at managing pain, thromboprophylaxis, surgical antimicrobial prophylaxis and preventing postoperative nausea and vomiting (PONV). Older persons often have altered pharmacokinetics and pharmacodynamics, making them more susceptible to adverse drug reactions and side effects. For pain management, opioids should be used cautiously due to the increased risk of gastrointestinal side effects, sedation, delirium and respiratory depression, with consideration given to non-opioid analgesics such as acetaminophen (paracetamol) or regional anaesthesia techniques (Abdulla et al. 2013; Schofield et al. 2022); refer to Chap. 8. Thromboprophylaxis must be tailored to the individual, with careful assessment of renal function, weight and bleeding risk, and may include low-molecular-weight heparin, unfractionated heparin or mechanical compression devices (Bartlett et al. 2020). Surgical antimicrobial prophylaxis should be guided by local infection rates and the patient's renal function, as older persons are at greater risk for antimicrobial toxicity and resistance. Additionally, preventing PONV in this population requires an individualised approach, with the use of antiemetics that have a favourable side effect profile in older persons and attention to factors such as polypharmacy, and comorbidities like dementia, which may alter the response to standard treatments (Stephenson et al. 2020; Gan et al. 2020). These considerations are essential for optimising postoperative recovery while minimising complications in older persons undergoing surgery.

References

Abdulla A, Bone M, Adams N, Elliott AM, Jones D, Knaggs R, Martin D, Sampson EL, Schofield P (2013) Evidence-based clinical practice guidelines on management of pain in older people. Age Ageing 42(2):151–153

Ackland GL, Patel A, Abbott TEF, Begum S, Dias P, Crane DR, Somanath S, Middleditch A, Cleland S, Gutierrez Del Arroyo A, Brealey D, Pearse RM (2024) Discontinuation vs. continuation of renin–angiotensin system inhibition before non-cardiac surgery: the SPACE trial. Eur Heart J 45(13):1146–1155

ADS-ANZCA (2022) Perioperative diabetes guidelines and hyperglycaemia guidelines. https://www.diabetessociety.com.au/wp-content/uploads/2023/03/ADS-ANZCA-Perioperative-Diabetes-and-Hyperglycaemia-Guidelines-Adults-November-2022-v2-Final.pdf. Accessed 18 Dec 2024

American Diabetes Association (2024) American Diabetes Association standards of care. Diabetes Care 43(2):S244-257,S301-302.

Australian Institute of Health and Welfare (2024) Chronic musculoskeletal conditions: osteoporosis and minimal trauma fractures. https://www.aihw.gov.au/reports/chronic-musculoskeletal-conditions/osteoporosis. Accessed 18 Dec 2024

Bartlett MA, Mauck KF, Stephenson CR, Ganesh R, Daniels PR (2020) Perioperative venous thromboembolism prophylaxis. Mayo Clin Proc 95(12):2775–2798

Bell S, Rennie T, Marwick CA, Davey P (2018) Effects of peri-operative nonsteroidal anti-inflammatory drugs on post-operative kidney function for adults with normal kidney function. Cochrane Database Syst Rev 11(11):CD011274

Ben-Schlomo Y, Darweesh S, Llibre-Guerra J (2024) The epidemiology of Parkinson's disease. Lancet 403(10423):283–292

Bongiovanni T, Lancaster E, Ledesma Y, Whitaker E, Steinman MA, Allen IE, Auerbach A, Wick E (2021) Systematic review and meta-analysis of the association between non-steroidal anti-inflammatory drugs and operative bleeding in the perioperative period. J Am Coll Surg 232(5):765–790.e1

Brody DJ, Gu Q (2020) Antidepressant use among adults: United States, 2015-2018. https://www.cdc.gov. Accessed 23 Dec 2024

Buchbinder R, Glennon V, Johnston RV, Brennan SE, Fong C, Edward May S, O'Neill S, Smitham P, Trevena L, Whittaker G, Wluka A, Whittle SL (2023) Australian recommendations on perioperative use of disease-modifying anti-rheumatic drugs in people with inflammatory arthritis undergoing elective surgery. Intern Med J 53(7):1248–1212

Bui T, Fitzpatrick B, Forrester T, Gu G, Hill C, Mulqueen C, Penno J, Munro C, Mellor Y (2022) Standard of practice in surgery and perioperative medicine for pharmacy services. J Pharm Pract Res 52(2):139–158

Centre for Perioperative Care (2021) Guideline for perioperative care for people with diabetes mellitus undergoing elective and emergency surgery. https://cpoc.org.uk/guidelines-resources/guidelines. Accessed 18 Dec 2024

Clinical Excellence Commission (2018) Guidelines on perioperative management of anticoagulant and antiplatelet agents. https://www.cec.health.nsw.gov.au/__data/assets/pdf_file/0006/458988/Guidelines-on-perioperative-management-of-anticoagulant-and-antiplatelet-agents.pdf. Accessed 23 Dec 2024

Dooley MJ, Van de Vreede M, Tan E (2008) Patient-completed medication histories versus those obtained by a pharmacist in a pre-admission clinic. J Pharm Pract Res 38(3):216–218

Douketis JD, Spyropoulos AC, Murad MH, Arcelus JI, Dager WE, Dunn AS, Fargo RA, Levy JH, Samama CM, Shah SH, Sherwood MW, Tafur AJ, Tang LV, Moores LK (2022) Perioperative management of antithrombotic therapy. Chest 162(5):e207–e243

Drenth-van Maanen AC, Wilting I, Jansen PAF (2020) Prescribing medicines to older people-How to consider the impact of ageing on human organ and body functions. Br J Clin Pharmacol 86(10):1921–1930

Dumurgier J, Tzourio C (2020) Epidemiology of neurological diseases in older adults. Rev Neuro (Paris) 176(9):642–648

Duprey MS, Devlin JW, Griffith JL, Travison TG, Briesacher BA, Jones R, Saczynski JS, Schmitt EM, Gou Y, Marcantonio ER, Inouye SK (2022) Association between perioperative medication use and postoperative delirium and cognition in older adults undergoing elective noncardiac surgery. Anesth Analg 134(6):1154–1163

Feigin VL, Vos T, Alahdab F et al (2021) Burden of neurological disorders across the US from 1990-2017: a global burden of disease study. JAMA Neurol 78(2):165–176

Forget MF, McDonald EG, Shema AB, Lee TC, Wang HT (2020) Potentially inappropriate medication use in older adults in the preoperative period: a retrospective study of a noncardiac surgery cohort. Drugs Real World Outcomes 7:171–178

Forsyth MG, Clarkson DJ, O'Boyle CP (2018) A systematic review of the risk of postoperative bleeding with perioperative non-steroidal anti-inflammatory drugs (NSAIDs) in plastic surgery. Eur J Plast Surg 41:505–510

Gan TJ, Belani KG, Bergese S, Chung F, Diemunsch P, Habib AS, Jin Z, Kovac AL, Meyer TA, Urman RD, Apfel CC, Ayad S, Beagley L, Candiotti K, Englesakis M, Hedrick TL, Kranke P, Lee S, Lipman D, Minkowitz HS, Morton J, Philip BK (2020) Fourth consensus guidelines for the management of postoperative nausea and vomiting. Anesth Analg 131(2):411–448

Gao L, Maidment I, Matthews FE, Robinson L, Brayne C, on behalf of the Medical Research Council Cognitive Function and Ageing Study (2018) Medication usage change in older people (65+) in England over 20 years: findings from CFAS I and CFAS II. Age Ageing 47(2):220–225

GBD 2021 Rheumatoid Arthritis Collaborators (2023) Global, regional, and national burden of rheumatoid arthritis, 1990-2020, and projections to 2050: a systematic analysis of the Global Burden of Disease Study 2021. Lancet Rheumatol 5(10):e594–e610

George LJ, Senturk-Raif R, Hodgkinson M, Emmerton M, Larmour I (2011) Impact of a surgical preadmission clinic pharmacist on the quality of medication management from preadmission to discharge: a randomised controlled study. J Pharm Pract Res 41(3):212–216

Goodman SM, Springer BD, Chen AF, Davis M, Fernandez DR, Figgie M, Finlayson H, George MD, Giles JT, Gilliland J, Klatt B, MacKenzie R, Michaud K, Miller A, Russell L, Sah A, Abdel MP, Johnson B, Mandl LA, Sculco P, Turgunbaev M, Turner AS, Yates A Jr, Singh JA (2022) 2022 American College of Rheumatology/American Association of Hip and Knee Surgeons guideline for the perioperative management of antirheumatic medication in patients

with rheumatic diseases undergoing elective total hip or total knee arthroplasty. Arthritis Care Res (Hoboken) 74(9):1399–1408
Gu Q, Dillon CF, Eberhardt MS, Wright JD, Burt VL (2015) Preventive aspirin and other antiplatelet medication use among U.S. adults aged ≥ 40 years: data from the National Health and Nutrition Examination Survey, 2011-2012. Public Health Rep 130(6):643–654
Hale AR, Coombes ID, Stokes J, McDougall D, Whitfield K, Maycock E, Nissen L (2013) Perioperative medication management: expanding the role of the preadmission clinic pharmacist in a single centre, randomised controlled trial of collaborative prescribing. BMJ Open 3(7):e003027
Hales CM, Servais J, Martin CB, Kohen D (2019) Prescription drug use among adults aged 40–79 in the United States and Canada. NCHS Data Brief, no 347. National Center for Health Statistics, Hyattsville, MD
Halvorsen S, Mehilli J, Cassese S, Hall TS, Abdelhamid M, Barbato E, De Hert S, de Laval I, Geisler T, Hinterbuchner L, Ibanez B, Lenarczyk R, Mansmann UR, McGreavy P, Mueller C, Muneretto C, Niessner A, Potpara TS, Ristić A, Sade LE, Schirmer H, Schüpke S, Sillesen H, Skulstad H, Torracca L, Tutarel O, Van Der Meer P, Wojakowski W, Zacharowski K (2022) 2022 ESC guidelines on cardiovascular assessment and management of patients undergoing non-cardiac surgery: developed by the task force for cardiovascular assessment and management of patients undergoing non-cardiac surgery of the European Society of Cardiology (ESC) Endorsed by the European Society of Anaesthesiology and Intensive Care (ESAIC). Eur Heart J 43(39):3826–3924
Harbell MW, Dumitrascu C, Bettini L, Yu S, Thiele CM, Koyyalamudi V (2021) Anesthetic considerations for patients on psychotropic drug therapies. Neurol Int 13(4):640–658
Harnett J, McIntyre E, Adams J, Addison T, Bannerman H, Egelton L, Ma J, Zabakly L, Steel A (2023) Prevalence and characteristics of Australians complementary medicine product use, and concurrent use with prescription and over-the-counter medications-a cross sectional study. Nutrients 15(2):327
Hughes SG (1998) Prescribing for the elderly patient: why do we need to exercise caution? Br J Clin Pharmacol 46(6):531–533
Järvstråt L, Holm ACES, Lindh-Åstrand L, Hoffmann MJ, Fredrikson MG, Hammar ML (2015) Use of hormone therapy in Swedish women aged 80 years or older. Menopause 22(3):275–278
Jinjing W, Kang C, Xufei L, Xueqiong L, Xinye J, Miao Y, Jinping Z, Zhaohui L, Jingtao D, Yaolong C, Linong J, Yiming M (2021) Chinese clinical practice guidelines for perioperative blood glucose management. Diabetes Metab Res Rev 37(7):e3439
Kaine J, Tesser J, Takiya L, DeMasi R, Wang L, Snyder M, Soma K, Fan H, Bandi V, Wollenhaupt J (2020) Re-establishment of efficacy of tofacitinib, an oral JAK inhibitor, after temporary discontinuation in patients with rheumatoid arthritis. Clin Rheumatol 39(7):2127–2137
Kim S, Lee H, Park J, Kang J, Rahmati M, Rhee SY, Yon DK (2024) Global and regional prevalence of polypharmacy and related factors, 1997-2022: an umbrella review. Arch Gerontol Geriatr 124:105465
Kudoh A, Takase H, Takahira Y, Takazawa T (2004) Postoperative confusion increases in elderly long-term benzodiazepine users. Anesth Analg 99(6):1674–1678
Kwan Y, Fernandes OA, Nagge JJ, Wong GG, Huh JH, Hurn DA, Pond GR, Bajcar JM (2007) Pharmacist medication assessments in a surgical preadmission clinic. Arch Int Med 167(10):1034–1040
Lazo OLE, White PF, Lee C, Cruz Eng H, Matin JM, Lin C, Del Cid F, Yumul R (2024) Use of herbal medication in the perioperative period: Potential adverse drug interactions. J Clin Anaesth 95:111473
Lee PG, Halter J (2017) The pathophysiology of hyperglycemia in older adults: clinical considerations. Diabetes Care 40(4):444–452
Legrand M, Falcone J, Cholley B, Charbonneau H, Delaporte A, Lemoine A, Garot M, Joosten A, Meistelman C, Cheron-Leroy D, Rives JP, Pastene B, Dewitte A, Sigaut S, Danguy des Deserts M, Truc C, Boisson M, Lasocki S, Cuvillon P, Schiff U, Jaber S, Le Guen M, Caillard A, Bar S, Pereira de Souza Neto E, Colas V, Dimache F, Girardot T, Jozefowicz E, Viquesnel

S, Berthier F, Vicaut E, Gayat E (2024) Continuation vs discontinuation of renin-angiotensin system inhibitors before major noncardiac surgery: the stop-or-not randomized clinical trial. JAMA 332(12):970–978

Leung JM, Dzankic S, Manku K, Yuan S (2001) The prevalence and predictors of the use of alternative medicine in presurgical patients in five California hospitals. Anesth Analg 93:1062–1068

Mahanna-Gabrielli E, Schenning KJ, Deiner SG, Whittington RA (2023) Pro-con debate: Judicious benzodiazepine administration for preoperative anxiolysis in older patients. Anesth Analg 137(2):280–288

Marotti SB, Kerridge RK, Grimer MD (2011) A randomised controlled trial of pharmacist medication histories and supplementary prescribing on medication errors in postoperative medications. Anaesth Intensive Care 39(6):1064–1070

Masnoon N, Shakib S, Kalisch-Ellett L, Caughey GE (2017) What is polypharmacy? A systematic review of definitions. BMC Geriatr 17(1):230

MIMS Australia (2024) Vagifem low pessaries. https://app.emims.plus/medicineview?id=f8533f0c-1f20-41b1-9041-a53300fd7544&type=abbpi. Accessed 18 Dec 2024

Moug SJ, Stechman M, McCarthy K, Pearce L, Myint PK, Hewitt J (2016) Frailty and cognitive impairment: Unique challenges in the older emergency surgical patient. Ann R Coll Surg Engl 98(3):165–169

National Guideline Centre (UK) (2020) Evidence review for preoperative optimisation clinics in older adults: perioperative care in adults: evidence review D. National Institute for Health and Care Excellence (NICE), London

Oprea AD, Keshock MC, O'Glasser AY, Cummings KC 3rd, Edwards AF, Hunderfund AL, Urman RD, Mauck KF (2022a) Preoperative management of medications for neurologic diseases: Society for Perioperative Assessment and Quality Improvement consensus statement. Mayo Clinic Proc 97(2):375–396

Oprea AD, Keshock MC, O'Glasser AY, Cummings KC 3rd, Edwards AF, Zimbrean PC, Urman RD, Mauck KF (2022b) Preoperative management of medications for psychiatric diseases: Society for Perioperative Assessment and Quality Improvement consensus statement. Mayo Clin Proc 97(2):397–416

Pfeifer KJ, Selzer A, Mendez CE, Whinney CM, Rogers B, Simha V, Regan D, Urman RD, Mauck K (2021) Preoperative management of endocrine, hormonal, and urologic medications: Society for Perioperative Assessment and Quality Improvement (SPAQI) consensus statement. Mayo Clinic Proc 96(6):1655–1669

Poudel P, Yu J (2020) Geriatric rheumatology: the need for a separate subspecialty in the near future. Cureus 12(6):e8474

Pratley RE, Kanapka LG, Rickels MR, Ahmann A, Aleppo G, Beck R, Bhargava A, Bode BW, Carlson A, Chaytor NS, Fox DS, Goland R, Hirsch IB, Kruger D, Kudva YC, Levy C, McGill JB, Peters A, Philipson L, Philis-Tsimikas A, Pop-Busui R, Shah VN, Thompson M, Vendrame F, Verdejo A, Weinstock RS, Young L, Miller KM (2020) Effect of continuous glucose monitoring on hypoglycemia in older adults with type 1 diabetes. JAMA 323(23):2397–2406

Quek HW, Page A, Potter K, Etherton-Beer C (2023) Deprescribing considerations for older people in general practice. Aust J Gen Pract 52(4):173–180

RACGP-OA (2017) Osteoporosis risk assessment, diagnosis and management. https://healthybonesaustralia.org.au/wp-content/uploads/2022/10/oa-racgp-osteoporosis-clinical-guidelines-summary-ver-2018.pdf. Accessed 18 Dec 2024

Russell LA, Craig C, Flores EK, Wainaina JN, Keshock M, Kasten MJ, Hepner DL, Edwards AF, Urman RD, Mauck KF, Oprea AD (2022) Preoperative management of medications for rheumatologic and HIV diseases: Society for Perioperative Assessment and Quality Improvement (SPAQI) consensus statement. Mayo Clin Proc 97(8):1551–1571

Sahai SK, Balonov K, Bentov N, Bierle DMM, Browning LM, Cummings KC 3rd, Dougan BM, Maxwell M, Merli GJ, Oprea AD, Sweitzer B, Mauck KF, Urman RD (2022) Preoperative management of cardiovascular medications: a Society for Perioperative Assessment and Quality Improvement (SPAQI) consensus statement. Mayo Clin Proc 97(9):1734–1751

Schofield P, Dunham M, Martin D, Bellamy G, Francis SA, Sookhoo D, Bonacaro A, Hamid E, Chandler R, Abdulla A, Cumberbatch M, Knaggs R (2022) Evidence-based clinical practice guidelines on the management of pain in older people—a summary report. Br J Pain 16(1):6–13

Sim XL, Kwa CX, He Y, Ng KL, Sim EY, Abdullah HR (2023) Transforming the perioperative medicine care model: the Singapore experience. Anaesth Intensive Care 51(2):96–106. https://doi.org/10.1177/0310057X221114900

Spyropoulos AC, Brohi K, Caprini J, Samama CM, Siegal D, Tafur A, Verhamme P, Douketis JD, SSC Subcommittee on Perioperative and Critical Care Thrombosis and Haemostasis of the International Society on Thrombosis and Haemostasis (2019) Scientific and Standardization Committee Communication: guidance document on the periprocedural management of patients on chronic oral anticoagulant therapy: recommendations for standardized reporting of procedural/surgical bleed risk and patient-specific thromboembolic risk. J Thromb Haemost 17(11):1966–1972

Stephenson C, Mohabbat A, Raslau D, Gilman E, Wight E, Kashiwagi D (2020) Management of common postoperative complications. Mayo Clin Proc 95(11):2540–2554

Taylor DM, Barnes TRE, Young AH (2021) The Maudsley prescribing guidelines in psychiatry. Wiley Blackwell, Hoboken, NJ

Therapeutic Guidelines (2018) Parkinson disease. https://www.tg.org.au. Accessed 18 Dec 2024

Therapeutic Guidelines (2021) Dementia. https://tg.org.au. Accessed 23 Dec 2024

Thompson A, Fleischmann KE, Smilowitz NR, de Las Fuentes L, Mukherjee D, Aggarwal NR, Ahmad FS, Allen RB, Altin SE, Auerbach A, Berger JS, Chow B, Dakik HA, Eisenstein EL, Gerhard-Herman M, Ghadimi K, Kachulis B, Leclerc J, Lee CS, Macaulay TE, Mates G, Merli GJ, Parwani P, Poole JE, Rich MW, Ruetzler K, Stain SC, Sweitzer B, Talbot AW, Vallabhajosyula S, Whittle J, Williams KA Sr, Writing Committee Members (2024) 2024 AHA/ACC/ACS/ASNC/HRS/SCA/SCCT/SCMR/SVM guideline for perioperative cardiovascular management for noncardiac surgery: a report of the American College of Cardiology/American Heart Association Joint Committee on clinical practice guidelines. Circulation 150(19):e351–e442

UKCPA (2019a) Handbook of perioperative medicines—alendronic acid. https://periop-handbook.ukclinicalpharmacy.org/drug/alendronic-acid-alendronate/. Accessed 18 Dec 2024

UKCPA (2019b) Handbook of perioperative medicines—donepezil. https://periop-handbook.ukclinicalpharmacy.org/drug/donepezil/. Accessed 18 Dec 2024

UKCPA (2019c) Handbook of perioperative medicines—prednisolone. https://periop-handbook.ukclinicalpharmacy.org/drug/prednisolone/?highlight=prednisolone. Accessed 18 Dec 2024

UKCPA (2021) Handbook of perioperative medicines—diabetes overview. https://periop-handbook.ukclinicalpharmacy.org/note/diabetes-overview/. Accessed 18 Dec 2024

Widdifield J, Bernatsky S, Paterson JM, Gunraj N, Thorne JC, Pope J, Cividino A, Bombardier C (2013) Serious infections in a population-based cohort of 86,039 seniors with rheumatoid arthritis. Arthritis Care Res (Hoboken) 65(3):353–361

Woodcock T, Barker P, Daniel S, Fletcher S, Wass JAH, Tomlinson JW, Misra U, Dattani M, Arlt W, Vercueil A (2020) Guidelines for the management of glucocorticoids during the peri-operative period for patients with adrenal insufficiency: guidelines from the Association of Anaesthetists, the Royal College of Physicians and the Society for Endocrinology UK. Anaesthesia 75(5):654–663

World Health Organisation (2024) Traditional, complementary and integrative medicine. https://www.who.int/health-topics/traditional-complementary-and-integrative-medicine#tab=tab_1. Accessed 6 Oct 2024

Xu G, Liu B, Sun Y, Du Y, Snetselaar LG, Hu B, Bao W (2018) Prevalence of diagnosed type 1 and type 2 diabetes among US adults in 2016 and 2017: population based study. BMJ 2018:362

Zietlow KE, Wong S, Heflin MT, McDonald SR, Sickeler R, Devinney M, Blitz J, Lagoo-Deenadayalan S, Berger M (2022) Geriatric preoperative optimization: a review. Am J Med 135(1):39–48

Anaesthesia in the Older Person

7

Jill Van Acker and Ross Hanrahan

Take-Home Messages

- Growing surgical demand in older patients
  - Older adults are the fastest-growing population in healthcare due to increased life expectancy and medical advancements.
  - Older adults face higher perioperative risks due to age-related physiological decline and comorbidities.
- Physiological changes and anaesthetic considerations
  - Cardiovascular: increased vascular resistance, reduced beta-receptor responsiveness and higher risk of arrhythmias, more preload dependent and increased risk of labile blood pressure intraoperatively.
  - Respiratory: decreased lung elasticity, impaired ventilatory response and increased aspiration risk.

J. Van Acker (✉)
Department of Anaesthesia, Pain Management and Perioperative Medicine, North Canberra Hospital, Canberra Health Services, Canberra, ACT, Australia

ANZCA, Chapter of POM Board & Chapter of POM Advocacy & Policy Committee, Melbourne, VIC, Australia
e-mail: Jill.VanAcker@act.gov.au

R. Hanrahan
Department of Anaesthesia, Pain Management and Perioperative Medicine, North Canberra Hospital, Canberra Health Services, Canberra, ACT, Australia
e-mail: Ross.Hanrahan@act.gov.au

K.-Y. Tan et al. (eds.), *Mastering Geriatric Surgery*,
https://doi.org/10.1007/978-981-95-0665-1_7

  - Nervous system: reduced brain volume, altered pain perception and increased sensitivity to medications.
  - Renal and hepatic: declining kidney function affects drug clearance; reduced liver function alters metabolism.
  - Thermoregulation: older adults are prone to perioperative hypothermia.
- Pharmacological considerations
  - Age affects drug absorption, distribution, metabolism and excretion.
  - Increased sensitivity to anaesthetic drugs (propofol, opioids, benzodiazepines).
  - Lipophilic drugs accumulate in fat stores, prolonging their effects.
  - Renal impairment increases the risk of drug accumulation and toxicity.
- Preoperative assessment
  - Frailty and cognitive function: preoperative frailty and cognitive impairment assessments are critical for risk stratification.
  - Shared decision-making: patients, caregivers and clinicians must align expectations and treatment goals.
  - Prehabilitation: nutritional support, exercise and chronic disease optimisation improve outcomes.
- Anaesthetic management strategies
  - No single best anaesthetic technique; individualised plan based on patient-specific and procedure-specific risks.
  - Opioid-sparing strategies: regional anaesthesia and multimodal analgesia are preferred.
  - Intraoperative monitoring: blood pressure, depth of anaesthesia (EEG-guided), temperature monitoring to avoid hypothermia and neuromuscular monitoring are key.
- Postoperative care and risks
  - Delirium and cognitive dysfunction: a significant risk in older adults, minimised through careful medication use, orientation strategies and family involvement.
  - Pain management: balance between effective analgesia and minimising opioid-related complications.
- Importance of a multidisciplinary, patient-centred approach
  - Comprehensive, team-based care is essential for optimal perioperative outcomes.
  - Risk reduction strategies (early mobilisation, nutritional support, frailty management) are essential.

7.1 Introduction

Increasing age dependency ratio is a global trend, with older persons now representing the fastest-growing population in healthcare (Ludbrook 2022). Advancements in less invasive procedures and better techniques mean that older and sicker patients are offered surgical procedures they would not have been a decade ago (ANZCA n.d.). Older persons, therefore, undergo significantly higher rates of surgical and non-surgical procedures per population compared to other age groups (Mohanty et al. 2016). This trend is expected to place escalating demands on healthcare systems worldwide. Managing patients at the extremes of age presents significant challenges (Irwin et al. 2019; Mohanty et al. 2016). Increasing age, an independent perioperative risk factor, is not only associated with reduced reserve and increased vulnerability of multiple organ systems but also with an increasing prevalence of frailty, cognitive impairment and chronic disease burden (Irwin et al. 2019; Staheli and Rondeau 2023; Barnett 2022; Story et al. 2010). These factors require careful attention throughout the perioperative journey as they render this patient group especially susceptible to postoperative complications, functional decline and loss of independence. Postoperative complications, in general, pose a well-documented burden, being the third most common cause of death worldwide after ischaemic heart disease and stroke, leading to significant impact and cost to patients, the healthcare system and society as a whole (Nepogodiev et al. 2019). These costs are frequently underestimated as many complications are managed outside hospital settings, and indirect factors—such as diminished quality of life and loss of productivity—are often overlooked (Ludbrook 2022).

Perioperative care of the older person demands a proactive, patient-centred, collaborative, holistic team approach. Proactive risk assessment, optimisation and perioperative risk reduction strategies are vital to achieve optimal patient outcomes. It is further essential that shared decision-making is practised throughout the perioperative journey. Shared decision-making (SDM) is a collaborative process involving patients, carers and healthcare professionals. It integrates the patient's values, goals and preferences with the best available evidence on the benefits, risks and uncertainties of treatment to determine the most appropriate healthcare decision (ANZCA n.d.).

This chapter will outline the relevant changes in systems and organs with age that require consideration when formulating an anaesthesia plan.

7.2 Anaesthesia and Physiology in the Older Person

Ageing is accompanied by a gradual decline in functional reserve across all organ systems. Even in healthy older adults, physiological reserves are diminished. The degree of decline varies for each system and is influenced by genetics, lifestyle and preventive healthcare. Recognising these age-related physiological changes and their clinical implications, as outlined in Table 7.1, is crucial for developing a safe and effective anaesthesia plan (Mohanty et al. 2016; Irwin et al. 2019; Staheli and Rondeau 2023).

Table 7.1 Age-related system physiological changes and clinical implications

Organ system	Age-related changes	Clinical implications
Cardiovascular system	• Dysautonomia • Increased systemic vascular resistance due to stiffening, calcification and stenosis of arteries • Left ventricular hypertrophy/ myocardial diastolic dysfunction • Fibrotic remodelling of the cardiac conduction system • Pathological calcification and thickening of the aortic valve	• Labile blood pressure • Increased myocardial oxygen demand and reduced coronary perfusion ? increased risk of perioperative coronary ischaemia • Risk of ectopic beats and arrhythmias • Intolerant of even brief episodes of tachycardia or arrhythmias
Respiratory	• Flattening of the diaphragm, weakened intercostal muscles and chest wall stiffening • Reduced elasticity of lung parenchyma • An increase in alveolar airspace and physiological dead space with reduced surface area • Reduced response to hypoxia and hypercarbia • Weak pharyngeal muscles and reduced upper airway reflexes • On pulmonary function tests: reduced functional residual capacity, FEV1, vital capacity, diffusion capacity and increased A-a gradient	• Reduced inspiratory capacity • Less efficient gas exchange • Ventilation-perfusion mismatch • Increased work of breathing • Susceptibility to hypoventilation and adverse respiratory events • Increased risk of pulmonary aspiration
Nervous system	• Brain: loss of volume, neuronal density and synapses • Regional reductions in neurotransmitters and neuroreceptors	• Altered pain response • Increased sensitivity to medications and their side effects • Increased vulnerability to perioperative neurocognitive disorders
Endocrine	• Impaired glucose tolerance	• Risk of intraoperative hyperglycaemia
Hepatic/renal	• Reduced renal mass and glomerular filtration rate • Blunted response to renin, angiotensin, aldosterone, vasopressin • Reduced hepatic mass and function • Reduced serum albumin levels	• Reduced drug metabolism and clearance • Increased risk of acute kidney injury • Larger free concentrations of highly protein-bound drugs
Thermoregulation	• Reduced muscle mass and vascular reactivity	• Prone to hypothermia

7.2.1 Cardiovascular System

Dysautonomia of ageing refers to age-related changes in autonomic function. Due to diminished beta-receptor responsiveness, which limits the tachycardic response, older adults rely more heavily on vascular tone and preload to maintain cardiac output (Staheli and Rondeau 2023; Barnett 2022). Additionally, systemic vascular resistance increases, and arterial compliance decreases due to the arteries' stiffening, stenosis and rigidity. These changes lead to a wider pulse pressure and labile blood pressure. The combination of dysautonomia and systemic vascular resistance changes increases the risk of significant intraoperative hypotension. This risk is further exacerbated in the context of reduced cardiac contractility, hypovolaemia aggravated by dehydration from fasting, the vasodilatory effects of anaesthetic agents, sympathetic blockade from neuraxial anaesthesia and the hemodynamic shifts associated with pneumoperitoneum (Staheli and Rondeau 2023; Barnett 2022).

Left ventricular hypertrophy, resulting from years of contracting against increased impedance, is worsened by chronic hypertension. This condition increases myocardial oxygen demand while reducing coronary perfusion. Consequently, older adults become more dependent on atrial filling during diastole (the 'atrial kick') to maintain adequate cardiac output. As a result, they are particularly intolerant of even brief episodes of tachycardia or arrhythmias, which can significantly compromise hemodynamic stability and increase their susceptibility to myocardial ischaemia or injury and diastolic heart failure (Staheli and Rondeau 2023).

Ageing of the cardiac conduction system involves fibrotic remodelling, which increases the risk of ectopic beats and arrhythmias, even in the absence of other underlying pathologies. Atrial fibrillation is the most common arrhythmia in older adults (Khurshid et al. 2023). It often presents atypically or without symptoms, making it more challenging to diagnose and manage effectively.

Chronic physiological stress on the aortic valve causes pathological calcification and thickening of the leaflets. Clinically significant aortic stenosis affects between 2% and 13% of patients over the age of 65, and many cases go undiagnosed (Staheli and Rondeau 2023).

Although not a normal part of ageing, coronary artery disease is more prevalent among older adults, placing them at an increased risk of perioperative coronary ischaemia.

7.2.2 Respiratory

A significant proportion of perioperative morbidity and mortality in older adults is attributed to perioperative pulmonary complications. This stems from a combination of factors, including age-related changes in the pulmonary system and thorax leading to reduced pulmonary function and diminished overall respiratory reserve (Table 7.1) (Staheli and Rondeau 2023; Corcoran and Hillyard 2011).

Additionally, ageing impairs the ventilatory response to hypercapnia and, more notably, hypoxaemia. The respiratory depressant effects of opioids, benzodiazepines and anaesthetic agents further exacerbate these deficits in the perioperative period, increasing the risk of adverse pulmonary outcomes. This highlights the importance of ensuring complete reversal of neuromuscular blockade at the end of surgery, conservative use of sedating medications, early postoperative mobilisation and chest physiotherapy (Barnett 2022; Berg et al. 1997).

Interestingly, older adults are also at an increased risk of pulmonary aspiration due to a combination of blunted ventilatory responses, weakened pharyngeal muscles and diminished upper airway reflexes, all of which compromise airway protection mechanisms (Staheli and Rondeau 2023; Barnett 2022).

Finally, higher prevalence of COPD and sleep-disordered breathing in the ageing population requires careful assessment and optimisation.

7.2.3 Nervous System

Age-related normal and pathological changes in the central and peripheral nervous systems result in an altered pain response and heightened sensitivity to medications and their side effects (Mohanty et al. 2016; Barnett 2022). These changes necessitate careful dosing adjustments for many intraoperative medications. Older adults typically require significant reduction in inhalational and intravenous anaesthetic dosages. Additionally, avoiding inappropriate medications, as outlined later in the chapter, is critical (By the 2023 American Geriatrics Society Beers Criteria® Update Expert Panel 2023).

The ageing brain loses volume, neuronal density and synapses, accompanied by regional reductions in neurotransmitters and neuroreceptors. While there is some debate about whether cerebral autoregulation changes with age, anaesthetic agents generally impair this mechanism. Therefore, protecting cerebral perfusion and oxygenation in the vulnerable ageing brain is crucial, especially in patients with pre-existing cognitive impairment (Berger et al. 2018; Partridge et al. 2022).

7.2.4 Renal

The glomerular filtration rate is reduced by 1 mm/min/m^2 annually after age 40, though individual decline rates may vary. Other comorbidities common in the older patient, like diabetes mellitus, hypertension and vasculopathy, can also negatively impact renal function. Older patients are less able to cope with a salt or water load due to a blunted response to renin, angiotensin, aldosterone and vasopressin (Staheli and Rondeau 2023; Mohanty et al. 2016). There is an increased risk of suffering perioperative acute kidney injury in a setting of increased vulnerability to nephrotoxic medications such as NSAIDs (Non Steroidal Anti-Inflammatory Drugs) or intravenous contrast, as well as increased sensitivity to dehydration and perioperative blood pressure lability. One also has to consider higher plasma concentrations of renally excreted intravenous agents (Staheli and Rondeau 2023; Barnett 2022).

7.2.5 Hepatic

Ageing is coupled with a reduction in hepatic mass and function, which results in slower metabolism of many intravenous anaesthetic agents. Additionally, lower serum albumin levels cause larger free-drug concentrations of highly protein-bound drugs like propofol (Barnett 2022; Mohanty et al. 2016).

7.2.6 Temperature Regulation

Ageing affects thermoregulation due to a reduction in heat production and insulation. Therefore, it is paramount to meticulously monitor intraoperative temperature and implement perioperative measures to prevent hypothermia (Staheli and Rondeau 2023; Mohanty et al. 2016; Barnett 2022).

7.2.7 Body Composition and Nutritional Status

Malnutrition occurs commonly in older patients and is associated with worse perioperative outcomes. Weight begins to decline in the sixth decade of life, though this depends on genetics, diet and physical activity (Mohanty et al. 2016).

Generally, a reduced total body water and muscle mass, associated with lower central compartment volume, affects the induction dose of many anaesthetic drugs. Loss of muscle mass and increased fat may result in prolonged clinical drug effects of lipid-soluble agents due to their larger volume of distribution (Staheli and Rondeau 2023).

7.3 Preoperative Assessment

The preoperative assessment for older patients should adhere to the general principles of any pre-anaesthesia evaluation. While advanced age alone should not be the sole indication for preoperative testing, specific consideration should be given to unique challenges associated with older adults (Parmar et al. 2021; Palaniappan et al. 2022). Age is an independent perioperative risk factor; however, much of the escalating risk related to age is due to the increased prevalence of comorbidities, frailty and varying degrees of cognitive impairment (Mohanty et al. 2016; Barnett 2022). The higher likelihood of urgent surgical presentations in this population further complicates preoperative planning. Patients residing in nursing homes may face logistical barriers that prevent attendance at preoperative evaluation clinics, limiting opportunities for thorough planning (Staheli and Rondeau 2023; Berger et al. 2018).

7.3.1 Assessment of Baseline Cognitive Function and Discussion of Perioperative Neurocognitive Disorders

Approximately 1 in 5 patients over the age of 65 have some degree of baseline cognitive impairment, a recognised risk factor for perioperative neurocognitive disorders (PND) (Staheli and Rondeau 2023). Perioperative neurocognitive disorders (NCDs), including postoperative delirium, delayed neurocognitive recovery and postoperative cognitive decline, pose significant challenges for older patients undergoing surgery. They are important because they are common, and the consequences are significant for patients and their family. Studies suggest that as many as 10–40% of older patients undergoing surgery develop a form of PND (Staheli and Rondeau 2023; Berger et al. 2018; Kong et al. 2022). The cognitive decline can persist for months or even years, adversely affecting independence, quality of life, the risk of developing dementia and long-term survival. Risk factors for PND include advanced age (>70 years), pre-existing cognitive dysfunction, depression, poor baseline functional status, electrolyte imbalances and a history of stroke (Berger et al. 2018).

The Brain Health Initiative advocates for a proactive approach, recommending a baseline preoperative cognitive assessment followed by implementing a risk reduction bundle (Berger et al. 2018). It is recommended that all patients aged 65 and over and those with risk factors for pre-existing cognitive impairment should have an objective evaluation of their baseline cognition using a brief screening tool (Berger et al. 2018). The Minicog is brief, ideally lending itself to use in the perioperative setting. If time permits, MMSE has higher sensitivity and specificity than Minicog but takes 4–5 times as long (Berger et al. 2018; Peden et al. 2021).

It is crucial to inform patients and their families about the potential risks of perioperative neurocognitive disorders (PNDs) during the preoperative evaluation. This discussion helps establish realistic expectations for postoperative recovery and enables advance planning to avoid critical decision-making in the weeks following surgery.

Evidence suggests that certain intraoperative anaesthetic or physiological variables may increase the risk of PND; however, there is currently insufficient literature to recommend a specific anaesthetic technique to mitigate this risk in older adults. A multifaceted approach incorporating several proactive measures, however, may reduce the incidence of perioperative neurocognitive disorders by 40%. These interventions are designed to support cognitive health and enhance overall outcomes for older surgical patients (Staheli and Rondeau 2023; Berger et al. 2018; Peden et al. 2021). Key elements of this approach include

1. **Avoidance or cautious use of certain medications (based on revised Beers criteria** By the 2023 American Geriatrics Society Beers Criteria® Update Expert Panel 2023)

   - Amiodarone
   - Antihistamines (first generation)
   - Centrally acting anticholinergics

- Antipsychotics
- Aspirin for primary prevention for those >80 years of age
- Benzodiazepines
- Diuretics
- Fluoxetine
- Methyldopa
- Nitrofurantoin
- Non-steroidal anti-inflammatory medications, including COX-2 inhibitors
- Tricyclic antidepressants
- Pethidine
- Corticosteroids
- Metoclopramide

2. **Meticulous temperature monitoring** to maintain normothermia
3. **Dose titration of anaesthetic agents** to achieve the minimum effective dose and avoid overdosing
    - Monitoring of age-adjusted end-tidal MAC levels
    - Use of EEG-based brain monitoring to assess the depth of anaesthesia
4. **Optimise cerebral perfusion**
5. **Attention to sleep and nutrition hygiene**
6. **Ensuring glasses and hearing aids are available**
7. **Frequent orientation to time and place**
8. **Family engagement**
9. **Regular orientation strategies**

7.3.2 Assessment of Frailty

Frailty is now recognised as a significant risk factor for complications in both elective and emergency surgical patients. A measurable clinical syndrome, frailty is defined as an age-related multidomain decline in physiological reserve and function resulting in an increased vulnerability to stressors. It is a predictor of poorer perioperative outcomes, including mortality, perioperative neurocognitive disorder, increased length of hospital stay and long-term functional decline (Mohanty et al. 2016; Barnett 2022; Makary et al. 2010; Kim et al. 2014; Thillainadesan et al. 2021). Therefore, careful assessment for frailty is required to inform tailored care plans and preoperative risk discussion (Pollock et al. 2015; The Royal Australian College of General Practitioners 2019). There is some suggestion that surgical outcomes may be improved by optimising the patient's preoperative condition and physiological reserve with a prehabilitation program that covers smoking cessation, exercise prescription, optimisation of nutritional status and multidisciplinary, proactive postoperative care, but further research is required (Irwin et al. 2019; Gupta and Gan 2016; Ng et al. 2015).

Frailty assessment, using validated tools such as the Clinical Frailty Score, therefore plays a vital role in risk stratification and supports shared decision-making during the preoperative phase (Makary et al. 2010; Hall et al. 2017). The score is easy to use, time-efficient and used in many centres.

7.3.3 Preoperative Testing

There is no consensus on standardised preoperative testing guidelines for non-cardiac surgery, irrespective of age. Instead, preoperative testing should be tailored to the patient's comorbidities and potential anticipated medical and surgical perioperative complications (Staheli and Rondeau 2023; Chung et al. 2009).

7.4 Anaesthesia and Pharmacology in the Older Person

Tailoring anaesthetic pharmacology for older patients requires addressing both universal physiological changes inherent in ageing and the heightened interindividual variation resulting from a higher prevalence of chronic conditions. Even among individuals of the same chronological age, physiological condition can differ substantially (Pollock et al. 2015; The Royal Australian College of General Practitioners 2019). Compounding this variability are impaired homeostatic mechanisms, diminished physiological reserve and diverse comorbid conditions. Consequently, tailoring the anaesthetic approach is essential to minimise adverse drug effects and prevent iatrogenic injury (Onder et al. 2013; Mangoni and Jackson 2004).

Pharmacological considerations may be categorised under pharmacokinetic and pharmacodynamic factors, sometimes characterised as '*what the body does to the drug*' and '*what the drug does to the body*'.

7.4.1 Pharmacokinetic Changes

7.4.1.1 Absorption

Polypharmacy, confusing medication instructions, omitted over-the-counter drugs and variable compliance necessitate extra vigilance to ensure the preoperative medication record accurately reflects the patient's actual intake. The same factors bear consideration in postoperative planning. Written communication, diligence, patience and the involvement of a family member are a critical foundation to effective pharmacotherapy. Medications not taken when they should, or taken inappropriately through failed communication, is a simple modifiable risk (Hermon and Williams 2013).

While intravenous medications avoid absorptive changes, the practitioner should be aware that advanced age is associated with slower gastric emptying, reduced peristalsis and delayed colonic transit, all of which may affect both the rate and extent of absorption of orally administered drugs (McLean and Le Couteur 2004;

Bender 1968; Marathe et al. 2000). Comorbidities such as diabetes or Parkinson's disease may affect motility, right heart failure or impaired gastric blood flow may impair medication absorption.

Reduced liver mass and hepatic perfusion in older patients may result in medications subject to extensive first-pass metabolism (e.g. morphine, tapentadol) achieving higher plasma levels following oral administration than may be seen in younger patients with more effective first-pass clearance (Baillie et al. 1989; Klotz 2009). By comparison, oral oxycodone has lower first-pass metabolism and thus less subject to this effect.

In healthy ageing, cardiac output is generally preserved. Comorbid cardiac conditions reducing cardiac output may accelerate wash-in of volatile anaesthetics; however, onset of clinical effect may be slowed by alveolar ventilation–perfusion mismatch and decreased cerebral perfusion (Dodds et al. 2014). Overall, in older patients the equilibrium between brain and end-tidal volatile concentrations is slower, and corresponding EEG changes occur later than in younger patients (Dodds et al. 2014; Fragen and Dunn 1996; Cortínez et al. 2008). While onset is slower, pharmacodynamic factors result in significantly greater sensitivity in older patients to volatile agents (see below).

Transdermal medication absorption can be compromised by lower skin water content limiting the uptake of hydrophilic molecules, and by decreased vascularity impairing systemic absorption (De Mello et al. 2024).

7.4.1.2 Distribution

Anaesthetic drug pharmacokinetics follow a three-compartment model: a central compartment (V1) into which intravenous medications are directly administered, and two further distribution compartments. The fast distribution compartment (V2) represents well-perfused tissues (muscles, organs), whereas a slower distribution compartment (V3) represents poorly perfused tissues, including fat (Coetzee and Absalom 2023). Offset of effect following bolus of many anaesthetic drugs (propofol, fentanyl) reflects redistribution to the fast component.

Older patients have decreased lean body mass (V2) and total body water, but increased body fat (V3). The central compartment is relatively unaffected by age. A smaller fast distribution compartment may delay the offset of medications following bolus injection, but a larger slow distribution compartment with high capacity to absorb lipophilic drugs predisposes to drug accumulation and a slow elimination half-life (Coetzee and Absalom 2023). Most anaesthetic drugs are lipophilic (Table 7.2), resulting in an increased overall volume of distribution and prolonged elimination. Conversely, decreased body water and lean mass may lead to higher plasma levels of water-soluble drugs (Dodds et al. 2014).

Protein binding affects both drug distribution and pharmacological effects. As it is the unbound fraction of a drug which determines its activity and toxicity, heavily protein-bound drugs can be significantly impacted by changes affecting their bound and unbound fractions (see Table 7.3). Major binding proteins include albumin, with an affinity for acidic drugs, and alpha-1-acid glycoprotein, with an affinity for basic drugs. Albumin is far more abundant and some drugs (e.g. fentanyl) bind to

Table 7.2 Lipophilic and hydrophilic classification of common anaesthetic medications

Lipophilic medications	Hydrophilic medications
• Propofol • Benzodiazepines • Fentanyl, alfentanil, sufentanil • Volatile anaesthetics (desflurane < sevoflurane < isoflurane)	• Neuromuscular blocking drugs • Morphine

Table 7.3 Highly protein-bound anaesthetic medications and their binding protein (Sear 2011)

Drug	Binding protein (% bound)
Midazolam	Albumin (98%)
Alfentanil	Alpha-1-acid glycoprotein (90%)
Fentanyl	Alpha-1-acid glycoprotein (80%)
Remifentanil	Alpha-1-acid glycoprotein (70%)
Lignocaine	Alpha-1-acid glycoprotein (65%)

both. Serum albumin levels decline with age, whereas alpha-1-acid glycoprotein levels remain relatively stable in health (Grandison and Boudinot 2000). In the presence of inflammation, alpha-1-acid glycoprotein rises as an acute phase reactant, whereas albumin falls (Gulhar et al. 2025). Ageing-associated decline in albumin levels thus results in an increased unbound active fraction of midazolam with increased clinical effect.

7.4.1.3 Metabolism and Excretion

Ageing-associated decline in liver mass, hepatic blood flow and enzyme function affects medications subject to significant hepatic metabolism or biliary excretion (Dodds et al. 2014; Thürmann 2020). Clearance of high hepatic extraction ratio medications (e.g. morphine, fentanyl, ketamine) directly relates to liver blood flow, which declines by around 10% per decade. Liver function tests correlate poorly with hepatic enzymatic drug metabolism and are unreliable in assessing hepatic drug handling (Thürmann 2020).

Renal function declines progressively with age and is reliably assessed with creatinine clearance calculation. Vecuronium, rocuronium and pancuronium elimination is prolonged in renal impairment, whereas elimination of atracurium and cisatracurium is organ independent. Morphine's metabolite morphine-6-glucuronide accumulates in renal impairment and may lead to respiratory depression and sedation. Non-steroidal anti-inflammatory drugs are potentially nephrotoxic, and care should be taken in the presence of pre-existing renal impairment (Chowdhury and McLure 2022) (Table 7.4).

Table 7.4 Pharmacokinetic implications of ageing-associated physiological changes (Klotz 2009)

Physiological changes	Pharmacokinetic consequences
Absorption	
Increased gastric pH – Decreased acid secretion – PPI use	Potentially decreased absorption
Altered gastric motility	Delayed or reduced absorption of oral medications
Distribution	
Changes in body composition – Increased body fat – Decreased lean body mass – Decreased total body water	Increased volume of distribution and half-life of lipophilic drugs
Decreased serum albumin	Increased active fraction of albumin-bound drugs
Metabolism	
Age-related reduction in hepatic blood flow	Reduced elimination of high extraction ratio medications
Excretion	
Age-related reduction in glomerular filtration rate	Reduced elimination of renally cleared medications

7.4.2 Pharmacodynamic Changes

Pharmacodynamics describes the relationship between drug concentration and effect. While drug concentration is measured in the plasma, actual drug effect is reliant on effect sites within the central and peripheral nervous system. Older patients have a well-established increased susceptibility to drugs acting on the central nervous system. Brain mass declines with age, gamma-aminobutyric acid (GABA) neurons and receptors also decline, and are accompanied by compensatory upregulation of inhibitory function in the older person (Dodds et al. 2014). Susceptibility to volatile anaesthetics increases, leading to a decline in MAC of around 6% for each decade of age (Dodds et al. 2014). Sensitivity to propofol is also increased by around 30–50% in 75-year-old patients compared to 25-year-old patients (Andres et al. 2019).

Opioid receptor density and binding affinity decline, as do muscarinic and nicotinic acetylcholine receptors. Decreased homeostatic cardiovascular and neuroendocrine mechanisms, combined with reduced functional reserve, may also serve to amplify drug effects (Table 7.5).

Table 7.5 Summary of pharmacological considerations and suggested adjustments to anaesthetic medications in older patients (Dodds et al. 2014; Andres et al. 2019; Prostran et al. 2016; Gourkanti et al. 2024; Wang et al. 2018; Gragasin et al. 2012)

Drug class	Pharmacological considerations in older patients	Suggestions
Benzodiazepines	Increased sensitivity Increased risk of delirium	Decrease dose or avoid altogether 20% dose reduction in ASA 3 50% dose reduction in ASA 4 75% dose reduction in 90-year-old
Propofol	Increased sensitivity Decreased clearance Reduced sympathetic and vascular tone and reduced baroreceptor reflex lead to increased hypotension Synergistic reduction in blood pressure in the presence of ACE inhibitors or angiotensin II receptor antagonists	20% induction dose reduction delivered over slower speed 30–50% reduction in infusion rate Use target-controlled infusion Use EEG monitoring Stop infusion early to allow timely recovery
Volatile anaesthetics	Increased pharmacodynamic susceptibility Decreased vascular tone and reduced baroreceptor response lead to increased hypotension Synergistic reduction in blood pressure in the presence of ACE inhibitors or angiotensin II receptor antagonists	Use age-adjusted MAC Begin reducing early to allow timely recovery Use EEG monitoring
Opioids	Age-related prolonged half-life of morphine, hydromorphone and methadone Increased pharmacodynamic sensitivity to analgesic, sedative and respiratory depressant effects Renal impairment risks accumulation of toxic metabolites from morphine and pethidine Remifentanil onset of effect and recovery prolonged	'Start low and go slow' Maximise non-opioid medications Use target-controlled infusion for remifentanil Caution with long-acting opioids Oxycodone's half-life is less affected by age than morphine
Non Depolarising Neuromusculur blocking agents (NDNMB)	Amino steroids effect prolonged in altered hepatic or renal function Atracurium and cisatracurium organ-independent elimination not prolonged with age Increased sensitivity to effect	Longer redosing interval Neuromuscular monitoring Ensure fully reversed at the end of procedure
Suxamethonium	Prolonged duration due to decreased serum cholinesterase levels	Ensure complete resolution prior to extubation
Dexmedetomidine	Prolonged clearance	33% dose reduction

7.5 Anaesthetic Technique

There is insufficient evidence to support a single anaesthetic approach for all older persons. As previously outlined, the physiological changes associated with normal ageing must be considered when designing an individualised anaesthetic plan (Mohanty et al. 2016; Staheli and Rondeau 2023; Barnett 2022). Similarly, while no definitive evidence suggests that regional anaesthesia is superior to general anaesthesia when used as the primary modality for surgical anaesthesia, regional anaesthesia may benefit specific patient populations and procedures (Mohanty et al. 2016).

7.5.1 Perioperative Pain Management

Multimodal or opioid-sparing analgesic strategies are strongly recommended for older adults to optimise pain management while minimising potential risks. When appropriate, these strategies should incorporate regional anaesthesia to improve pain control, alongside careful adjustments to drug dosages to account for age-related physiological changes in the nervous, hepatic and renal systems (Staheli and Rondeau 2023).

In older patients, opioids, in particular, exhibit increased potency due to reduced metabolic clearance and heightened neurological sensitivity. Additionally, older individuals are more susceptible to opioid-related side effects. As mentioned before, the respiratory response to hypoxia and hypercarbia is blunted, increasing the risk of opioid-induced hypoventilation and apnoea. When opioids are required, they should be initiated at low doses and titrated carefully based on the patient's clinical response.

7.6 Anaesthetic Monitoring of Older Patients Undergoing Surgery

Monitoring standards for older patients should follow the same principles as for patients of any age (Klein et al. 2021; ANZCA 2017). Nevertheless, an appreciation of the physiological changes accompanying ageing, their clinical implications and the increased prevalence of comorbidities warrants a higher index of suspicion than typical for a younger patient.

7.6.1 Blood Pressure Monitoring

For reasons mentioned above, physiological factors place older patients at greater risk of intraoperative haemodynamic lability. 2024 AHA/ACC Perioperative Cardiovascular Management guidelines provide general perioperative recommendations to maintain intraoperative mean arterial pressure (MAP) =60–65 mmHg or systolic blood pressure (SBP) =90 mmHg to reduce myocardial injury risk

(Thompson et al. 2024). Note is made, though, that higher targets may be preferred in older patients in the setting of chronic hypertension.

Individualising blood pressure targets to the patient's usual preoperative baseline reduces postoperative organ dysfunction (Futier et al. 2017). A usual recommendation is to maintain blood pressure within 20% of baseline value, within the limits of MAP >60 mmHg and SBP <160 mmHg (Dodds et al. 2014; Meng et al. 2018; Griffiths et al. 2014). Blood pressure targets should also be tailored to individual patient comorbidities (e.g. renal impairment) and the planned procedure (Kim et al. 2023; Wu et al. 2017). Take care to avoid mistaking preoperative 'white-coat' hypertension for the patient's normal baseline blood pressure. Ideally ambulatory blood pressures or stable ward blood pressures should be compared to gain a complete picture.

When determining the need for invasive blood pressure monitoring, it is important to consider the potential for rapid haemodynamic changes. As induction is a high-risk period for hypotension, it is prudent to insert the arterial line before induction if one is required. Comparison between invasive and non-invasive blood pressure measurements across age groups reveal a declining correlation with advancing age, potentially reflecting increased arterial stiffness (Liu et al. 2016). The method of blood pressure measurement can also affect observed variability; for example, during hypotension, non-invasive readings are often higher than radial intra-arterial measurements, while during hypotension they tend to be lower (Wax et al. 2011). Non-invasive continuous blood pressure monitoring is also hampered by physiological changes in elderly vessels and does not appear to be as reliable as invasive monitoring in this population (Xu et al. 2022).

Risk of unstable arrhythmias in older patients may justify invasive blood pressure monitoring; however, stable arrhythmias such as atrial fibrillation alone do not necessitate it as modern non-invasive blood pressure cuffs can reliably measure blood pressure in the presence of such arrhythmias (Pecha et al. 2023; Li et al. 2023; Lakhal et al. 2015).

7.6.2 Depth of Anaesthesia

Minimum alveolar concentration (MAC) reflects a clinically defined end point of spinal cord-mediated movement and declines by around 6% per decade of age (Eger 2001). MAC-Aware (suppression of a voluntary response to verbal commands) decreases proportionally, and the relationship between MAC and MAC-Aware remains consistent with age (Eger 2001). Care should be taken to ensure an appropriately age-adjusted target is used.

Propofol target-controlled infusions targeting plasma levels (TCIp) consider pharmacokinetic aspects of ageing, but do not directly address pharmacodynamic factors. Compared to younger patients, older patients show greater susceptibility to propofol, exhibiting EEG and hypnotic responses at lower plasma concentrations (Schnider et al. 1999). Effect site-guided TCIs (TCIe) such as Schnider and Eleveld address pharmacodynamic factors through models derived using EEG and Bispectral

Index (BIS) data to assess drug effect, but applicability of these measures in an older population is not straightforward (Schnider et al. 1999; Eleveld et al. 2018). BIS and Entropy were developed from data derived from young and middle-aged patients. Brain changes associated with age are reflected in the EEG, and analysis suggests processed EEG indices may increase by around 2 points per decade of age (Obert et al. 2021). There is increasing evidence that older brains may yield higher processed EEG readings, leading to a tendency for excessive anaesthetic dosing with processed EEG-guided anaesthesia (Berger et al. 2018; Purdon et al. 2015; Biggs et al. 2022; Ebensperger et al. 2025).

This observation is supported by non-EEG-based measures of anaesthetic depth. On induction, older patients are observed to experience loss of consciousness at higher BIS (70 vs 58) and State Entropy (71 vs 55) than younger patients, and return of consciousness at procedure end occurs at lower effect site concentrations in older patients than younger patients (Lysakowski et al. 2009). Similarly, a cohort study assessing older patients under volatile anaesthesia found that despite higher age-adjusted volatile concentrations, BIS levels were higher in older patients (Ni et al. 2019).

Systematic review and meta-analysis of randomised controlled trials have demonstrated that targeting a lighter BIS (50 vs 35) is associated with reduced risk of postoperative delirium (Sumner et al. 2023). EEG burst suppression, a pattern of high-voltage activity alternating with periods of electrical silence, has also been found to be an independent risk factors for postoperative delirium (Fritz et al. 2016; Park et al. 2025; Ma and Bebawy 2021).

Taken together, the use of EEG monitoring to titrate depth of anaesthesia with a goal of minimising burst suppression and targeting a lighter processed EEG index (~50) is supported. The American Society for Enhanced Recovery supports the use of intraoperative EEG to reduce risk of awareness, but concludes there is insufficient evidence to recommend its use for the prevention of postoperative delirium (POD) or postoperative cognitive dysfunction (POCD) (Chan et al. 2020). The Perioperative Brain Health Safety Initiative (Vacas et al. 2022) supports the use of intraoperative EEG monitoring and age-adjusted MAC as part of best practices, and the European Society of Anaesthesiology makes a weak recommendation for the use of intraoperative indexed-based EEG and burst suppression monitoring to decrease risk of POD on the basis of low-quality evidence (Aldecoa et al. 2023). The evidence for EEG monitoring for avoidance of postoperative cognitive dysfunction is conflicting, but evidence supportive of benefit does exist (Brook et al. 2024; Travica et al. 2023; Chan et al. 2013; Evered et al. 2021).

7.6.3 Positioning/Pressure Care

Due to changes in skin and circulation, joint stiffness and reduced range of motion, older patients are at increased risk of suffering perioperative nerve, joint and skin injury. A retrospective analysis of over 50,000 older adults treated for hip fractures found that 2.5% developed perioperative pressure injuries. Risk factors included malnutrition, hypoalbuminaemia, frailty, peripheral vascular disease and dementia (Tzen et al. 2023). Anaesthetic monitoring must include meticulous attention to positioning and pressure points, and regular reassessment during longer cases (Mohanty et al. 2016; Staheli and Rondeau 2023; Barnett 2022).

7.6.4 Temperature

Intraoperative hypothermia occurs 2.6 times more frequently in patients over 65 years of age than in patients aged 20–50 (Cho et al. 2022). Ageing-associated changes, including decreased body fat, muscle and subcutaneous tissue, reduced shivering and reduced vasoconstriction, limit the ability of older patients to self-regulate temperature. Hypothermia is independently associated with increased perioperative blood loss, adverse myocardial outcomes, surgical wound infection and hospital mortality (Karalapillai et al. 2013; Doufas 2003).

Take care to minimise exposure, monitor temperatures and actively warm the patients. Initiating warming prior to induction may be worth consideration.

7.6.5 Reversal of Neuromuscular Blockade

Neuromuscular blockade has an increased duration of effect in older patients, and older age is associated with an increased risk of prolonged neuromuscular block and related respiratory complications (Berg et al. 1997; Pandit et al. 2016). Neuromuscular monitoring to confirm adequate reversal (TOF >0.9) should be used whenever neuromuscular blockade has been used.

7.7 Conclusion

The anaesthetic management of older patients requires a thoughtful and tailored approach that considers age-related physiological changes, heightened susceptibility to perioperative complications and the increased prevalence of comorbidities.

Effective preoperative planning hinges on frailty assessment, cognitive evaluation and shared decision-making to align care with patient needs and risks. Safe intraoperative management depends on an in-depth understanding of age-related alterations in drug handling, proactive risk mitigation and the use of appropriate monitoring strategies to optimise patient safety.

Postoperative care should prioritise delirium prevention, effective pain management, early mobilisation and proactive anticipation and management of complications to help maintain functional independence. By integrating these principles into clinical practice, anaesthetists can enhance perioperative safety and contribute to better long-term outcomes for older patients.

References

Aldecoa C, Bettelli G, Bilotta F et al (2023) Update of the European Society of Anaesthesiology and Intensive Care Medicine evidence-based and consensus-based guideline on postoperative delirium in adult patients. Eur J Anaesthesiol. https://doi.org/10.1097/EJA.0000000000001876

Andres TM, McGrane T, McEvoy MD, Allen BFS (2019) Geriatric pharmacology. Anesthesiol Clin 37(3):475–492. https://doi.org/10.1016/j.anclin.2019.04.007

ANZCA (2017) PG(18)A guideline on monitoring during anaesthesia 2017

ANZCA (n.d.) The perioperative care framework document

Australian Commission on Safety and Quality in Health Care (n.d.) Shared decision making. https://www.safetyandquality.gov.au/our-work/partnering-consumers/shared-decision-making

Baillie SP, Bateman DN, Coates PE, Woodhouse KW (1989) Age and the pharmacokinetics of morphine. Age Ageing 18(4):258–262. https://doi.org/10.1093/ageing/18.4.258

Barnett S (2022) Anesthesia for the older adult. UpToDate

Bender AD (1968) Effect of age on intestinal absorption: implications for drug absorption in the elderly. J Am Geriatr Soc 16(12):1331–1339. https://doi.org/10.1111/j.1532-5415.1968.tb02776.x

Berg H, Viby-Mogensen J, Roed J et al (1997) Residual neuromuscular block is a risk factor for postoperative pulmonary complications A prospective, randomised, and blinded study of postoperative pulmonary complications after atracurium, vecuronium and pancuronium. Acta Anaesthesiol Scand 41(9):1095–1103. https://doi.org/10.1111/j.1399-6576.1997.tb04851.x

Berger M, Schenning KJ, Brown CH, Deiner SG, Whittington RA, Eckenhoff RG (2018) Best practices for postoperative brain health: recommendations from the Fifth International Perioperative Neurotoxicity Working Group. Anesth Analg 127(6):1406–1413. https://doi.org/10.1213/ANE.0000000000003841

Biggs D, Boncompte G, Pedemonte JC, Fuentes C, Cortinez LI (2022) The effect of age on electroencephalogram measures of anesthesia hypnosis: a comparison of BIS, Alpha Power, Lempel-Ziv complexity and permutation entropy during propofol induction. Front Aging Neurosci 14:910886. https://doi.org/10.3389/fnagi.2022.910886

Brook K, Agarwala AV, Li F, Purdon PL (2024) Depth of anesthesia monitoring: an argument for its use for patient safety. Curr Opin Anaesthesiol 37(6):689–696. https://doi.org/10.1097/ACO.0000000000001430

By the 2023 American Geriatrics Society Beers Criteria® Update Expert Panel (2023) American Geriatrics Society 2023 updated AGS Beers Criteria® for potentially inappropriate medication use in older adults. J Am Geriatr Soc 71(7):2052–2081. https://doi.org/10.1111/jgs.18372

Chan MTV, Cheng BCP, Lee TMC, Gin T (2013) BIS-guided anesthesia decreases postoperative delirium and cognitive decline. J Neurosurg Anesthesiol 25(1):33–42. https://doi.org/10.1097/ANA.0b013e3182712fba

Chan MTV, Hedrick TL, Egan TD et al (2020) American Society for Enhanced Recovery and Perioperative Quality Initiative Joint Consensus Statement on the role of neuromonitoring in perioperative outcomes: electroencephalography. Anesth Analg 130(5):1278–1291. https://doi.org/10.1213/ANE.0000000000004502

Cho SA, Yoon S, Lee SJ, Jee YS, Cho CK, Sung TY (2022) Clinical efficacy of short-term prewarming in elderly and adult patients: a prospective observational study. Int J Med Sci 19(10):1548–1556. https://doi.org/10.7150/ijms.77578

Chowdhury SR, McLure HA (2022) Chronic kidney disease and anaesthesia. BJA Educ 22(8):321–328. https://doi.org/10.1016/j.bjae.2022.03.005

Chung F, Yuan H, Yin L, Vairavanathan S, Wong DT (2009) Elimination of preoperative testing in ambulatory surgery. Anesth Analg 108(2):467–475. https://doi.org/10.1213/ane.0b013e318176bc19

Coetzee E, Absalom AR (2023) Pharmacokinetic and pharmacodynamic changes in the elderly. Anesthesiol Clin 41(3):549–565. https://doi.org/10.1016/j.anclin.2023.02.006

Corcoran TB, Hillyard S (2011) Cardiopulmonary aspects of anaesthesia for the elderly. Best Pract Res Clin Anaesthesiol 25(3):329–354. https://doi.org/10.1016/j.bpa.2011.07.002

Cortínez LI, Trocóniz IF, Fuentes R et al (2008) The influence of age on the dynamic relationship between end-tidal sevoflurane concentrations and bispectral index. Anesth Analg 107(5):1566–1572. https://doi.org/10.1213/ane.0b013e318181f013

De Mello T, Argenta DF, Caon T (2024) Revisiting the effect of aging on the transport of molecules through the skin. Pharm Res 41(6):1031–1044. https://doi.org/10.1007/s11095-024-03710-5

Dodds EC, Kumar CM, McLeod EG, McCartney C, Wildsmith T (2014) Oxford textbook of anaesthesia for the elderly patient. Oxford University Press

Doufas AG (2003) Consequences of inadvertent perioperative hypothermia. Best Pract Res Clin Anaesthesiol 17(4):535–549. https://doi.org/10.1016/S1521-6896(03)00052-1

Ebensperger M, Kreuzer M, Kratzer S, Schneider G, Schwerin S (2025. pii: S0007091225000224) Impact of age on the reliability of GE Entropy™ module indices for guidance of maintenance of anaesthesia in adult patients: a single-centre retrospective analysis. Br J Anaesth. https://doi.org/10.1016/j.bja.2024.11.050

Eger EI (2001) Age, minimum alveolar anesthetic concentration, and minimum alveolar anesthetic concentration-awake. Anesth Analg 93(4):947–953. https://doi.org/10.1097/00000539-200110000-00029

Eleveld DJ, Colin P, Absalom AR, Struys MMRF (2018) Pharmacokinetic–pharmacodynamic model for propofol for broad application in anaesthesia and sedation. Br J Anaesth 120(5):942–959. https://doi.org/10.1016/j.bja.2018.01.018

Evered LA, Chan MTV, Han R et al (2021) Anaesthetic depth and delirium after major surgery: a randomised clinical trial. Br J Anaesth 127(5):704–712. https://doi.org/10.1016/j.bja.2021.07.021

Fragen RJ, Dunn KL (1996) The minimum alveolar concentration (MAC) of sevoflurane with and without nitrous oxide in elderly versus young adults. J Clin Anesth 8:352–356

Fritz BA, Kalarickal PL, Maybrier HR et al (2016) Intraoperative electroencephalogram suppression predicts postoperative delirium. Anesth Analg 122(1):234–242. https://doi.org/10.1213/ANE.0000000000000989

Futier E, Lefrant JY, Guinot PG et al (2017) Effect of individualized vs standard blood pressure management strategies on postoperative organ dysfunction among high-risk patients undergoing major surgery: a randomized clinical trial. JAMA 318(14):1346. https://doi.org/10.1001/jama.2017.14172

Gourkanti B, Gratz I, Chaudhry D (2024) Geriatric anesthesia: a practical guide. Bentham Books

Gragasin FS, Bourque SL, Davidge ST (2012) Vascular aging and hemodynamic stability in the intraoperative period. Front Physiol 3. https://doi.org/10.3389/fphys.2012.00074

Grandison MK, Boudinot FD (2000) Age-related changes in protein binding of drugs: implications for therapy. Clin Pharmacokinet 38(3):271–290. https://doi.org/10.2165/00003088-200038030-00005

Griffiths R, Beech F, Brown A, Dhesi J, Foo I, Goodall J, Harrop-Griffiths W, Jameson J, Love N, Pappenheim K, White S (2014) Association of Anesthetists of Great Britain and Ireland. Perioperative care of the elderly 2014: Association of Anaesthetists of Great Britain and Ireland. Anaesthesia. 69(S1):81–98. https://doi.org/10.1111/anae.12524. PMID: 24303864.

Gulhar R, Ashraf MA, Jialal I (2025) Physiology, acute phase reactants. In: StatPearls. StatPearls Publishing. http://www.ncbi.nlm.nih.gov/books/NBK519570/. Accessed 25 Jan 2025

Gupta R, Gan TJ (2016) Preoperative nutrition and prehabilitation. Anesthesiol Clin 34(1):143–153. https://doi.org/10.1016/j.anclin.2015.10.012

Hall DE, Arya S, Schmid KK et al (2017) Association of a frailty screening initiative with postoperative survival at 30, 180, and 365 days. JAMA Surg 152(3):233. https://doi.org/10.1001/jamasurg.2016.4219

Hermon R, Williams PAH (2013) A study on information induced medication errors. In: Proceedings of the 2nd Australian eHealth Informatics and Security conference held on the 2nd–4th December 2013, Western Australia. https://doi.org/10.4225/75/57981E4131B42

Irwin MG, Ip KY, Hui YM (2019) Anaesthetic considerations in nonagenarians and centenarians. Curr Opin Anaesthesiol 32(6):776–782. https://doi.org/10.1097/ACO.0000000000000793

Karalapillai D, Story D, Hart GK et al (2013) Postoperative hypothermia and patient outcomes after major elective non-cardiac surgery. Anaesthesia 68(6):605–611. https://doi.org/10.1111/anae.12129

Khurshid S, Ashburner JM, Ellinor PT et al (2023) Prevalence and incidence of atrial fibrillation among older primary care patients. JAMA Netw Open 6(2):e2255838. https://doi.org/10.1001/jamanetworkopen.2022.55838

Kim S-W, Han HS, Jung H-W et al (2014) Multidimensional frailty score for the prediction of postoperative mortality risk. JAMA Surg 149(7):633. https://doi.org/10.1001/jamasurg.2014.241

Kim B, Sangha G, Singh A, Bohringer C (2023) The effect of intraoperative hypotension on postoperative renal function. Curr Anesthesiol Rep 13(3):181–186. https://doi.org/10.1007/s40140-023-00564-2

Klein AA, Meek T, Allcock E et al (2021) Recommendations for standards of monitoring during anaesthesia and recovery 2021: guideline from the Association of Anaesthetists. Anaesthesia 76(9):1212–1223. https://doi.org/10.1111/anae.15501

Klotz U (2009) Pharmacokinetics and drug metabolism in the elderly. Drug Metab Rev 41(2):67–76. https://doi.org/10.1080/03602530902722679

Kong H, Xu L, Wang D (2022) Perioperative neurocognitive disorders: a narrative review focusing on diagnosis, prevention, and treatment. CNS Neurosci Ther 28(8):1147–1167. https://doi.org/10.1111/cns.13873

Lakhal K, Ehrmann S, Martin M et al (2015) Blood pressure monitoring during arrhythmia: agreement between automated brachial cuff and intra-arterial measurements. Br J Anaesth 115(4):540–549. https://doi.org/10.1093/bja/aev304

Li Y, Wang B, Fan F et al (2023) Impact of atrial fibrillation on the accuracy of oscillometric blood pressure monitoring in ICU patients from a large real-world database. J Hypertens. https://doi.org/10.1097/HJH.0000000000003408

Liu B, Li Q, Qiu P (2016) Comparison between invasive and non-invasive blood pressure in young, middle and old age. Blood Press 25(3):155–161. https://doi.org/10.3109/08037051.2015.1110935

Ludbrook GL (2022) The hidden pandemic: the cost of postoperative complications. Curr Anesthesiol Rep 12(1):1–9. https://doi.org/10.1007/s40140-021-00493-y

Lysakowski C, Elia N, Czarnetzki C et al (2009) Bispectral and spectral entropy indices at propofol-induced loss of consciousness in young and elderly patients. Br J Anaesth 103(3):387–393. https://doi.org/10.1093/bja/aep162

Ma K, Bebawy JF (2021) Electroencephalographic burst-suppression, perioperative neuroprotection, postoperative cognitive function, and mortality: a focused narrative review of the literature. Anesth Analg. https://doi.org/10.1213/ANE.0000000000005806

Makary MA, Segev DL, Pronovost PJ et al (2010) Frailty as a predictor of surgical outcomes in older patients. J Am Coll Surg 210(6):901–908. https://doi.org/10.1016/j.jamcollsurg.2010.01.028

Mangoni AA, Jackson SHD (2004) Age-related changes in pharmacokinetics and pharmacodynamics: basic principles and practical applications. Br J Clin Pharmacol 57(1):6–14. https://doi.org/10.1046/j.1365-2125.2003.02007.x

Marathe PH, Wen Y, Norton J, Greene DS, Barbhaiya RH, Wilding IR (2000) Effect of altered gastric emptying and gastrointestinal motility on metformin absorption. Br J Clin Pharmacol 50(4):325–332. https://doi.org/10.1046/j.1365-2125.2000.00264.x

McLean AJ, Le Couteur DG (2004) Aging biology and geriatric clinical pharmacology. Pharmacol Rev 56(2):163–184. https://doi.org/10.1124/pr.56.2.4

Meng L, Yu W, Wang T, Zhang L, Heerdt PM, Gelb AW (2018) Blood pressure targets in perioperative care: provisional considerations based on a comprehensive literature review. Hypertension 72(4):806–817. https://doi.org/10.1161/HYPERTENSIONAHA.118.11688

Mohanty S, Rosenthal RA, Russell MM, Neuman MD, Ko CY, Esnaola NF (2016) Optimal perioperative management of the geriatric patient: a best practices guideline from the

American College of Surgeons NSQIP and the American Geriatrics Society. J Am Coll Surg 222(5):930–947. https://doi.org/10.1016/j.jamcollsurg.2015.12.026
Nepogodiev D, Martin J, Biccard B et al (2019) Global burden of postoperative death. Lancet 393(10170):401. https://doi.org/10.1016/S0140-6736(18)33139-8
Ng TP, Feng L, Nyunt MSZ et al (2015) Nutritional, physical, cognitive, and combination interventions and frailty reversal among older adults: a randomized controlled trial. Am J Med 128(11):1225–1236.e1. https://doi.org/10.1016/j.amjmed.2015.06.017
Ni K, Cooter M, Gupta DK et al (2019) Paradox of age: older patients receive higher age-adjusted minimum alveolar concentration fractions of volatile anaesthetics yet display higher bispectral index values. Br J Anaesth 123(3):288–297. https://doi.org/10.1016/j.bja.2019.05.040
Obert DP, Schweizer C, Zinn S et al (2021) The influence of age on EEG-based anaesthesia indices. J Clin Anesth 73:110325. https://doi.org/10.1016/j.jclinane.2021.110325
Onder G, Van Der Cammen TJM, Petrovic M, Somers A, Rajkumar C (2013) Strategies to reduce the risk of iatrogenic illness in complex older adults. Age Ageing 42(3):284–291. https://doi.org/10.1093/ageing/aft038
Palaniappan S, Soiza RL, Duffy S, Moug SJ, Myint PK, The Older People's Surgical Outcomes Collaborative (OPSOC), The Emergency Laparoscopic, Laparotomy Scottish Audit (ELLSA) (2022) Comparison of the clinical frailty score (CFS) to the National Emergency Laparotomy Audit (NELA) risk calculator in all patients undergoing emergency laparotomy. Color Dis 24(6):782–789. https://doi.org/10.1111/codi.16089
Pandit J, Athanassoglou V, Lee L (2016) Neuromuscular blockade in the elderly patient. J Pain Res 9:437. https://doi.org/10.2147/JPR.S85183
Park SK, Han DW, Chang CH, Jung H, Kang H, Song Y (2025) Association between intraoperative electroencephalogram burst suppression and postoperative delirium: a systematic review and meta-analysis. Anesthesiology 142(1):107–120. https://doi.org/10.1097/ALN.0000000000005255
Parmar KL, Law J, Carter B et al (2021) Frailty in older patients undergoing emergency laparotomy: results from the UK Observational Emergency Laparotomy and Frailty (ELF) study. Ann Surg 273(4):709–718. https://doi.org/10.1097/SLA.0000000000003402
Partridge JSL, Moonesinghe SR, Lees N, Dhesi JK (2022) Perioperative care for older people. Age Ageing 51(8):afac194. https://doi.org/10.1093/ageing/afac194
Pecha S, Kirchhof P, Reißmann B (2023) Perioperative arrhythmias. Dtsch Ärztebl Int. https://doi.org/10.3238/arztebl.m2023.0052
Peden CJ, Miller TR, Deiner SG et al (2021) Improving perioperative brain health: an expert consensus review of key actions for the perioperative care team. Br J Anaesth 126(2):423–432. https://doi.org/10.1016/j.bja.2020.10.037
Pollock RD, Carter S, Velloso CP et al (2015) An investigation into the relationship between age and physiological function in highly active older adults. J Physiol 593(3):657–680. https://doi.org/10.1113/jphysiol.2014.282863
Prostran M, Vujovic KS, Vuckovic S et al (2016) Pharmacotherapy of pain in the older population: the place of opioids. Front Aging Neurosci 8. https://doi.org/10.3389/fnagi.2016.00144
Purdon PL, Pavone KJ, Akeju O et al (2015) The ageing brain: age-dependent changes in the electroencephalogram during propofol and sevoflurane general anaesthesia. Br J Anaesth 115:i46–i57. https://doi.org/10.1093/bja/aev213
Schnider TW, Minto CF, Shafer SL et al (1999) The influence of age on propofol pharmacodynamics. Anesthesiology 90(6):1502–1516. https://doi.org/10.1097/00000542-199906000-00003
Sear J (2011) Bonding, binding and isomerism. Anaesth Intensive Care Med 12(4):160–165. https://doi.org/10.1016/j.mpaic.2010.12.013
Staheli B, Rondeau B (2023) Anesthetic considerations in the geriatric population. StatPearls Publishing. https://www.ncbi.nlm.nih.gov/books/NBK572137/
Story DA, Leslie K, Myles PS et al (2010) Complications and mortality in older surgical patients in Australia and New Zealand (the REASON study): a multicentre, prospective, observational study. Anaesthesia 65(10):1022–1030. https://doi.org/10.1111/j.1365-2044.2010.06478.x

Sumner M, Deng C, Evered L et al (2023) Processed electroencephalography-guided general anaesthesia to reduce postoperative delirium: a systematic review and meta-analysis. Br J Anaesth 130(2):e243–e253. https://doi.org/10.1016/j.bja.2022.01.006

The Royal Australian College of General Practitioners (2019) RACGP aged care clinical guide (Silver Book), 5th edn. RACGP. https://www.racgp.org.au/silverbook

Thillainadesan J, Mudge AM, Aitken SJ et al (2021) The prognostic performance of frailty for delirium and functional decline in vascular surgery patients. J Am Geriatr Soc 69(3):688–695. https://doi.org/10.1111/jgs.16907

Thompson A, Fleischmann KE, Smilowitz NR et al (2024) AHA/ACC/ACS/ASNC/HRS/SCA/SCCT/SCMR/SVM guideline for perioperative cardiovascular management for noncardiac surgery: a report of the American College of Cardiology/American Heart Association Joint Committee on Clinical Practice Guidelines. Circulation 150(19):e351. https://doi.org/10.1161/CIR.0000000000001285

Thürmann PA (2020) Pharmacodynamics and pharmacokinetics in older adults. Curr Opin Anaesthesiol 33(1):109–113. https://doi.org/10.1097/ACO.0000000000000814

Travica N, Lotfaliany M, Marriott A et al (2023) Peri-operative risk factors associated with post-operative cognitive dysfunction (POCD): an umbrella review of meta-analyses of observational studies. J Clin Med 12(4):1610. https://doi.org/10.3390/jcm12041610

Tzen YT, Sambandam S, Delmore B, Wang J, Chu A, Wukich DK (2023) Clinical risk factors of perioperative pressure injury in older adult patients with a hip fracture. Adv Skin Wound Care 36(12):642–650. https://doi.org/10.1097/ASW.0000000000000068

Vacas S, Canales C, Deiner SG, Cole DJ (2022) Perioperative brain health in the older adult: a patient safety imperative. Anesth Analg. https://doi.org/10.1213/ANE.0000000000006090

Wang C, Zhang H, Fu Q (2018) Effective dose of dexmedetomidine as an adjuvant sedative to peripheral nerve blockade in elderly patients. Acta Anaesthesiol Scand 62(6):848–856. https://doi.org/10.1111/aas.13087

Wax DB, Lin HM, Leibowitz AB (2011) Invasive and concomitant noninvasive intraoperative blood pressure monitoring. Anesthesiology 115(5):973–978. https://doi.org/10.1097/ALN.0b013e3182330286

Wu X, Jiang Z, Ying J, Han Y, Chen Z (2017) Optimal blood pressure decreases acute kidney injury after gastrointestinal surgery in elderly hypertensive patients: a randomized study. J Clin Anesth 43:77–83. https://doi.org/10.1016/j.jclinane.2017.09.004

Xu Z, Chen H, Zhou H et al (2022) Comparison of noninvasive continuous arterial blood pressure measured by NICAP with arterial line in elderly patients. BMC Geriatr 22(1):108. https://doi.org/10.1186/s12877-022-02803-3

Pain Control in the Older Person

8

Ashutosh Joshi and Thuy Bui

Take-Home Messages

- Chronic pain after undergoing surgery is common in older adults, reduces their quality of life, and is linked to problems like falls, frailty, cognitive decline, sleep problems, and emotional challenges.
- Factors like changes in how pain is felt with age, misconceptions about pain being a normal part of aging, provider knowledge gaps, multiple health issues, medicine intolerance, and cognitive decline often result in pain being overlooked or poorly treated in older adults.
- Managing pain in older adults effectively requires a multimodal approach that combines nondrug methods (e.g., exercise, CBT) with medications and other medical procedures to reduce side effects and improve outcomes.

8.1 Introduction

Chronic pain is more prevalent in older adults than in younger individuals (Gibson and Lussier 2012). It is estimated that around 25% of older adults living in the community experience chronic pain, and this number can reach as high as 80% in residential care settings (Blyth et al. 2001; Stompor et al. 2019). Chronic pain

A. Joshi (✉)
Department of Anaesthesia, Khoo Teck Puat Hospital, Singapore, Republic of Singapore
e-mail: Ashutosh.joshi@ktph.com.sg

T. Bui
Pharmacy Department, Alfred Health, Melbourne, VIC, Australia
e-mail: t.bui@alfred.org.au

K.-Y. Tan et al. (eds.), *Mastering Geriatric Surgery*,
https://doi.org/10.1007/978-981-95-0665-1_8

significantly impacts quality of life and independence and has been associated with adverse health outcomes, such as falls, frailty, cognitive decline, dementia, sleep problems, and emotional distress (Duong et al. 2005; Welsh et al. 2020).

Chronic pain in older adults differs in several ways from that in the general population, making it a distinct area of study. Older adults are not only more likely to suffer from chronic pain, but they also tend to experience types of pain that are uncommon in younger people, such as postherpetic neuralgia and spinal stenosis. Moreover, older adults may perceive pain differently, have multiple comorbidities, possess fewer physiological reserves, and are frequently prescribed multiple medications. These unique factors must be considered when managing chronic pain in an older person.

Table 8.1 Common diseases causing pain

Somatic/musculoskeletal
– Facet joint pain—cervical, lumbar
– Improper positioning in the bedbound
– Rheumatoid arthritis, osteoarthritis
– Occult fracture, failure of old prosthetics
– Compression fractures due to osteoporosis
– Contractures
– Bedsores
Neuropathic
– Spinal stenosis—cervical, lumbar
– Post surgical—hernia, breast, thoracic surgeries
– Poststroke pain
– Lower limb pain due to claudication/peripheral vascular disease
– Neuropathies—diabetic, phantom limb
– Postherpetic neuralgia
– Trigeminal neuralgia
Visceral
– Mesenteric ischemia
– Cancer

8.2 Epidemiology of Chronic Pain

The aging process predisposes older adults to the development of chronic pain. The prevalence rates of pain in older adults vary from 25% to 80% (Blyth et al. 2001; Stompor et al. 2019). The common causes of chronic pain are musculoskeletal conditions, peripheral vascular disease, cancer, and neuropathic pain (Huang et al. 2020). Table 8.1 highlights the typical causes of pain in later life. Arthritis and conditions related to it are the leading contributors to chronic pain among older adults. Additionally, neuropathic pain linked to diabetes and herpes zoster is prevalent in this age group and can be equally or even more debilitating than musculoskeletal pain. Cancer pain arises from the tumor infiltrating or compressing surrounding tissues, or from widespread physical changes due to hormones secreted by the tumor. It may also result from diagnostic procedures and treatments used to address the cancer. For instance, a breast tumor might cause localized acute pain, which could be treated with surgery and chemotherapy. However, chemotherapy can lead to long-lasting painful neuropathies, and surgical complications, such as chronic lymphedema, may also contribute to persistent pain in cancer survivors.

Risk factors for developing chronic pain include older age, female sex, lower socioeconomic status, severe pain, multiple sites of pain, genetic predisposition, and smoking (van Hecke et al. 2013; Mills et al. 2019; Larsson et al. 2017). Additionally, mental health conditions such as anxiety, depression, and catastrophic thinking are often associated with chronic pain (van Hecke et al. 2013; Mills et al. 2019). However, the exact nature of the relationship between chronic pain and these psychological factors remains unclear.

Chronic postsurgical pain (CPSP) is a frequently observed complication among older adults undergoing surgery. The incidence is reported to be as high as 35% and factors such as preoperative anxiety, depression, orthopedic procedures, and heightened acute postoperative pain as linked to elevated risk of CPSP (Jin et al. 2023).

8.3 Changes in Pain Physiology

Pain transmission and perception are likely to be altered in older adults, although the mechanisms underlying these changes remain poorly understood. Current evidence suggests that aging is associated with widespread modifications in the pain pathways, affecting both the peripheral and central nervous systems.

In the peripheral nervous system, aging is linked to neuronal loss, reduced nerve fiber density, decreased conduction velocity, and changes in neurochemical composition (Gibson and Farrell 2004). Similar changes are observed in the central nervous system, including neuronal loss within the neocortex and hippocampus, specifically the locus coeruleus and substantia nigra that are involved in nociceptive processing (Gibson and Farrell 2004). Given that pain perception is partially dependent on the balance between excitatory and inhibitory pathways, these anatomical and physiological changes in the nervous system likely influence pain perception in older adults.

Psychophysical studies have explored whether older adults experience more or less pain. Generally, the pain threshold tends to increase in older adults when stimuli are brief, less spatially extensive, and located at peripheral cutaneous or visceral sites. This suggests that older individuals may have a reduced ability to sense acute pain, potentially increasing their risk of injury (Gibson and Farrell 2004). Conversely, when exposed to more intense stimuli for longer durations, older adults may exhibit increased pain perception and prolonged hyperalgesia (Lane and Smith 2018). While the clinical significance of this finding remains unclear, it raises the possibility that older adults may experience heightened pain under certain conditions.

8.4 Challenges and Barriers in Managing Chronic Pain in Older Persons

Managing chronic pain in older adults presents distinct challenges due to a variety of factors as listed in Table 8.2. Common issues like impaired vision, hearing loss, and cognitive decline can hinder accurate pain assessment. Cognitively impaired seniors are at a higher risk for pain being underassessed and undertreated. Their pain may manifest through behavioral changes, such as aggression or lethargy, as well as nonverbal cues like groaning or grimacing. These symptoms complicate pain management, requiring extra time from healthcare providers, familiarity with pain-related behaviors, and informed clinical judgment.

Beliefs about pain in older adults can also pose obstacles to effective assessment and treatment. Misconceptions, such as viewing pain as a normal aspect of aging, fear of addiction, or adopting stoic attitudes that prevent them from reporting pain or seeking treatment, are common (Lane and Smith 2018). Additionally, the presence of multiple health conditions and the use of numerous medications limit treatment options. For example, nonsteroidal anti-inflammatory drugs (NSAIDs) may be contraindicated in those with heart failure, kidney disease, or those on anticoagulants like warfarin. Age-related physiological changes also impact how drugs are processed, further complicating pain management. Reduced kidney function, for

Table 8.2 Challenges of pain assessment in the older person

Acceptance of pain as normal part of aging and underreporting
Sensory and cognitive impairment
Comorbidities
Provider's belief that there is no pain if patient does not complaint
Fear of addiction
Difference in assessment of pain by patient, caregiver, and provider

instance, affects the elimination of opioids, necessitating dosage adjustments and close monitoring for side effects.

Healthcare providers also contribute to the underassessment and undertreatment of pain in various ways (Borsheski and Johnson 2014). Distrust in patient-reported pain, a lack of routine assessments, and limited pain education can result in inadequate care. Concerns about causing harm, the subjectivity of pain, and limited knowledge of pain management tools and medication side effects further hinder effective treatment. Provider biases, such as fears about dependence, addiction, and legal consequences, add to the challenges. Despite the relatively low risk of addiction in older adults without a history of substance abuse, tools like the opioid risk tool can help identify potential opioid misuse through routine screening (Webster and Webster 2005).

8.5 Goals of Pain Assessment in Older Persons

8.5.1 Establishing a Diagnosis

A critical goal of pain assessment is to establish an accurate diagnosis. For patients with secondary chronic pain conditions, a precise diagnosis may enable targeted treatments, such as joint replacement for knee osteoarthritis or non-pharmacological interventions (Reid et al. 2015). In contrast, primary chronic pain conditions (e.g., fibromyalgia) may lack specific treatments or interventions. In addition to identifying the source of pain, it is also crucial to exclude serious or life-threatening conditions, such as infections or malignancies.

8.5.2 Evaluating Pain Severity

As mentioned, older adults may deny having pain but acknowledge "soreness," "aching," or "discomfort." In such cases, reframing the question—such as asking, "Do you hurt anywhere?" or "What is stopping you from walking?"—can help clarify the presence or absence of pain (Schofield 2018).

In older adults, self-reporting is the gold standard for assessing severity of pain. Tools like the Numerical Rating Scale and Categorical Pain Scale are widely used in clinical and research settings and have been validated for both acute and chronic pain (Schofield 2018). However, the ability of patients to utilize these scales can vary.

Studies have shown that patients with mild to moderate cognitive impairment retain a good understanding of pain scales, with approximately 80% demonstrating comprehension. For those with severe cognitive impairment, comprehension decreases to about 60% (Pautex et al. 2006). Among those who understand the scales, both inter- and intra-rater reliability have been shown to be high (Pautex et al. 2006). Therefore, self-reporting is still considered the standard for most patients with cognitive impairment.

However, self-reporting is not suitable for patients who cannot comprehend the pain scales or are nonverbal. Behavioral pain assessment tools are used in such cases. Commonly used scales for this purpose include the Pain in Advanced Dementia (PAINAD) scale and the Checklist of Nonverbal Pain Indicators (CNPI) (Schofield 2018). The PAINAD scale has five specific indicators: breathing, vocalization, facial expression, body language, and consolability. The score is an indicator of pain being present and is not indicative of severity of pain. The "score" can be helpful in evaluating treatment interventions over time.

8.5.3 Assessing the Impact of Pain

Chronic pain can severely affect an individual's quality of life, including their physical and emotional well-being. Therefore, it is essential to assess not only the pain itself but also its impact on physical, emotional, and social functioning, both in clinical and research settings (Hadjistavropoulos et al. 2007; Turk et al. 2003).

Multidimensional pain assessment tools have been developed to capture comprehensive information, including pain quality and its effect on activities such as walking and sleep (see Table 8.3). While these tools can be useful, their practicality in a busy clinical environment may be limited. In such cases, even a brief inquiry into how pain affects daily activities—like walking, household tasks, mood, and sleep—can provide valuable insights into the severity and impact of pain.

For patients with cognitive impairments, these multidimensional tools may not be appropriate. A triangulated approach that includes patient self-report, observation of behaviors, and information from caregivers is recommended when assessing pain in cognitively impaired older adults (Snow and Shuster 2006). Although several observational tools have been proposed for this population, none have been universally validated for clinical use (Hadjistavropoulos et al. 2007).

The proper use of validated pain scales, including those that are easy to use, translated for non-English speakers, and adapted for visual impairments, is

Table 8.3 Multidimensional pain assessment tools (Hadjistavropoulos et al. 2007)

Short-form McGill Pain Questionnaire (SF-MPQ)
Functional pain scale
Pain disability index
Brief pain inventory
Geriatric pain measure
Multidimensional pain inventory
Western Ontario and McMaster Universities Osteoarthritis Index (WOMAC)
Arthritis Impact Measurement Scale (AIMS)

essential. However, it is also important to engage patients in discussions about their pain experiences through open-ended questions, as pain assessment should not rely solely on standardized tools.

8.5.4 Addressing Attitudes and Beliefs

Attitudes and beliefs can pose significant barriers to effective pain management in older adults. These may include normalizing pain as a part of aging, increased stoicism, reluctance to be a burden, and concerns about using analgesics (e.g., fears of tolerance, addiction, and side effects) (Cousins et al. 2004). Perceived control over pain strongly influences the choice of coping strategies patients engage when attempting to manage their pain. Patients who perceive little or no control over their pain more often engage in emotion-focused coping (vs. problem-focused coping) and passive coping strategies (vs. active), which have both been linked to poorer psychological adjustment in all age groups (Hadjistavropoulos et al. 2007). Recognizing and addressing these attitudes and beliefs is crucial to optimizing pain management and improving the quality of life for older adults.

8.6 Approach to Pain Management in Older People

A broad spectrum of treatment options exists to ameliorate pain in older adults, ranging from nonpharmacological methods to pharmacological therapies and invasive techniques. A multimodal strategy is often effective and advised for managing pain in older adults. Nonpharmacological treatments can be broadly categorized into physical and psychosocial approaches. Physical methods encompass activities such as exercise, acupuncture, and transcutaneous electrical nerve stimulation (TENS). Psychosocial approaches include educational programs focused on self-management, cognitive-behavioral therapy (CBT), mindfulness meditation, music therapy, guided imagery, and progressive muscle relaxation techniques. Given the reduced therapeutic index of many medications in older adults, these nonpharmacological strategies are particularly important in managing pain in this group. This section will focus on key considerations when using medications and interventional pain management techniques for older adults.

8.7 Acute Management of Postoperative Pain in Older Persons

The primary goal in the acute management of postoperative pain is to enhance physical function and optimize recovery, rather than eliminating pain. This approach applies equally to older adults, who require a tailored pain management strategy. A multimodal approach, utilizing both pharmacological and nonpharmacological interventions, should be used, with the choice of analgesics based on the reported or

Table 8.4 Approach to acute management of postoperative pain in older persons

Mild pain[a]	Moderate pain[a]	Severe pain[a]
Nonpharmacological treatment such as physical therapy (e.g. splinting, dressings, positioning), physiotherapy exercises, psychological approaches (e.g. relaxation, education, music)		
Paracetamol ± NSAID taken regularly	Paracetamol ± NSAID taken regularly ± Opioid (oral) when required	Paracetamol ± NSAID taken regularly ± Opioid (oral or PCA) when required Consider referral to anesthesiologist or acute pain service for analgesic infusions or regional anesthesia techniques

NSAID nonsteroidal anti-inflammatory drugs, *PCA* patient-controlled analgesia

[a] Use validated assessment tools to determine severity and impact of pain

anticipated severity of pain (see Table 8.4). Combining analgesics with complementary mechanisms can produce synergistic effects to enhance pain control, reduce opioid use, and minimize side effects. The optimal multimodal analgesic regimen should be determined based on several factors, including the type and severity of pain (e.g., acute, nociceptive, or neuropathic), patient characteristics (e.g., comorbidities, organ dysfunction), and pharmacological properties of the chosen analgesics (e.g., side effects, pharmacokinetics). For further details on different analgesic medications, refer to Sect. 8.8.

Oral analgesics are generally preferred due to their convenience, ease of use, and relatively stable plasma concentrations. However, parenteral administration, such as through a patient-controlled analgesia (PCA) device or regional anesthesia techniques, may be necessary for rapid onset or localized effect. These specialized analgesic regimens require additional equipment, labor, technical expertise, and monitoring (American Geriatrics Society Panel on Pharmacological Management of Persistent Pain in Older Persons 2009). The timing of analgesic administration is also critical. Regular dosing is recommended for persistent pain, while pro re rata dosing is preferable for breakthrough and pre-emptive pain management before physical activity or invasive procedures.

Regional analgesic techniques, including neuraxial and peripheral nerve blocks, provide exceptional efficacy for perioperative anesthesia and pain management. These methods, often complemented by indwelling catheters for continuous medication delivery, surpass traditional parenteral analgesics, particularly in managing postoperative dynamic pain (Pasero et al. 2005). However, the development of definitive guidelines for older patients remains limited due to inconsistent study protocols. When incorporated into multimodal pain management strategies, regional techniques contribute to reduced opioid consumption, shorter hospital stays, earlier ambulation, improved bowel function, and enhanced postoperative mental status (Pasero et al. 2005).

Epidural analgesia, employing local anesthetics, opioids, or their combination, offers superior control of both dynamic and resting pain compared to systemic opioids. Its benefits include decreased opioid requirements, attenuation of surgical stress responses, and enhanced bowel motility, particularly with thoracic-level placements (Kehlet and Holte 2001). Studies have demonstrated that epidural analgesia improves functional exercise capacity and health-related quality of life following colonic surgery compared to systemic opioid use (Carli et al. 2002). Positive outcomes, such as better pain control, earlier mobilization, improved gastrointestinal motility, and increased protein and calorie intake, were observed in the patients randomized to the epidural group. Researchers attributed these improvements in bowel function, which reduce nausea and encourage eating, to the effects of local anesthetics. Commonly used combinations, such as 0.2% ropivacaine and 2 mcg/mL fentanyl, provide effective analgesia while minimizing side effects like hypotension and urinary retention. Patient-controlled epidural analgesia (PCEA) has been shown to decrease the need for pain medication compared to continuous epidural infusion following major abdominal surgery (Standl et al. 2003). However, no standardized protocol has been established for older adults. In our practice, we commonly use a combination of a local anesthetic and an opioid, with background infusion rates of 3–6 mL/h, bolus doses of 2–3 mL, and a lockout interval of 15–20 min. To mitigate risks of complications such as hematomas or infections, epidural catheters should generally be removed within 7 days. Combining epidural with parenteral analgesics is discouraged to simplify drug titration and side effect management.

Peripheral nerve blocks, available as single-shot or continuous catheter techniques, deliver targeted, unilateral pain control with reduced opioid consumption and faster recovery times, all without necessitating a Foley catheter. These techniques are suitable for a wide range of surgical procedures, including upper and lower extremity surgeries (e.g., brachial plexus blocks and sciatic nerve block), abdominal interventions (e.g., transversus abdominis plane and rectus sheath blocks), and thoracic operations (e.g., paravertebral blocks). Ultrasound guidance has enhanced the precision and safety of these procedures. Compared to general or neuraxial anesthesia, peripheral nerve blocks are associated with reduced postoperative nausea, lower opioid consumption, shorter recovery unit stays, and improved patient satisfaction (Hadzic et al. 2005). For older adults, special considerations include vigilant monitoring for catheter-related complications, local anesthetic toxicity, and fall risks due to motor blockade. It is important to highlight the consideration of local anesthetic concentrations in older adults as their lower serum protein levels can result in elevated plasma concentrations of the anesthetic. Additionally, hepatic and renal impairments should be taken into account as they can reduce the body's capacity to metabolize the medication and lower the threshold for local anesthetic toxicity. Ropivacaine is often favored for prolonged use due to its lower cardiac and central nervous system toxicity profile. Ensuring proper caregiver education and providing oral analgesics for emergencies are crucial for safe home care management in case patients are discharged with indwelling nerve block catheters.

8.8 Pharmacological Strategies

Pharmacological pain management in older adults requires a tailored approach due to age-related physiological, pharmacodynamic, and pharmacokinetic changes. Comorbidities, polypharmacy, and geriatric syndromes can increase the risk of adverse drug reactions. As older patients are often excluded from clinical trials, evidence for analgesic use in this group is limited (McLachlan et al. 2011). Below is an overview of key pharmacological strategies and considerations.

8.8.1 Nonopioid Analgesics

Acetaminophen (paracetamol) is a first-line treatment for mild to moderate nociceptive pain in older adults (American Geriatrics Society Panel on Pharmacological Management of Persistent Pain in Older Persons 2009; Schug et al. 2020; Abdulla et al. 2013). When used at recommended doses (3–4 g/day), it has a favorable side-effect profile and can reduce opioid needs (American Geriatrics Society Panel on Pharmacological Management of Persistent Pain in Older Persons 2009; Schug et al. 2020; Abdulla et al. 2013). However, the impact of frailty and aging on paracetamol clearance and the risk of hepatotoxicity remains inconsistent (American Geriatrics Society Panel on Pharmacological Management of Persistent Pain in Older Persons 2009; Schug et al. 2020; Abdulla et al. 2013; Mitchell et al. 2011). Long-term use at maximum doses was associated with transient elevations in alanine aminotransferase levels but not liver failure or dysfunction (Kuffner et al. 2006). Recent guidelines recommend dose adjustments for those who are malnourished, have hepatic impairment, or a history of alcohol abuse (American Geriatrics Society Panel on Pharmacological Management of Persistent Pain in Older Persons 2009; Abdulla et al. 2013).

NSAIDs (e.g., ibuprofen, naproxen) are effective for inflammatory pain, such as osteoarthritis. When combined with paracetamol, NSAIDs can enhance pain relief and reduce opioid use (American Geriatrics Society Panel on Pharmacological Management of Persistent Pain in Older Persons 2009; Schug et al. 2020; Abdulla et al. 2013). The choice of NSAID depends on availability, route of administration, adverse effects, and duration of action (see Table 8.5).

Older adults are particularly susceptible to gastrointestinal, renal, and cardiovascular adverse effects from NSAIDs. Selective COX-2 inhibitors (e.g., celecoxib) may be considered for those at higher gastrointestinal risk due to their lack of antiplatelet effects (Munsterhjelm et al. 2006) and lower incidence of upper gastrointestinal issues (Jarupongprapa et al. 2013). Celecoxib is also associated with a lower risk of renal dysfunction, hypertension, and heart failure exacerbation (Schug et al. 2020; Zhang et al. 2006). Both selective and nonselective NSAIDs, however,

Table 8.5 Half-life and adverse effects of nonselective and selective NSAIDs (American Geriatrics Society Panel on Pharmacological Management of Persistent Pain in Older Persons 2009; Schug et al. 2020; Younan et al. 2013)

<table>
<tr><th>NSAIDs</th><th>Half-life (hours)</th><th>Gastrointestinal effects</th><th>Renal effects</th><th>Cardiovascular and cerebrovascular effects</th></tr>
<tr><td colspan="2">Nonselective</td><td rowspan="4">• Dyspepsia, gastroduodenal ulcers, gastrointestinal bleeding
• Celecoxib may be preferred
• Greater risk with nonselective than selective COX-2
• Nonselective: greatest risk with piroxicam and ketorolac, lowest risk with ibuprofen</td><td rowspan="4">• Edema, electrolyte imbalance, reduced glomerular filtration rate, acute kidney injury
• Celecoxib or naproxen may be preferred
• Common perioperatively due to hypovolemia, hypotension, other nephrotoxins</td><td rowspan="4">• Edema, hypertension, myocardial infarction, stroke, and other thrombotic events
• Naproxen, ibuprofen, or celecoxib may be preferred
• Avoid diclofenac (highest risk), and post-CABG surgery
• Short-term use (<7 days) after noncardiac surgery does not increase risk</td></tr>
<tr><td>Diclofenac
Ibuprofen
Indomethacin
Ketoprofen
Ketorolac
Mefenamic acid
Naproxen
Piroxicam
Sulindac</td><td>2.3
1.8–2
4.5
1.6–4
5.3
2
12–17
50
16–18</td></tr>
<tr><td>Selective COX-2 inhibitors (coxibs)</td><td></td></tr>
<tr><td>Celecoxib
Meloxicam
Parecoxib</td><td>11
15–20
22 min; valdecoxib 8</td></tr>
</table>

increased the risk of cardiovascular and cerebrovascular thrombotic events, with naproxen and celecoxib having the lowest risk (Trelle et al. 2011).

Regular use of nonselective NSAIDs, especially ibuprofen, may negate low-dose aspirin's protective effects (Reed et al. 2018). For localized pain, topical NSAIDs may be preferred due to reduced systemic absorption and gastrointestinal risks (Honvo et al. 2019). In older adults with gastrointestinal risk factors (see Box 8.1) switching to a coxib or adding a gastrointestinal protective agent (e.g., proton pump inhibitor) may help reduce upper gastrointestinal complications (Schug et al. 2020; Scheiman and Fendrick 2005; Targownik et al. 2008; Massó González et al. 2010). NSAIDs should be used at the lowest effective dose for the shortest duration, close monitoring for adverse effects (American Geriatrics Society Panel on Pharmacological Management of Persistent Pain in Older Persons 2009).

Box 8.1 Risk Factors for NSAID Major Gastrointestinal Complications (Schug et al. 2020; Scheiman and Fendrick 2005; Targownik et al. 2008; Massó González et al. 2010)

- NSAID factors
  - Nonselective greater risk than selective COX-2 inhibitors
  - (ketorolac > piroxicam > ketoprofen > naproxen > indomethacin > meloxicam > diclofenac > ibuprofen > celecoxib)
  - Higher dose
  - Longer duration
  - Longer half-life or slow-release formulation
- Patient factors
  - >65 years
  - History of upper gastrointestinal bleed or peptic ulcer disease or perforation
  - *Helicobacter pylori* infection
  - Concurrent illness/comorbidities (e.g., severe rheumatoid arthritis, heart disease)
  - Concomitant drugs (anticoagulants/antiplatelets, selective serotonin/noradrenaline reuptake inhibitors, corticosteroids, smoking)

8.8.2 Opioid Analgesics

Opioids are commonly used for moderate to severe pain, especially in cancer, post-surgical recovery, or severe osteoarthritis. Older adults typically require lower opioid doses, about half those needed by younger individuals, to achieve the same level of pain relief (Schug et al. 2020; Gupta and Avram 2012). This difference is attributed to age-related pharmacodynamic changes and increased sensitivity, rather than differences in pharmacokinetics (Gupta and Avram 2012). However, opioids in older adults require close monitoring due to risks of sedation, confusion, constipation, falls, and respiratory depression. Vigilant monitoring of sedation level can mitigate respiratory depression, while constipation can be managed with aperients, adequate fluid and oral intake, and mobilization. Although limited studies exist on the effects of opioids on delirium in older adults (Schug et al. 2020), appropriate opioid use is generally linked to better cognitive outcomes, while undertreated postoperative pain may worsen cognitive function (Morrison and Siu 2000; Lynch et al. 1998).

Short-acting opioids like morphine are preferred over long-acting ones for opioid-naïve or frail older adults due to the risk of accumulation and toxicity (Schug et al. 2020). The choice of opioid should be individualized based on patient characteristics and opioid properties (see Table 8.6). Combining opioids with simple analgesics or adjunct medications (e.g., antidepressants, anticonvulsants), or opioid rotation can reduce the need for high opioid doses and minimize side effects.

Table 8.6 Comparison of atypical and conventional opioids (Schug et al. 2020; Faculty of Pain Medicine, Australian and New Zealand College of Anaesthetists 2021; Nielsen et al. 2016; Ashley and Dunleavy 2024)

	Available routes of administration	Unit converted from	OME conversion factor (mg/day)	Metabolism and excretion	Comments
Atypical opioids					
Tramadol	Oral Parenteral	mg/day	0.2	• Hepatic metabolism via CYP3A4 and CYP2D6 to more potent metabolite (M1) • Tramadol and metabolites are renally excreted	• Activity at mu-opioid receptors and inhibits reuptake of noradrenaline and serotonin • Age >75 years, 300 mg/day; age ≥75 years, 400 mg/day; risk of delirium in older adults • Less effective as sole agent for moderate to severe pain • Effective for neuropathic pain Lower risk of respiratory depression and constipation compared to conventional opioids • Reduce dose and extend dosing interval in renal impairment • Reduce dose in severe liver impairment • Risk of serotonin syndrome and seizure with other serotonergic or seizure-threshold-lowering drugs • Drug interactions with CYP3A4 and 2D6 inducers or inhibitors; variable response in patients with CYP2D6 polymorphism

(continued)

Table 8.6 (continued)

	Available routes of administration	Unit converted from	OME conversion factor (mg/day)	Metabolism and excretion	Comments
Tapentadol	Oral	mg/day	0.3	• Hepatic metabolism predominantly via glucuronidation to inactive metabolites • Tapentadol and metabolites are renally excreted	• Activity at mu-opioid receptors and inhibits reuptake of noradrenaline • Less gastrointestinal adverse effects than conventional opioids • Effective for neuropathic pain • Reduce dose in moderate liver impairment • Not recommended by the manufacturer in severe renal or liver impairment due to the lack of studies
Buprenorphine	Sublingual Transdermal Parenteral	mcg/day mcg/h mg/day	0.04 2 75	• Hepatic metabolism via CYP3A4 (to inactive or less active metabolites) • Biliary and renal excretion of metabolites	• Unique activity at opioid receptors—strong affinity and slow dissociation from mu-receptor and antagonist at kappa receptor • Ceiling effect for respiratory depression and not analgesia • May need higher doses of naloxone to reverse respiratory depression • Suitable alternative opioid when enteral route is not available • No dose adjustment in renal impairment • Use with caution in severe liver impairment • Potential drug interactions with CYP3A4 inducers or inhibitors

Conventional opioids					
Codeine	Oral Parenteral	mg/day mg/day	0.13 0.25	• Hepatic metabolism via glucuronidation, CYP2D6 to morphine, and CYP3A4 to inactive metabolite • Codeine and metabolites are renally excreted	• Weak opioid, generally not recommended for acute pain • Drug interactions with CYP2D6 and CYP3A4 inducers or inhibitors; variable response in patients with CYP2D6 polymorphism • Use with caution in renal and liver impairment
Morphine	Oral Parenteral	mg/day mg/day	1 3	• Hepatic metabolism via glucuronidation to active metabolites—M6G (analgesia) and M3G (neurotoxic) • Metabolites are predominantly renally excreted	• Reduce dose and extend dosing interval in renal and liver impairment • Itch due to direct histamine release
Fentanyl	Buccal Parenteral Transdermal	mcg/day mcg/day mcg/hr	0.1 0.2 3	• Hepatic metabolism via CYP3A4 to inactive metabolites • Metabolites are renally excreted	• Potent opioid with rapid onset and lack of active metabolites • Use with caution in liver impairment • Drug interactions with CYP3A4 inducers or inhibitors
Oxycodone	Oral Parenteral	mg/day mg/day	1.5 3	• Hepatic metabolism via CYP3A4 (45%) and CYP2D6 (19%) to active metabolites • Oxycodone and metabolites are renally excreted	• Faster onset, more potent, longer duration of action, less concerning metabolites, and lower rates of adverse effects than morphine • Reduce dose in moderate to severe renal impairment • Drug interactions with CYP3A4 and 2D6 inducers or inhibitors; variable response in patients with CYP2D6 polymorphism

(continued)

Table 8.6 (continued)

	Available routes of administration	Unit converted from	OME conversion factor (mg/day)	Metabolism and excretion	Comments
Hydromorphone	Oral Parenteral	mg/day mg/day	5 15	• Hepatic metabolism by glucuronidation to inactive metabolite—H3G (neurotoxic) • Metabolites are renally excreted	• Alternative to morphine in renal impairment • Accumulation of metabolite may cause neuroexcitation and cognitive impairment • Use with caution in renal and liver impairment
Methadone	Oral Parenteral	mg/day mg/day	4.7[a] 13.5[a]	• Hepatic metabolism via CYP enzymes to inactive metabolites • Methadone and metabolites are excreted in feces and urine	• May have a role in chronic neuropathic pain owing to NMDA–receptor antagonism and monoamine reuptake inhibition • Potential for prolonged QT intervals and arrhythmias with high doses and concomitant risk factors, and drug interactions • No dose adjustment in renal impairment • Drug interactions with CYP enzyme inducers or inhibitors

OME oral morphine equivalent

[a] Seek specialist advice given complex pharmacokinetics

8.8.3 Local Anesthetics

Older adults may have increased sensitivity to local anesthetics due to age-related changes in drug clearance, nerve conduction, and spinal cord neuron density (Sadean and Glass 2003). Local anesthetics, such as bupivacaine, ropivacaine, or lignocaine, can be administered peripherally or centrally through single, intermittent, or continuous doses. For localized neuropathic pain, topical lidocaine (5% patches or gels) is effective and well-tolerated with minimal systemic effects (Finnerup et al. 2015).

8.8.4 Adjuvant Medications

Adjuvant medications are often helpful, particularly for neuropathic pain or pain refractory to conventional analgesics.

- **Antidepressants**: Tricyclic antidepressants (TCAs), such as amitriptyline, are effective for neuropathic pain but have significant anticholinergic side effects (e.g., sedation, confusion, constipation, dry mouth, increased risk of mortality and dementia). Nortriptyline may be the preferred TCA in older adults due to its reduced sedative and anticholinergic side effects compared to amitriptyline (Taylor et al. 2021). Selective serotonin-norepinephrine reuptake inhibitors (SNRIs), such as duloxetine and venlafaxine, offer a better side effect profile and are commonly used for neuropathic pain (e.g., diabetic neuropathy, fibromyalgia). Duloxetine has been shown to be both effective and safe for treating knee osteoarthritis in older adults (Chappell et al. 2009).
- **Anticonvulsants**: Gabapentinoids, including gabapentin and pregabalin, are effective for neuropathic pain but may cause dizziness, drowsiness, and gait disturbances, increasing fall risk. These should be started at low doses and titrated slowly. Both gabapentin and pregabalin are primarily excreted through the kidneys, necessitating dose adjustments in renal impairment. The lack of significant drug interactions with gabapentinoids may be advantageous compared to other anticonvulsants, such as carbamazepine, and certain analgesics.
- **Systemic alpha-2 agonists**: Clonidine and dexmedetomidine are selective alpha-2 adrenoceptor agonists that produce analgesia through the dorsal horn of the spinal cord and peripheral mechanisms. Dexmedetomidine is typically administered via continuous infusion intraoperatively or the intensive care unit for sedation and analgesia. Perioperative use of clonidine has been investigated as an adjuvant to both general and regional anesthesia, as well as in the postoperative period, to enhance analgesia with systemic, spinal, or peripheral opioids, reduce opioid consumption, and prolong the analgesic effects of local anesthetics (Tryba and Gehling 2002). The primary adverse effects of sedation and hypotension limit the dosing and use in older adults.
- **Ketamine**: An NMDA-receptor antagonist is indicated for the treatment of pain associated with central sensitization, including severe acute pain, neuropathic

pain, and opioid-resistant pain (Schug et al. 2020). Older patients are more susceptible to the cognitive adverse effects of ketamine, such as hallucinations or vivid dreams, which can be mitigated by lower doses within the usual pain management dose range (0.1–0.3 mg/kg bolus or hourly infusion).
- **Salmon calcitonin and bisphosphonates**: Calcitonin is a hormone produced by the thyroid gland that lowers blood calcium levels by inhibiting osteoclast activity in bones and reducing renal reabsorption of calcium and phosphate. It also exerts analgesic effects through serotonergic pathways in the central nervous system. Salmon calcitonin reduces acute phantom limb pain (Neumüller et al. 2023), alleviates acute pain, and improves mobilization after recent osteoporotic vertebral compression fractures (Boucher et al. 2020), and in early treatment of complex regional pain syndrome (CRPS) (Harden et al. 2022). Common adverse effects include nausea, facial flushing, diarrhea, abdominal pain, and fatigue. Bisphosphonates are an alternative option to reduce pain in acute osteoporotic vertebral compression fractures and CRPS (Tzschentke 2021).

8.8.5 Corticosteroids

Corticosteroids are used for inflammatory pain, such as arthritis or spinal stenosis, and perioperative administration reduces postoperative pain and analgesic requirements. However, their use in the perioperative setting is more frequently for other indications, such as the prophylaxis of postoperative nausea and vomiting or to decrease swelling following throat or maxillofacial surgery (Schug et al. 2020). Long-term oral use should be avoided due to risks such as osteoporosis, diabetes, and gastrointestinal ulcers. For localized pain, intra-articular or epidural steroid injections may be preferred as they target specific areas but carry risks of infection, tissue damage, and potentially elevate blood glucose.

8.8.6 Muscle Relaxants

Muscle relaxants, such as baclofen, orphenadrine, cyclobenzaprine, and methocarbamol, are occasionally used for musculoskeletal pain but are limited in older adults due to the risk of sedation, confusion, and falls. These should be used sparingly and for short durations to minimize adverse effects.

8.8.7 Other Considerations

- **Polypharmacy**: Older patients are at higher risk of drug interactions due to the higher number of medications they typically take. Drug interactions may either potentiate or reduce the efficacy of pain medications or increase the risk of side effects, requiring careful monitoring and management.

- **Renal and hepatic function**: Age-related decline in renal and hepatic function may necessitate adjustments to pain medications. For example, opioids, NSAIDs, and gabapentinoids may require dose reductions or be avoided altogether in impaired renal or hepatic function to prevent accumulation and adverse effects.
- **Cognitive function**: Cognitive impairment, including delirium and confusion, is common in older adults. Medications with central nervous system effects, such as opioids, TCAs, and gabapentinoids, should be used cautiously to avoid exacerbating cognitive decline, confusion, delirium, or increasing falls risk.

8.9 Regular Review of Analgesia

The pharmacological management of pain in older adults should be individualized, considering comorbidities, renal and hepatic function, cognitive status, and potential adverse effects. Nonopioid analgesics are preferred for mild to moderate pain, with opioids reserved for more severe cases at the lowest effective dose. Adjuvant therapies, including antidepressants and anticonvulsants, are crucial for neuropathic pain. Although procedure-specific postoperative pain management guidelines exist, they are not specifically tailored for older adults (The European Society of Regional Anaesthesia and Pain Therapy 2024). Regular review and adjustment of analgesics are necessary to minimize side effects and optimize pain relief in this vulnerable population.

Short-term analgesia initiated following surgical procedures should be reassessed regularly, tapering or discontinuing medications when appropriate. The increasing recognition of the harms associated with opioids has led to governmental and institutional initiatives promoting prudent prescribing to minimize persistent opioid use and adverse outcomes (Australian Commission on Safety and Quality in Health Care 2022). Similar to antimicrobial stewardship, opioid or analgesic stewardship should be applied in older adults (Australian Commission on Safety and Quality in Health Care 2022), balancing the benefits of pain relief with the potential risks. In some cases, prolonged opioid use may be necessary, especially when other treatments are not well tolerated, to improve physical function and quality of life. It is essential to engage patients and their families in the development of a comprehensive pain management plan, which should include clearly defined therapeutic goals, potential adverse effects, and the expected duration of treatment.

8.10 Interventional Strategies

While medications can effectively manage chronic pain in many older adults, some may experience dose-limiting side effects like sedation, and others may not achieve sufficient pain relief even with therapeutic doses of analgesics. For these individuals, interventional pain treatments offer a safe and effective alternative. Common procedures and indications for older persons are listed in Table 8.7. Principles of successful pain interventions include identifying and treating the pain generator as well as modifying or blocking the nociceptive pathway.

Table 8.7 Common procedures and indications

Target region	Procedure	Indications
Peripheral nerves	• Iliohypogastric/ Ilioinguinal (II/IH) nerve block • II/IH pulsed radio frequency ablation	• Postoperative pain following hernia surgeries • Ilioinguinal and iliohypogastric neuralgia
	(TAP) Transversus abdominis plane block	• Postoperative pain following abdominal surgeries • Chronic abdominal wall pain
	• Intercostal nerve block • ICN pulsed radiofrequency ablation	• Chest wall surgery • Chest wall trauma • Post herpetic neuralgia • Chest wall tumors • Intercostal neuralgia
Spinal structures	Cervical nerve root block	• Cervical radiculopathy • Cervical degenerative disk disease • Cervical disk herniation • Cervical spinal stenosis • Cervical post laminectomy (failed neck) surgery syndrome • Cancer-related pain
	Diagnostic: • Cervical MBB (medial branch blocks)	Diagnostic MBB: • Persistent and disabling axial neck and/or upper back pain or suspected cervicogenic headache • Lack of evidence for disc herniation and radiculitis causing pain • Lack of obvious evidence for discogenic pain
	Therapeutic: • Facet joint injection • Radiofrequency ablation of MBB	Therapeutic: • Therapeutic modalities are applied based on the diagnosis established with a positive response to controlled diagnostic blocks, with a criterion standard of 80% pain relief and the ability to perform prior painful movements without significant pain
	Lumbar, caudal epidural, transforaminal injections	• Lumbar radiculopathy • Lumbar degenerative disk disease • Lumbar disk herniation • Lumbar spinal stenosis • Lumbar post laminectomy (failed back) surgery syndrome • Lumbar vertebral compression fractures • Cancer-related pain

(continued)

Table 8.7 (continued)

Target region	Procedure	Indications
	Diagnostic: • Lumbar (MBB) medial branch blocks	Diagnostic: • Somatic or nonradicular low back pain • Lack of evidence, for either discogenic or sacroiliac joint pain • Lack of painful disc herniation or evidence of radiculitis
	Therapeutic: • Facet joint injection • Radiofrequency ablation of MBB	Therapeutic: • Diagnosis established with a positive response to controlled diagnostic blocks, with a criterion standard of 80% pain relief and the ability to perform prior painful movements without significant pain
	Neurolytic blocks • Coeliac plexus • Superior hypogastric • Ganglion impar	• Cancer pain
Major joints	Knee: • Intra-articular injection: steroids, Monovisc® • Genicular nerve radio frequency ablation	• Osteoarthritis • Other arthritis, e.g., rheumatoid
	Hip joint denervation	• Osteoarthritis • Intra-articular cartilage degeneration • Labral tears • Loose bodies • Avascular necrosis • Metastatic pain
	SIJ (sacroiliac joint): • SIJ steroid injection • SIJ denervation	• Sacroiliitis: ankylosing spondylitis • Capsular/synovial disruption • Ligamentous/tendon disruptions

8.10.1 Identifying/Treating the Pain Generator

- ***Nerve block*** (Fig. 8.1): Injecting a local anesthetic to temporarily block the transmission of chronic pain or pain originating from the sympathetic nervous system can sometimes help predict the outcomes of nerve destruction procedures. Nerve blocks are performed for two purposes: diagnostic and therapeutic. Diagnostic nerve blocks differentiate among the mechanisms that may be responsible for the patient's persistent pain. Therapeutic nerve blocks provide longer pain relief after the diagnosis is made. Steroid injections are the most common types of interventional treatment options. Injection of a local anesthetic with steroids can provide symptom relief and functional improvement (Joshi and Bin 2021). Although generally safe, excessive use of steroids can cause side effects such as

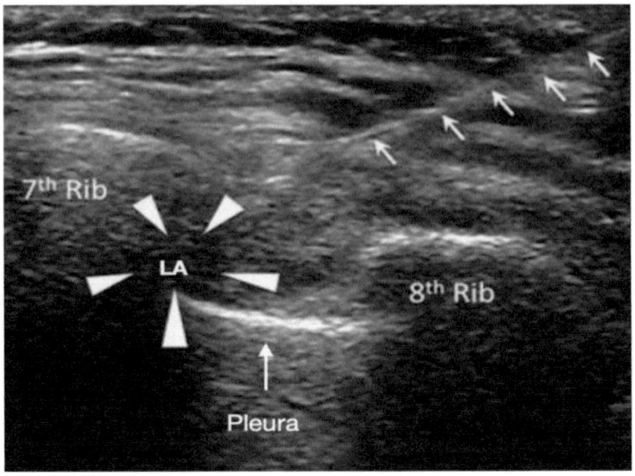

Fig. 8.1 Sonographic image of diagnostic intercostal nerve block in a patient with intercostal neuralgia. The local anesthetic (LA) is deposited at the caudal aspect of rib and depression of pleura is observed during the injection. Needle trajectory (white arrows)

osteoporosis and worsening of pre-existing diabetes/hypertension. Strategies to minimize side effects from steroid injections include (Mattie et al. 2019)

- Lowest possible steroid injections in a year, preferably <3
- Avoid performing a series of injections separated by 1 week
- Repeat injections only if patients had significant pain and functional benefits
- Avoid high-dose injections (>40 mg triamcinolone equivalent)

8.10.2 Blocking the Nociceptive Pathway

- ***Conventional radiofrequency (RF) ablation*** (Figs. 8.2 and 8.3): The primary objective of conventional radiofrequency (RF) is to elevate the temperature around neural tissue, causing irreversible nerve damage and interrupting the nociceptive pathway. By altering or disrupting pain signals from their source, this technique provides significant pain relief. While it does not directly address the underlying causes of pain, the long-lasting analgesia achieved through RF can alleviate complications associated with chronic pain, such as sleep disturbances, poor hygiene, mood disorders, and functional limitations. It also supports patients in resuming normal daily activities.
- Currently, RF is performed percutaneously by inserting an insulated needle with an active metallic tip near the targeted nerve pathway (Cosman et al. 2014). The high-frequency alternating current delivered through the active tip induces molecular oscillation, generating friction within the tissue and creating lesions in the nerve fibers. These lesions effectively block the transmission of nociceptive signals from the pain source.
- ***Pulsed radiofrequency*** (Fig. 8.4): Pulsed radiofrequency (RF) is a less invasive option with a lower complication rate compared to conventional RF, though the exact mechanism of its pain-relieving effects remains unclear. This technique

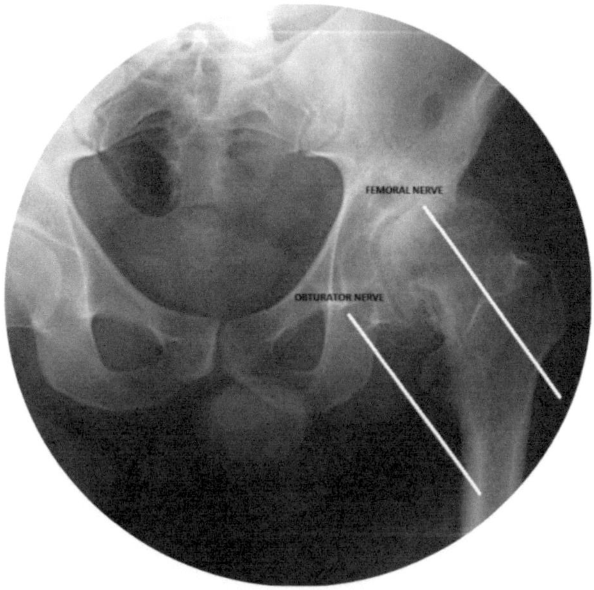

Fig. 8.2 Pelvis X-ray (anteroposterior): targets for femoral and obturator nerve articular branches block

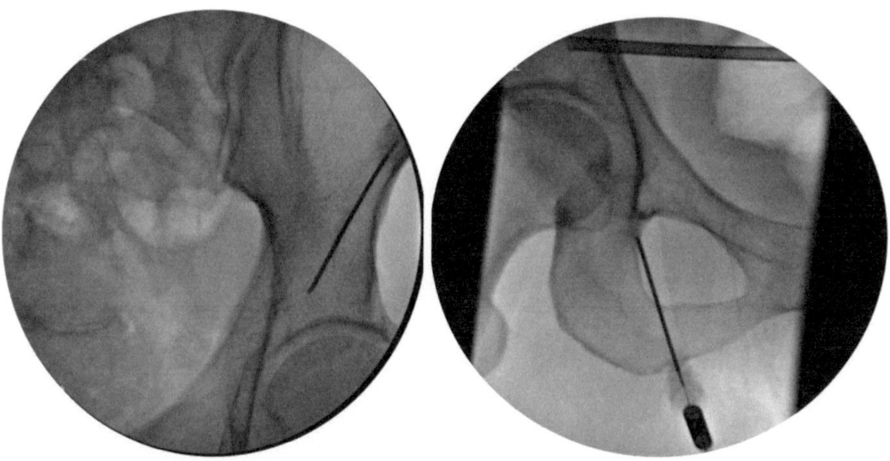

Fig. 8.3 Conventional radiofrequency of articular branches of hip joint for osteoarthritis pain

creates strong electric fields by delivering short bursts of current lasting 20 ms, typically at a frequency of two pulses per second. Between pulses, a cooling period of 480 ms allows heat to dissipate, preventing the temperature from exceeding 42 °C, which is below the threshold for neurodestruction (Chong and Joshi 2022). As a result, pulsed RF is not believed to cause protein denaturation or neural tissue damage.

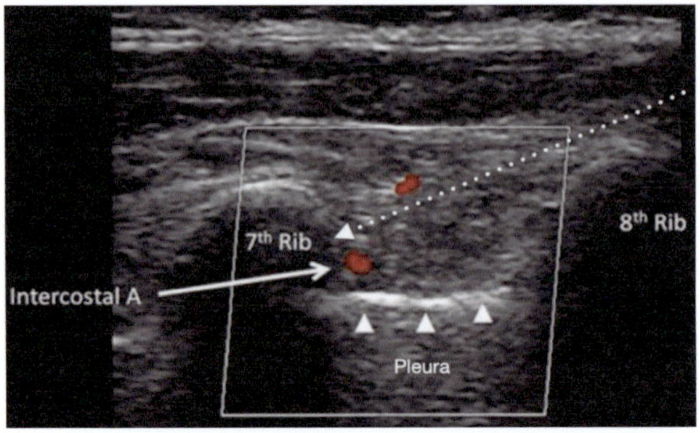

Fig. 8.4 A case of intercostal neuralgia post trauma. Pulsed radiofrequency electrode (dotted arrow) is placed next to the intercostal nerve avoiding the vessels

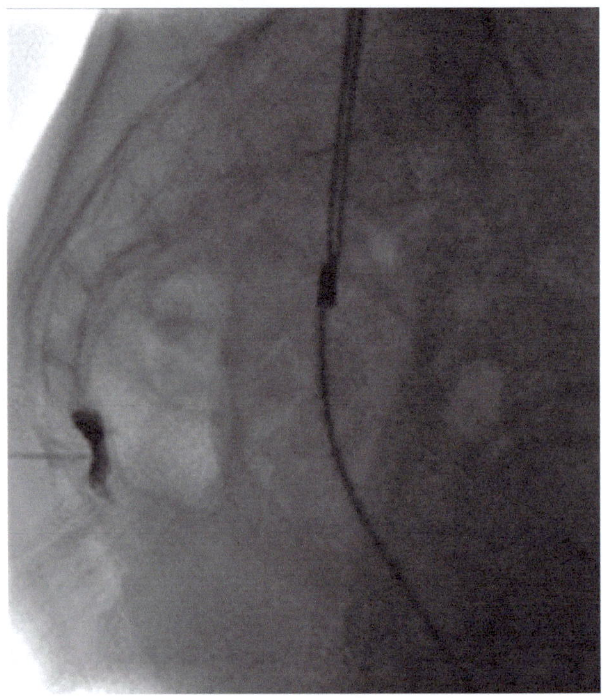

Fig. 8.5 Ganglion impar block for perineal pain due to rectal carcinoma. Lateral projection during fluoroscopic neurolysis of ganglion impar

- Potential mechanisms behind its effects may include structural changes in the nerve, modulation of gene expression, and immunomodulatory actions (Erdine et al. 2009; Vallejo et al. 2013; Ren et al. 2018). Common applications include treating neuralgia in the iliohypogastric, ilioinguinal, and intercostal nerves.
- ***Chemical neurolysis*** (Fig. 8.5): Chemical neurolytic techniques are typically considered a last-resort option for managing severe, intractable pain syndromes. Due to their destructive nature, these methods are most commonly used in cancer pain management, particularly for patients with terminal illnesses. Unlike radio-

frequency techniques, the extent of tissue damage caused by chemical neurolysis is less predictable, and unintended spread to nontargeted areas can result in serious complications, such as neurological deficits, tissue necrosis, or vascular injury and spasm.

- The neurolytic effects of phenol are achieved through protein coagulation, which leads to neural tissue destruction and Wallerian degeneration. Effective concentrations for neurolysis range from 4% to 10% (Benzon and Raj 2008). Common clinical applications of chemical neurolysis include splanchnic nerve blocks for abdominal cancer pain, superior hypogastric plexus blocks for pelvic cancer pain, and ganglion impar blocks for pain associated with rectal or colon cancer.

8.11 Conclusion

There is some evidence suggesting that older patients might have a lower threshold for acute pain, but chronic pain can be more intense for them. As a result, the idea that older adults experience less pain is outdated. Chronic pain is common in this population but often goes unnoticed and untreated. To improve healthcare, it is essential to better recognize these issues. Managing pain in older patients can be challenging due to factors such as cognitive impairment, age-related or disease-related organ dysfunction, and potential drug interactions. Therefore, healthcare providers need to be mindful of how these factors impact patient care. While pharmacotherapy is often utilized in managing pain, using multimodal regimen that also includes interventions, physical therapy, and cognitive-behavioral therapy provides an opportunity to reduce medication dosage and potential side effects.

References

Abdulla A, Adams N, Bone M, Elliott AM, Gaffin J, Jones D, Knaggs R, Martin D, Sampson L, Schofield P (2013) British Geriatric Society. Guidance on the management of pain in older people. Age Ageing 42(Suppl 1):i1–i57

American Geriatrics Society Panel on Pharmacological Management of Persistent Pain in Older Persons (2009) Pharmacological management of persistent pain in older persons. J Am Geriatr Soc 57(8):1331–1346

Ashley C, Dunleavy A (2024) The renal drug database. Taylor & Francis Group, London. https://www.renaldrugdatabase.com.acs.hcn.com.au. Accessed 8 Dec 2024

Australian Commission on Safety and Quality in Health Care (2022) Opioid analgesic Stewardship in acute pain clinical care standard, Acute care edn. ACSQHC, Sydney

Benzon HT, Raj PP (2008) Raj's practical management of pain, 4th edn. Mosby-Elsevier, Philadelphia, xix, 1319

Blyth FM, March LM, Brnabic AJ, Jorm LR, Williamson M, Cousins MJ (2001) Chronic pain in Australia: a prevalence study. Pain 89(2–3):127–134

Borsheski R, Johnson QL (2014) Pain management in the geriatric population. Mo Med 111(6):508–511

Boucher E, Rosgen B, Lang E (2020) Efficacy of calcitonin for treating acute pain associated with osteoporotic vertebral compression fracture: an updated systematic review. CJEM 22(3):359–367

Carli F, Phil M, Mayo N et al (2002) Epidural analgesia enhances functional exercise capacity and health related quality of life after colonic surgery. Results of a randomized trial. Anesthesiology 97(3):540–549

Chappell AS, Ossanna MJ, Liu-Seifert H, Iyengar S, Skljarevski V, Li LC, Bennett RM, Collins H (2009) Duloxetine, a centrally acting analgesic, in the treatment of patients with osteoarthritis knee pain: a 13-week, randomized, placebo-controlled trial. Pain 146(3):253–260

Chong CCW, Joshi A (2022) The pathophysiology of neuropathic pain. In: de Castro J, El Miedany Y (eds) Advances in chronic and neuropathic pain. Contemporary rheumatology. Springer, Cham. https://doi.org/10.1007/978-3-031-10687-3_4

Cosman ER Jr, Dolensky JR, Hoffman RA (2014) Factors that affect radiofrequency heat lesion size. Pain Med 15(12):2020–2036

Cousins MJ, Brennan F, Carr DB (2004) Pain relief: a universal human right. Pain 112(1–2):1–4

Duong BD, Kerns RD, Towle V, Reid MC (2005) Identifying the activities affected by chronic nonmalignant pain in older veterans receiving primary care. J Am Geriatr Soc 53(4):687–694

Erdine S, Bilir A, Cosman ER, Cosman ER Jr (2009) Ultrastructural changes in axons following exposure to pulsed radiofrequency fields. Pain Pract 9(6):407–417

Faculty of Pain Medicine, Australian and New Zealand College of Anaesthetists (2021) Opioid dose equivalence calculation table PS01 (PM) (Appendix) 2021. https://www.anzca.edu.au/getattachment/6892fb13-47fc-446b-a7a2-11cdfe1c9902/PS01(PM)-(Appendix)-Opioid-Dose-Equivalence-Calculation-Table. Accessed 8 Dec 2024

Finnerup NB, Attal N, Haroutounian S, McNicol E, Baron R, Dworkin RH, Gilron I, Haanpää M, Hansson P, Jensen TS, Kamerman PR, Lund K, Moore A, Raja SN, Rice AS, Rowbotham M, Sena E, Siddall P, Smith BH, Wallace M (2015) Pharmacotherapy for neuropathic pain in adults: a systematic review and meta-analysis. Lancet Neurol 14(2):162–173

Gibson SJ, Farrell M (2004) A review of age differences in the neurophysiology of nociception and the perceptual experience of pain. Clin J Pain 20(4):227–239

Gibson SJ, Lussier D (2012) Prevalence and relevance of pain in older persons. Pain Med 13(Suppl 2):S23–S26

Gupta DK, Avram MJ (2012) Rational opioid dosing in the elderly: dose and dosing interval when initiating opioid therapy. Clin Pharmacol Ther 91(2):339–343

Hadjistavropoulos T, Herr K, Turk DC, Fine PG, Dworkin RH, Helme R et al (2007) An interdisciplinary expert consensus statement on assessment of pain in older persons. Clin J Pain 23(1 Suppl):S1–S43

Hadzic A, Williams BA, Karaca PE et al (2005) For outpatient rotator cuff surgery nerve block anesthesia provides superior same-day recovery over general anesthesia. Anesthesiology 102:1001–1007

Harden RN, McCabe CS, Goebel A, Massey M, Suvar T, Grieve S, Bruehl S (2022) Complex regional pain syndrome: practical diagnostic and treatment guidelines, 5th edition. Pain Med 23(Suppl 1):S1–S53

Honvo G, Leclercq V, Geerinck A, Thomas T, Veronese N, Charles A, Rabenda V, Beaudart C, Cooper C, Reginster JY, Bruyère O (2019) Safety of topical non-steroidal anti-inflammatory drugs in osteoarthritis: outcomes of a systematic review and meta-analysis. Drugs Aging 36(Suppl 1):45–64

Huang YL, Tsay WI, Her SH, Ho CH, Tsai KT, Hsu CC et al (2020) Chronic pain and use of analgesics in the elderly: a nationwide population-based study. Arch Med Sci 16(3):627–634

Jarupongprapa S, Ussavasodhi P, Katchamart W (2013) Comparison of gastrointestinal adverse effects between cyclooxygenase-2 inhibitors and non-selective, non-steroidal anti-inflammatory drugs plus proton pump inhibitors: a systematic review and meta-analysis. J Gastroenterol 48(7):830–838

Jin J, Zhang T, Xiong X et al (2023) A prospective study of chronic postsurgical pain in elderly patients: incidence, characteristics and risk factors. BMC Geriatr 23:289. https://doi.org/10.1186/s12877-023-04006-w

Joshi A, Bin WH (2021) Epidural Steroid Injections. In: Munk PL, Babu SB (eds) Interventional radiology in palliative care. Medical radiology. Springer, Cham. https://doi.org/10.1007/978-3-030-65463-4_10

Kehlet H, Holte K (2001) Effect of postoperative analgesia on surgical outcome. Br J Anaesth 87(1):62–72

Kuffner EK, Temple AR, Cooper KM, Baggish JS, Parenti DL (2006) Retrospective analysis of transient elevations in alanine aminotransferase during long-term treatment with acetaminophen in osteoarthritis clinical trials. Curr Med Res Opin 22(11):2137–2148

Lane P, Smith D (2018) Culture, ageing and the construction of pain. Geriatrics (Basel) 3(3):40

Larsson C, Hansson EE, Sundquist K, Jakobsson U (2017) Chronic pain in older adults: prevalence, incidence, and risk factors. Scand J Rheumatol 46(4):317–325

Lynch EP, Lazor MA, Gellis JE, Orav J, Goldman L, Marcantonio ER (1998) The impact of postoperative pain on the development of postoperative delirium. Anesth Analg 86(4):781–785

Massó González EL, Patrignani P, Tacconelli S, García Rodríguez LA (2010) Variability among nonsteroidal antiinflammatory drugs in risk of upper gastrointestinal bleeding. Arthritis Rheum 62(6):1592–1601

Mattie R, Miller DC, Smith C (2019) On behalf of the spine intervention society's patient safety C. annual maximum dose of epidural steroid injection. Pain Med 20(10):2069–2070

McLachlan AJ, Bath S, Naganathan V, Hilmer SN, Le Couteur DG, Gibson SJ, Blyth FM (2011) Clinical pharmacology of analgesic medicines in older people: impact of frailty and cognitive impairment. Br J Clin Pharmacol 71(3):351–364

Mills SEE, Nicolson KP, Smith BH (2019) Chronic pain: a review of its epidemiology and associated factors in population-based studies. Br J Anaesth 123(2):e273–e283

Mitchell SJ, Hilmer SN, Murnion BP, Matthews S (2011) Hepatotoxicity of therapeutic short-course paracetamol in hospital inpatients: impact of ageing and frailty. J Clin Pharm Ther 36(3):327–335

Morrison RS, Siu AL (2000) A comparison of pain and its treatment in advanced dementia and cognitively intact patients with hip fracture. J Pain Symptom Manag 19(4):240–248

Munsterhjelm E, Niemi TT, Ylikorkala O, Neuvonen PJ, Rosenberg PH (2006) Influence on platelet aggregation of i.v. parecoxib and acetaminophen in healthy volunteers. Br J Anaesth 97(2):226–231

Neumüller J, Lang-Illievich K, Brenna CTA, Klivinyi C, Bornemann-Cimenti H (2023) Calcitonin in the treatment of phantom limb pain: a systematic review. CNS Drugs 37(6):513–521

Nielsen S, Degenhardt L, Hoban B, Gisev N (2016) A synthesis of oral morphine equivalents (OME) for opioid utilisation studies. Pharmacoepidemiol Drug Saf 25(6):733–737

Pasero C, Rakel B, McCaffery M (2005) Postoperative pain management in the older adult. In: Gibson SJ, Weiner DK (eds) Pain in older persons, vol 35. IASP Press, Seattle, pp 377–395

Pautex S, Michon A, Guedira M, Emond H, Le Lous P, Samaras D et al (2006) Pain in severe dementia: self-assessment or observational scales? J Am Geriatr Soc 54(7):1040–1045

Reed GW, Abdallah MS, Shao M, Wolski K, Wisniewski L, Yeomans N, Lüscher TF, Borer JS, Graham DY, Husni ME, Solomon DH, Libby P, Menon V, Lincoff AM, Nissen SE (2018) Effect of aspirin coadministration on the safety of celecoxib, naproxen, or ibuprofen. J Am Coll Cardiol 71(16):1741–1751

Reid MC, Eccleston C, Pillemer K (2015) Management of chronic pain in older adults. BMJ 350:h532

Ren H, Jin H, Jia Z, Ji N, Luo F (2018) Pulsed radiofrequency applied to the sciatic nerve improves neuropathic pain by Down-regulating the expression of calcitonin gene-related peptide in the dorsal root ganglion. Int J Med Sci 15(2):153–160

Sadean MR, Glass PS (2003) Pharmacokinetics in the elderly. Best Pract Res Clin Anaesthesiol 17(2):191–205

Scheiman JM, Fendrick AM (2005) Practical approaches to minimizing gastrointestinal and cardiovascular safety concerns with COX-2 inhibitors and NSAIDs. Arthritis Res Ther 7(Suppl 4):S23–S29

Schofield P (2018) The assessment of pain in older people: UK National Guidelines. Age Ageing 47(Suppl_1):i1–i22

Schug SA, Palmer GM, Scott DA, Alcock M, Halliwell R, Mott JF, APM:SE Working Group of the Australian and New Zealand College of Anaesthetists and Faculty of Pain Medicine (2020) Acute pain management: scientific evidence, 5th edn. ANZCA & FPM, Melbourne

Snow AL, Shuster JL Jr (2006) Assessment and treatment of persistent pain in persons with cognitive and communicative impairment. J Clin Psychol 62(11):1379–1387

Standl T, Burmeister M-A, Ohnesorge H et al (2003) Patient-controlled epidural analgesia reduces analgesic requirements compared to continuous epidural infusion after major abdominal surgery. Can J Anesth 50:258–264

Stompor M, Grodzicki T, Stompor T, Wordliczek J, Dubiel M, Kurowska I (2019) Prevalence of chronic pain, particularly with neuropathic component, and its effect on overall functioning of elderly patients. Med Sci Monit 25:2695–2701

Targownik LE, Metge CJ, Leung S, Chateau DG (2008) The relative efficacies of gastroprotective strategies in chronic users of nonsteroidal anti-inflammatory drugs. Gastroenterology 134(4):937–944

Taylor DM, Barnes TRE, Young AH (2021) The Maudsley prescribing guidelines in psychiatry, 14th edn. Wiley Global Research (STMS), Australia

The European Society of Regional Anaesthesia and Pain Therapy (2024) Better postoperative pain management. https://esraeurope.org/prospect/. Accessed 8 Dec 2024

Trelle S, Reichenbach S, Wandel S, Hildebrand P, Tschannen B, Villiger PM, Egger M, Jüni P (2011) Cardiovascular safety of non-steroidal anti-inflammatory drugs: network meta-analysis. BMJ 342:c7086

Tryba M, Gehling M (2002) Clonidine—a potent analgesic adjuvant. Curr Opin Anaesthesiol 15(5):511–517

Turk DC, Dworkin RH, Allen RR, Bellamy N, Brandenburg N, Carr DB et al (2003) Core outcome domains for chronic pain clinical trials: IMMPACT recommendations. Pain 106(3):337–345

Tzschentke TM (2021) Pharmacology of bisphosphonates in pain. Br J Pharmacol 178(9):1973–1994

Vallejo R, Tilley DM, Williams J, Labak S, Aliaga L, Benyamin RM (2013) Pulsed radiofrequency modulates pain regulatory gene expression along the nociceptive pathway. Pain Physician 16(5):E601–E613

van Hecke O, Torrance N, Smith BH (2013) Chronic pain epidemiology and its clinical relevance. Br J Anaesth 111(1):13–18

Webster LR, Webster RM (2005) Predicting aberrant behaviors in opioid-treated patients: preliminary validation of the opioid risk tool. Pain Med 6:432–442

Welsh TP, Yang AE, Makris UE (2020) Musculoskeletal pain in older adults: a clinical review. Med Clin North Am 104(5):855–872

Younan M, Atkinson T, Fudin J. A Practical Approach to Discontinuing NSAID Therapy Prior to a Procedure. Pract Pain Manag. 2013;13(10). https://www.medcentral.com/pain/chronic/practical-approach-discontinuing-nsaid-therapy-prior. Accessed 6 Aug 2025

Zhang J, Ding EL, Song Y (2006) Adverse effects of cyclooxygenase 2 inhibitors on renal and arrhythmia events: meta-analysis of randomized trials. JAMA 296(13):1619–1632

9 Cognitive Impairment and Surgical Care in Geriatric Patients

Boon-Hian Tan

Take-Home Messages

- Cognitively impaired older persons are commonly at risk of perioperative delirium and resultant adverse outcomes.
- Delirium can be prevented by proactive identification, with the comprehensive geriatric assessment leading to comprehensive, consolidated, and coordinated multidisciplinary management.
- Most psychotropic medications can be discontinued safely in the perioperative setting and generally do not require an increase in dose after treatment of delirium. The decision to discontinue, however, needs to be weighed against the risk of a behavioral flare.
- There are delirium-causing medications with high anticholinergic burden that should be avoided, substituted, or tapered in older persons undergoing surgery.
- A high index of suspicion of POCD is required for early intervention and will improve healthcare outcomes.
- The mainstay of delirium management requires addressing the underlying causes of delirium and nonpharmacological measures.

B.-H. Tan (✉)
Department of Geriatric Medicine, Sengkang General Hospital, Singapore, Singapore
e-mail: tan.boon.hian@singhealth.com.sg

K.-Y. Tan et al. (eds.), *Mastering Geriatric Surgery*,
https://doi.org/10.1007/978-981-95-0665-1_9

9.1 Introduction and Epidemiology

Cognitive impairment is common condition affecting older persons going for surgery, affecting more than half of older persons undergoing surgery. The incidence of POCD can go as high as 50% in the general surgery wards and up to 82% in patients in the intensive care unit (Inouye et al. 2014). Despite being mostly preventable, it has led to billions of dollars in healthcare costs and adverse healthcare outcomes of functional decline, prolonged hospitalizations, readmissions, and mortality.

This chapter aims firstly to define POCD, followed by discussions pertaining to the mechanism of action, its risk factors, precipitants, and how we can prevent and manage it.

9.2 Definitions

Various terms can be found when reviewing cognitive impairment in the perioperative setting in older persons (White et al. 2019; Brodier and Cibelli 2021; Needham et al. 2017). They include

1. **Major and mild neurocognitive disorder** (NCD)—Under the Diagnostic and Statistical Manual of Mental Disorders, Fifth Edition (DSM V), they are chronic conditions of insidious decline in at least one of the six domains of cognition, namely memory, executive function, attention, language, perceptual-motor, and social cognition.

   In a major neurocognitive disorder, otherwise known as dementia, the cognitive loss has resulted in a downstream loss of function (e.g., a person who previously could cook forgets the steps to cook complex dishes), and in a mild NCD, the function is yet to be affected. These deficits in cognition need to be supported by finding deficits in objective testing, such as with a Mini Mental State Examination (MMSE). Mild NCD can progress to major NCDs.
2. **Delirium**—As defined by DSM V, delirium is an acutely occurring condition with disturbances in cognition, in particular, attention [such as counting from 20 to 1 on the Abbreviated Mental Test (AMT)] and awareness. It is a medical emergency as it suggests an underlying cause with resultant morbidity and mortality. Classic definitions of delirium suggest a degree of reversibility. Delirium is further subdivided into

   (a) **Hyperactive delirium**: This manifests in a state of hyperarousal, increased and aberrant motor activity, or restlessness and prominent inattention. Some may hallucinate.
   (b) **Hypoactive delirium**: This manifests in a state of inactivity, poor arousal, and some may be near comatose. This is the more dangerous form of delirium as it is less readily detectable and can be misinterpreted as a sleeping patient.
   (c) **Mixed delirium**: This has components of both hyperactive and hypoactive delirium.

9.2.1 Postoperative Cognitive Dysfunction (POCD) or Decline

Postoperative cognitive dysfunction is synonymous with postoperative cognitive decline and is divided based on timing into the following:

1. **Preexisting cognitive impairment** (either mild or major NCD).
2. **Postoperative delirium**—This is an area of contention and the timings vary, and is the subject of continual research and should be revised when future guidelines are available. Nonetheless,
    (a) Literature describes a range of 24–96 h (Needham et al. 2017); 2–5 days (Jin et al. 2020) and within 7 days.
    (b) The cutoff of 7 days is supported by
        - *Epidemiologically*—With meta-analyses of POCD showing higher incidence of delirium at 7 days (23%) decreasing to 16% at 1 month and 3% at 1 year (Huang et al. 2025).
        - *Biologically*—A raised cerebrospinal fluid amyloid beta 42 ratio at day 7 postoperatively was associated with a linear risk and severity of postoperative delirium (Fan et al. 2025).
        - *Management*—Nonpharmacological trials often define interventions by day 7 postoperatively (Zhao et al. 2024b).
        - *Drug trials*—Drug trials on sevoflurane (Cao et al. 2023) were able to demonstrate the natural history of POCD showing the cumulative incidence of delirium plateaus after day 7.
        - *Prediction models*—A newly developed Pre-Interventional Preventive Risk Assessment (PIPRA) algorithm (Reeve et al. 2025) with an area under the receiver operating characteristic curve of 0.77 was able to predict postoperative delirium for the first 7 days, which was correlated with mortality, intensive care unit use, and increasing care needs (Reeve et al. 2025).
3. **Delayed neurocognitive recovery**—Defined as delirium lasting up to 30 days.
4. **Postoperative neurocognitive disorder**—Defined as delirium lasting up to a year. Patients eventually are defined as major NCD (dementia) if the cognition continues to not improve or worsen.

9.3 Mechanisms of Action of Postoperative Cognitive Dysfunction

The exact biological mechanisms of precipitating POCD are not completed elucidated. Current hypotheses (Maldonado 2013; Aldecoa et al. 2024) include (1) direct effects of anesthesia leading to Tau protein hyperphosphorylation, a marker of neuronal damage and neuronal death; (2) activation of an inflammatory cascade of cytokines from microglia or circulating inflammatory cells arising from tissue damage,

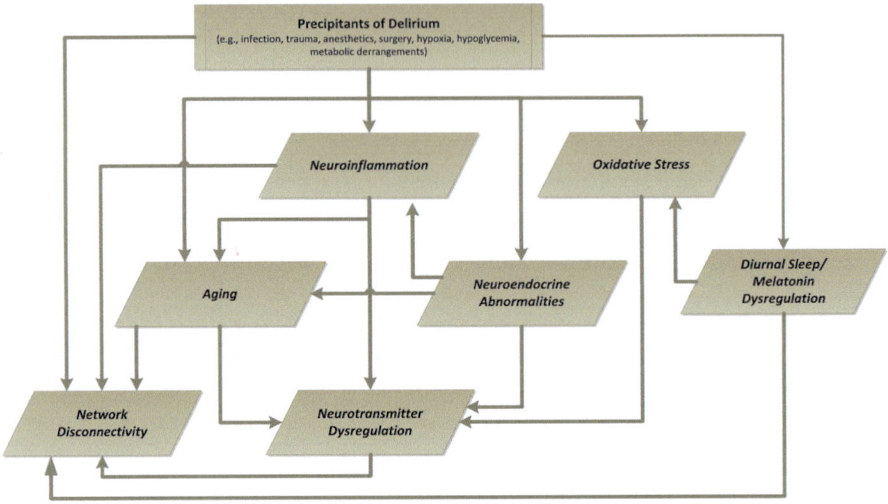

Fig. 9.1 Neuroendocrinological pathways of delirium. (Adapted from Maldonado JR. Neuropathogenesis of delirium: review of current etiologic theories and common pathways, Am J Geriatr Psychiatry. 2013 Dec;21(12):1190–222)

surgical stress, or lipopolysaccharide stimulation; and (3) alterations in secretions of neuroendocrine hormones and its interactions with the sleep–wake cycle. It is additionally postulated that these pathways interact with each other to produce the delirium phenotype (Fig. 9.1).

It is more likely that POCD is associated with multiple risk factors and causes as it is seen in nonsurgical animal and human studies. This observation has implications on the efficacy and evidence in the prevention and the amelioration of POCD and is relevant to trialed medications in later sections.

The above putative mechanisms assume the absence of postoperative stroke. Perioperative stroke is a known and direct cause of postoperative cognitive and functional impairment after surgery, which has implications on the prognosis of short-term and long-term recovery. In practical terms, family members often describe the patient having a "step-wise" and permanent decline in cognition and function after a prolonged stay in hospital, for example, after a procedure, a stay in the intensive care unit, or after a fall. Such strokes may be covert or overt and is usually appreciated in neuroimaging done retrospectively.

9.4 Risk Factors and Precipitants of Postoperative Cognitive Impairment

As the pathogenesis of delirium is via interaction of various pathways, it follows that no single risk factor is predictive of delirium, but it is the combination and synergism of multiple risk factors crossing a cognitive threshold that causes delirium.

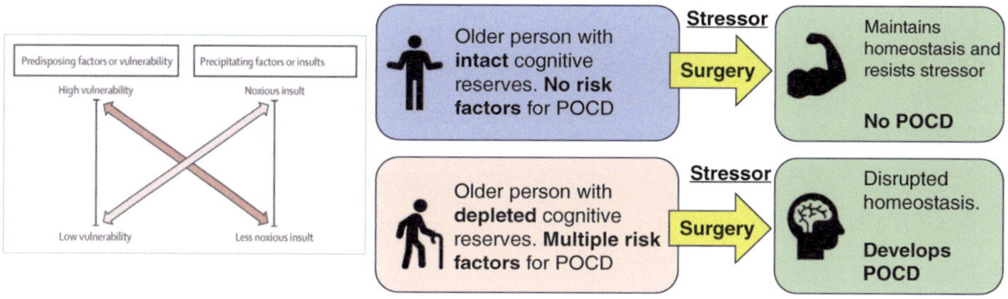

Fig. 9.2 Model of development of postoperative cognitive dysfunction in older persons with different cognitive reserves. *POCD* postoperative cognitive dysfunction. (Diagrams adapted from Inouye et al., Delirium in elderly people. Lancet. 2014 Mar 8;383(9920):911–22)

Conceptually, every older person is thought to have intrinsic capacity, a summation of an individual's physical and mental capacities. Focusing on the mental capacities, it can be imagined as a cognitive reserve bank of which can be reduced with each risk factor. When challenged with a stressor ("precipitant") to cognition such as surgery or a postoperative infection, the older person will have one of two outcomes: (1) maintain homeostasis or (2) have his reserves overwhelmed and develop POCD. The less the cognitive reserves (Inouye et al. 2014), the less severe a stressor (e.g., use of an anticholinergic medication) needs to be, to precipitate delirium (Fig. 9.2).

The risk factors (Needham et al. 2017; Sadeghirad et al. 2023; He et al. 2024) are shown in Fig. 9.3. They are divided into predisposing (usually present preoperatively) and precipitating risk factors (otherwise also known as a "stressor").

Predisposing Risk Factors		Precipitating Risk Factors ('Stressors') intraoperative or postoperative
Age	Frailty	Intra-operative Cumulative time with low bispectral index values Variance in blood pressure Hypothermia Greater intra-operative infusion volume Longer duration of operation -Postoperative- Environmental factors Inadequately controlled pain Sleep disturbance Use of physical restraints Use of bladder catheterization Constipation Sensory impairment Infection (any) Polypharmacy Substance withdrawal Metabolic derangements Hypoxia Acidosis Electrolyte derangements Hypoglycemia Dehydration Acute blood loss /anemia Hypotension
Low education level	Poor functional status or immobility	
Comorbidities (Charlson Comorbidity Scale >2), vascular risk factors , renal impairment, Alcoholism or cigarette smoking	Preexisting cognitive impairment (Mild or Major Neurocognitive Disorder) and previous delirium	
Severe illness (American Society of Anesthesiologists Score)	Depression	
Emergency surgery	Malnutrition or Low body mass index	
Type of surgery: Hip fracture, aortic aneurysm repair, non cardiac thoracic surgery, frontal craniectomy	Sensory impairment (Visual or hearing)	
Abnormal laboratory values: glucose, sodium and potassium; anaemia, hypoxia or hypercarbia	Polypharmacy – especially current anticholinergics, antihistamine, benzodiazepine or antipsychotic use	
Preoperative infection		
Acute retention of urine, constipation, or indwelling catheter		

Fig. 9.3 Risk factors and precipitants of delirium

9.5 Management of Postoperative Cognitive Impairment

We suggest the management of postoperative cognitive impairment as follows and is divided into the following phases:

9.5.1 Preoperative Phase

The focus in this phase is the **identification of at-risk patients** and **prevention** (Peden et al. 2021).

9.5.1.1 Identification of At-Risk Patients

In patients with the abovementioned relevant risk factors, the patient's baseline cognition should be assessed. The cognitive history is to be taken from a reliable informant and should cover the six cognitive domains of memory, executive function, attention, language, perceptual-motor, and social cognition. Upon completion of the cognitive history, the assessor should be able to visualize how the patient would interact and behave when in the outpatient setting. In the absence of delirium, mental state testing in the form of AMT, MMSE, or other forms of neurocognitive tests should be performed. The main purpose of assessing the cognition is to diagnose preoperative cognitive impairment and determine the patient's risk factor for developing POCD.

Cognitive assessment is part of a larger assessment: The cognitive assessment should not be conducted in silo, but as part of a comprehensive geriatric assessment (CGA) that identifies a comprehensive list of medical, geriatric, functional, and social problems (Fig. 9.4), following which the list is curated and consolidated based on clinical priorities and geriatric principles of management (Mohanty et al. 2016). This plan is subsequently communicated and coordinated with the entire healthcare team to allow work in tandem. This includes the surgeons, the anesthesiologists, other specialists (e.g., cardiologists, medical oncologists), nurses, and the allied health team members.

CGA allows individualized care: The CGA is useful also in leading the managing physician to know the patient in a patient-centered manner and provide individu-

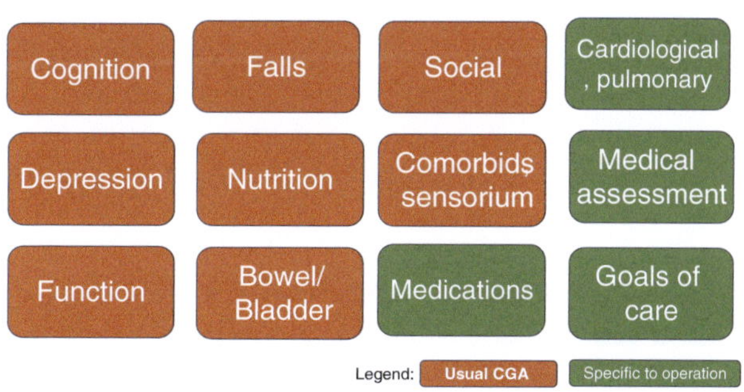

Fig. 9.4 Comprehensive geriatric assessment (CGA)

alized care (Mohanty et al. 2016). In Guidelines from the Association of Anesthetists, there are recommendations that assume a preoperative CGA leading to such care. In particular, they emphasize the needs for (a) tailored management and follow-up, (b) involvement of carers throughout the perioperative process, (c) trained staff and geriatric champions within the anesthesiologic department who can manage cognitive impaired older persons, (d) multidisciplinary involvement of allied health and other specialists, and (e) equality of medical treatment rigor of medical and cognitive assessment between cognitively impaired and noncognitively impaired older persons.

9.5.1.2 Evidence-Based Prevention of POCD

1. *Geriatrician-led programs*: Evidence-wise, geriatrician-led co-management or Enhanced Recovery After Surgery (ERAS) protocols have been shown to reduce POCD (Scott et al. 2023; Mohanty et al. 2016; American Geriatrics Society Expert Panel (AGS) 2015; NELA Project Team 2023). Both management models employ principles of the CGA as it would identify problems proactively for management before the problems occur. Current guidelines suggest the early involvement of a geriatrician and/or geriatric assessment in patients aged 65 years and above in perioperative setting and this is evidence-based in multiple prospective studies involving older persons in oncological, orthopedic, and other noncardiac surgeries. In detail, geriatric co-management addresses components such as the acute and chronic medical conditions, geriatric syndromes in particular frailty, malnutrition and polypharmacy, functional optimization, mood behavior and sleep, social and familial support (Fig. 9.4).
2. *Prehabilitation*: Prehabilitation, which can be read in detail in other sections of this book, has been shown to help reduce POCD and improve overall hospital and clinical outcomes. Unless in urgent situations requiring immediate surgery, older persons should undergo prehabilitation to optimize their outcomes. Prehabilitation increases the older person's physical and cognitive reserves, that is, intrinsic capacity, and makes the older person more resilient to stressors such as surgery, anesthesia, blood loss, and unforetold intraoperative events, against downstream adverse health outcomes.
3. *Nonpharmacological measures*: Many variations of these geriatric care bundles exist and these bundles are grounded in the management concepts found in the Hospital Elder Life Program (HELP) program (Inouye et al. 2014). The important components of the bundle involve empowering nurses with appropriate means to monitor, screen, and intervene in older persons. Key categories include orientation and cognitive stimulation, nutrition, hydration, elimination, early mobilization, and ensuring safety, with protocols for assessment and escalation. An example of a delirium care bundle in Sengkang General Hospital is provided (Fig. 9.5). Having a hospital-wide bundle empowers nurses to act as first responders to prevent and escalate care for POCD.
4. *Cognitive training*: Cognitive training (Zhao et al. 2024a) as part of a postoperative delirium care bundle has been shown to reduce POCD under cognitive stimulation and cognitive orientational activities. There is currently increasing

Cognitive Stimulation	Reality orientation
	Therapeutic activities
Early Mobilisation	Minimise restraint use
	Review / prompt doctor to review unnecessary tubes and lines
	Sit out of bed if appropriate
	Supervised ambulation (to toilet whenever possible)
	Refer to Physiotherapy (if appropriate)
Addressing Sensory Impairment	Help patient to put on glasses (if available)
	Help patient to put on hearing aid (if available)
	Use amplifier if without hearing aid
Encouraging oral intake	Maintain oral hygiene
	Keep dentures clean & assist to put on for meals
	Assistance for those with poor oral intake, aspiration risk or unable to feed independently
	Refer to Speech Therapy (if appropriate)
	Refer to dietitian (if appropriate)
Bladder and Bowel Care	Monitor Bowel movements, inform doctor if No Bowel Open > 2 days
	Timed toileting / voiding every-34 hours if continent
	Do bladder scan if not passing urine > 8 hours (see 4.3 below)
	Aim to wean off diaper if not indicated
Ensure Safety	Falls precaution with bed exit alarm activated

Fig. 9.5 Delirium care bundle

evidence that cognitive training, preoperatively (e.g., 4 weeks prior to operation), whether with face-to-face or remotely via use of software applications (computer or handphone), can reduce POCD, albeit this is a field under active investigation.

5. *No benefit of a single pharmacological agent*: Pharmacologically, there no evidence of benefit in the use of specific medications to prevent POCD. Medications trialed include antipsychotics such as haloperidol and risperidone, sleep-aids such as melatonin, ramelteon, and benzodiazepines, anti-inflammatory agents such as steroids and nonsteroidal inflammatory agents, as well as cognitive enhancers. As there is no evidence of benefit with the real risk of harm, the author considers the prescription of these medications in the sole context of POCD prevention harmful by adding to the burden of care, polypharmacy, and risk of side effects (Aldecoa et al. 2024; White et al. 2019; AGS 2015).

   The success of prevention of POCD with nonpharmacological measures in comparison to a specific pharmacological agent is in support of the theory that there are multiple biochemical pathways leading to POCD. Logically, it follows that the management of a patient with nascent POCD requires a patient-centered approach with a detailed medical and surgical assessment, and targeting individualized root causes of that patient's POCD. For example, should a patient be found to be septic (e.g., from an obstructed colon), early access to appropriate antibiotics with source control is necessary to manage POCD.

6. *Psychotropic medication management*: We refer to published recommendations (Fig. 9.6, Aldecoa et al. 2024; White et al. 2019).

   Cholinesterase inhibitors can inhibit interact with muscle relaxants, prolonging the effects of depolarizing neuromuscular blocking drugs and impairing the effects of nondepolarizing neuromuscular blocking drugs. They are typically activating medications and would lead to a need to increase the dose of anesthe-

	Half-life; hr	Recommendation/effect
Cholinesterase inhibitors		
Galantamine	7	Discontinue[a] day before surgery
Rivastigmine	9	Discontinue[a] day before surgery
Donepezil	70	Not recommended
Memantine	60–100	Care with ketamine, anticholineric and dopaminergic drugs
Gingko biloba	4–6	Monitor blood loss
		Use atracurium; neostigmine may be ineffective/prolong neuromuscular blockade
		Use sugammadex to reverse rocuronium and vecuronium
Drugs used to modify non-cognitive symptoms in dementia		
SSRIs	Various	Risk of serotonin syndrome with fentanyl, ondansetron, tramadol
Cognitive stimulants	Various	Antagonise hypnotic anaesthetic drugs
Benzodiazepines ± antipsychotics	Various	Potentiate neuro- and cardio-depressant effects of anaesthetic drugs

SSRI, selective serotonin reuptake inhibitor.

Fig. 9.6 Potential drug-drug interactions between psychotropic medications and anaesthesia. (Adapted from White et al., Guidelines for the peri-operative care of people with dementia: Guidelines from the Association of Anaesthetists. Anaesthesia. 2019 Mar;74(3):357–372)

sia to achieve sedation. In perioperative patients, poor oral intake and cardiac events are major and common complications that can be worsened with cholinesterase inhibitors. As these medications are for symptoms and not disease-modifying, if the medication can be suspended, it should be withheld until the patient is postoperative, has no cardiac events, and is eating well. Memantine can be withheld especially in neurosurgical procedures due to the risk of precipitating seizures and has interactions with ketamine, amantadine, and dextromethorphan. Ginko has an increased risk of worsening bleeding. While it would make sense to suspend cognitive enhancers prior to surgery, it needs to be weighed against the risk of a neuropsychiatric flare (e.g., hallucinations in Lewy body dementia).

For patients on benzodiazepines, they have the potential to interact with anesthesiologic agents and its abrupt cessation in a patient on long-term use can lead to withdrawal and delirium tremens. Antipsychotics, if not needed, can be suspended perioperatively as it would worsen sedation and precipitate hypoactive delirium but needs to be weighed against the risk of behavioral flare especially in patients with psychosis. There is also a black-box warning that antipsychotics can increase the risk of cardiovascular events. Antidepressants acting via serotoninergic pathways can precipitate serotonin syndrome when given together with high doses of tramadol or fentanyl.

7. *Medications with anticholinergic burden (ACB)*: The anticholinergic burden (Boustani et al. 2008) is a concept describing the summative anticholinergic properties of medications administered to the patient. A high ACB is predictive of POCD and adverse healthcare outcomes. The decision to withhold such medications is balanced against the indication, whether suitable alternatives exist (e.g., substitution of anarex for paracetamol), and risk of withdrawal (e.g., rebound insomnia in patients using tricyclic antidepressants for sleep). Figure 9.7 shows a list of medications with high ACB in common use and possible alternatives to consider (AGS 2015; Boustani et al. 2008)

Purpose of medications	Medication names	Alternatives to use
Behaviour control in Behavioural and Psychological Symptoms of Dementia or Delirium	• First-generation antipsychotics: chlorpromazine, thioridazine • Newer generation antipsychotics: Olanzapine, Risperidone	• Address underlying causes at all times; Consider non-pharmacological agents as first line e.g. earplugs for *other* patients for REM-sleep behaviour disorder vocalization • In Intensive Care Unit, appropriate sedation if extubated with physical restraints as needed. • If behaviour at risk of harm, chemical restraints include quetiapine, haloperidol and lorazepam.
Sleep aids	• Tricyclic antidepressants: amitriptyline, doxepin, imipramine* • Benzodiazepines: alprazolam, diazepam, lorazepam, midazolam*# • Non-benzodiazepine hyponotics : zolpidem, zaleplon*# • Antihistamines: Chlorpheniramine cyproheptadine, diphenhydramine, hydroxyzine	• Treat underlying cause e.g. pain dyspnea itch or depression • Melatonin
Muscle relaxants	• Skeletal muscle relaxants: Orphenadrine/Anarex , cyclobenzaprine, tizanidine*	• Address underlying cause.
Pain	• Skeletal muscle relaxants: Orphenadrine/Anarex , cyclobenzaprine, tizanidine* • Pethidine	• 1st line: Paracetamol; In specific situations e.g. hip fracture or immediate perioperatively, consider nerve blocks or catheters (e.g. Fascia Iliaca blocks) to avoid opioid use;Topical medications such as ketoprofen gels or plasters; In vertebral fractures consider intranasal calcitonin as adjunct • Opioids may be necessary, of which fentanyl and oxycodone are less delirium-causing.
Abdominal Pain	• H2-receptor antagonists: cimetidine, ranitidine • Antispasmodics: hyoscyamine, scopolamine	• Address underlying cause including constipation, retention of urine and interventional management of source of pain; See pain section
Antiemetics	• Promethazine	• Treat underlying cause • Ondansetron, Metoclopramide
Mood treatment/ Depression	• Paroxetine*	• Consider non-pharmacological agents as first line • Selective serotonin reuptake inhibitors except fluoxetine
Itch	• Antihistamines: Chlorpheniramine cyproheptadine, diphenhydramine, hydroxyzine	• Treat underlying cause e.g. Antiparastics e.g. malathion if cause is due to scabies; Consider topical emollients with or without steroid components; Fexofenadine, cetirizine and loratadine
Urinary frequency	• Oxybutynin	• Treat underlying cause include need for catheterization for urinary obstruction and constipation., consider Solifenacin , mirabegron
Diarrhea	• Antispasmodics: hyoscyamine, scopolamine*	• Treat underlying cause e.g. spurious diarrheal in constipation, feeds -related, infections • Loperamide e.g. high output stoma post-colectomy

Fig. 9.7 Medications with high anticholinergic burden, and recommended alternatives. * Medication may need to be tapered; # to be continued in patients taking long term and tapered due to risk of delirium tremens. (Medication list adapted from Boustani et al., and American Geriatrics Society Expert Panel on Postoperative Delirium in Older Adults. Postoperative delirium in older adults: best practice statement from the American Geriatrics Society)

9.5.2 Operative Phase

During an operation, two variables directly affect outcomes of POCD, namely **depth of anesthesia** and **intraoperative events**.

Anesthesia: Various anesthesiologic agents have been trialed, with most studies looking into dexmedetomidine (summarized in Aldecoa et al. 2024; White et al. 2019). Inhalational versus intravenous agents and regional versus general anesthesia have also been looked at. The summary of the evidence in these studies is that while there is a suggestion that dexmedetomidine can reduce POCD, use of this medication needs to be weighed against the clinical context and the risks of bradycardia and hypotension. Other agents trialed have yet to be proven to be effective in the prevention of POCD. In conclusion, we do not currently have evidence suggesting whether the mode (inhalation versus intravenous) or intent (general versus regional) or the agent itself is useful for preventing POCD or would worsen dementia.

Titration of the depth of anesthesia, monitored through modalities such as processed EEG, has been shown to reduce POCD. This is not surprising as a key geriatric principle of "go low, go slow" is being practiced here—in that one should use the lowest titrated dose of a medication needed to achieve anesthesia due to the often-depleted cognitive reserves of older persons.

Intraoperative events: The clinical status of the older person undergoing surgery can change rapidly. Events such as hypotension and hypothermia, and nascent medical events such as myocardial infarction and stroke and nascent surgical events such as soilage of the abdominal cavity, can precipitate POCD (Aldecoa et al. 2024; White et al. 2019). This highlights the need to optimize the preoperative cardiovascular assessment and patient-centered intraoperative management and monitoring. There have been attempts to investigate if types of surgery affect POCD outcomes, in particular laparoscopy versus laparotomy, and currently there is no evidence favoring any modality of surgery in preventing POCD. The choice of modality of surgery should be clinically guided.

Older persons with cognitive impairment are sensitive to changes in their sleep–wake cycle, their environment, and their mealtime habits. There are recommendations (Fig. 9.8; White et al. 2019) with the aims of mimicking the patient's original home environment and schedule as much as possible, as part of person-centered care of older persons with cognitive impairment.

9.5.3 Postoperative Phase

The focus of the postoperative phase is **optimization** and **rehabilitation**.

POCD is known to lead to adverse healthcare outcomes, including prolonged length of stay, functional decline, institutionalization, and mortality, and such outcomes are more likely to occur in older persons undergoing emergency surgery.

Dementia friendly environment	Person centred approach
Have a large-face clock and written and pictorial signages indicating locations of important places e.g. toilets, operating theater	Allow the case to be the first in the operating theatre list to minimize fasting, changes to sleep wake and medication cycles.
A quiet environment minimizing unnecessary noise including drip alarms	Allow carers/relative to be in recovery room before induction and emergence
Provide gauze rolls to grip onto	Allow access to comforters (personal pillows, soft toys, blankets etc.)
Use natural/natural effect lighting	Enable the person to sit upright if possible
Use color contrasts to aid identification	Have staff wear legible name and role badges to ease Identification
Provide easy assess to callbell	Staff to speak slowly, legibly and in the patient's native language and with pocket talkers if necessary
	Simplify communications but provide as needed, detailed explanation of what is happening
	Remove visual and hearing aids only when necessary
	Avoid restraints. Instead hide lines and tubes if possible e.g under clothing or with a towel or dressing.

Fig. 9.8 Recommendations for person-centred management of older persons with cognitive impairment in the perioperative setting. (Adapted from White et al., Guidelines for the peri-operative care of people with dementia: Guidelines from the Association of Anaesthetists. Anaesthesia. 2019 Mar;74(3):357–372)

This is due to the observation that patients undergoing emergency surgery are not optimized, and they also have other medical problems that electively operated patients do not have (e.g., electrolyte imbalances, sepsis, functional decline), and such problems often do not completely resolve despite appropriate surgical management and source control.

In the postoperative phase, priority therefore needs to be given to the most pressing medical problem(s), without which the amelioration of geriatric syndromes, the functional recovery, and the rehabilitation cannot occur. Unresolved medical issues can precipitate or prolong POCD. For example, if a patient in hypoactive delirium (e.g., from hypoglycemia) is fed during his drowsy state, there is a risk of aspiration pneumonia that can perpetuate delirium. Yet the treatment of this patient is related to feeding, in the form of intravenous glucose replacement, and withholding diabetic medications.

The index of suspicion of POCD should be high especially in patients with risk factors. Proactive and early detection leading to timely management of POCD leads to improved healthcare outcomes. In the setting of nascent POCD in the postoperative setting, the following approach is recommended (Fig. 9.9). The principles of management are similar to management of nonsurgical causes of delirium, namely (a) Identify all causes of delirium, (b) treat all possible causes of delirium, including withholding medications with ACB, and (c) supportive care to allow recovery and prevention of future episodes while ensuring safety. It is clear, given the multifactorial nature of POCD, that there is no single medication that can resolve delirium.

There have been preliminary studies done on markers of systemic inflammation, neuronal and cellular injury, plasticity, and cholinesterase concentrations to see if it can predict POCD. It, however, remains that there are no biomarkers that can

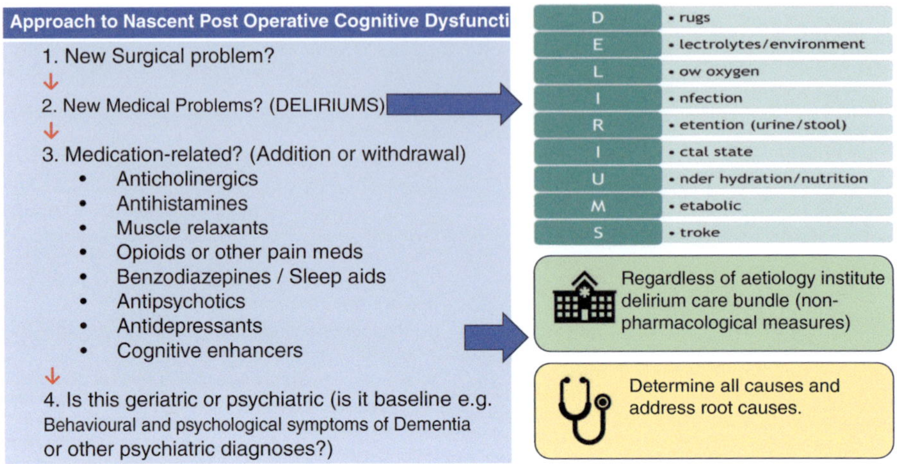

Fig. 9.9 Approach to postoperative cognitive dysfunction

accurately predict POCD, and thus diagnosis of POCD remains based on clinical assessment alone.

Holistic postoperative care, either via geriatrician-led management or via protocol-related postoperative bundles, improves healthcare outcomes, including POCD. An example of guideline-based care is described in detail in ERAS Guidelines Part 2 (Scott et al. 2023). The preoperative delirium care bundle should be continued.

Sedatives such as antipsychotics, antidepressants, and sleep aids should be used only as a last resort (White et al. 2019) and may precipitate other problems (e.g., Haloperidol in Parkinson's disease will worsen Parkinsonism and the sedation may cause aspiration pneumonia). We are more likely to use such sedatives if (a) there has been a long-standing history of behavioral problems in the setting of dementia or other psychiatric illness; (b) if there is a risk of harm to the patient, for example, lines or drains; or (c) there is harm to healthcare staff (e.g., physical violence). Medications should only be used when nonpharmacological measures fail. Choices of medications include quetiapine (6.25 mg), lorazepam (0.5 mg), and haloperidol (0.5 mg) and should be given as a single dose as much as possible. Exceptions exist for care of POCD in the intensive care unit or in severe agitation, which would warrant the use of higher dosages or the use of different medications. Regardless, deliberate usage of anticholinergic or antihistaminergic medications for sedation in older persons with POCD is harmful.

Acknowledgments The author thanks the Geriatric Perioperative Service team in Sengkang Hospital, the Department of Geriatric Medicine, the Department of General Surgery, and the Department of Nursing for their support of this chapter.

References

Aldecoa C, Bettelli G, Bilotta F, Sanders RD, Aceto P, Audisio R, Cherubini A, Cunningham C, Dabrowski W, Forookhi A, Gitti N, Immonen K, Kehlet H, Koch S, Kotfis K, Latronico N, MacLullich AMJ, Mevorach L, Mueller A, Neuner B, Piva S, Radtke F, Blaser AR, Renzi S, Romagnoli S, Schubert M, Slooter AJC, Tommasino C, Vasiljewa L, Weiss B, Yuerek F, Spies CD (2024) Update of the European Society of Anaesthesiology and Intensive Care Medicine evidence-based and consensus-based guideline on postoperative delirium in adult patients. Eur J Anaesthesiol 41(2):81–108. https://doi.org/10.1097/EJA.0000000000001876. Epub 2023 Aug 30

American Geriatrics Society Expert Panel on Postoperative Delirium in Older Adults (2015) Postoperative delirium in older adults: best practice statement from the American Geriatrics Society. J Am Coll Surg. 220(2):136–48.e1. https://doi.org/10.1016/j.jamcollsurg.2014.10.019. Epub 2014 Nov 14

Boustani M, Campbell N, Munger S, Fox C (2008) Impact of anticholinergics on the aging brain: a review and practical application. Aging Health 4:311–320. https://doi.org/10.2217/1745509X.4.3.311

Brodier EA, Cibelli M (2021) Postoperative cognitive dysfunction in clinical practice. BJA Educ 21(2):75–82. https://doi.org/10.1016/j.bjae.2020.10.004. Epub 2020 Dec 24

Cao SJ, Zhang Y, Zhang YX, Zhao W, Pan LH, Sun XD, Jia Z, Ouyang W, Ye QS, Zhang FX, Guo YQ, Ai YQ, Zhao BJ, Yu JB, Liu ZH, Yin N, Li XY, Ma JH, Li HJ, Wang MR, Sessler DI, Ma D, Wang DX, First Study of Perioperative Organ Protection (SPOP1) Investigators (2023) Delirium in older patients given propofol or sevoflurane anaesthesia for major cancer surgery: a multicentre randomised trial. Br J Anaesth 131(2):253–265. https://doi.org/10.1016/j.bja.2023.04.024. Epub 2023 Jun 4

Fan Q, Wang Y, Lu Z, Wang L, Yang X, Zheng Z, Dong H, Xiong L, Lei C (2025) Association between plasma amyloid-beta 42 ratio and postoperative delirium in elderly patients undergoing major abdominal surgery: secondary analysis of a randomized controlled trial. Brain Behav 15(4):e70501. https://doi.org/10.1002/brb3.70501

He M, Zhu Z, Jiang M, Liu X, Wu R, Zhou J, Chen X, Liu C (2024) Risk factors for postanesthetic emergence delirium in adults: a systematic review and meta-analysis. J Neurosurg Anesthesiol 36(3):190–200. https://doi.org/10.1097/ANA.0000000000000942. Epub 2023 Nov 2

Huang WWY, Fan S, Li WY, Thangavelu V, Saripella A, Englesakis M, Yan E, Chung F (2025) Prevalence of postoperative neurocognitive disorders in older non-cardiac surgical patients: a systematic review and meta-analysis. J Clin Anesth 103:111830. https://doi.org/10.1016/j.jclinane.2025.111830. Epub ahead of print

Inouye SK, Westendorp RG, Saczynski JS (2014) Delirium in elderly people. Lancet 383(9920):911–922. https://doi.org/10.1016/S0140-6736(13)60688-1. Epub 2013 Aug 28

Jin Z, Hu J, Ma D (2020) Postoperative delirium: perioperative assessment, risk reduction, and management. Br J Anaesth 125(4):492–504. https://doi.org/10.1016/j.bja.2020.06.063. Epub 2020 Aug 11

Maldonado JR (2013) Neuropathogenesis of delirium: review of current etiologic theories and common pathways. Am J Geriatr Psychiatry 21(12):1190–1222. https://doi.org/10.1016/j.jagp.2013.09.005

Mohanty S, Rosenthal RA, Russell MM, Neuman MD, Ko CY, Esnaola NF (2016) Optimal perioperative management of the geriatric patient: a best practices guideline from the American College of Surgeons NSQIP and the American Geriatrics Society. J Am Coll Surg 222(5):930–947. https://doi.org/10.1016/j.jamcollsurg.2015.12.026. Epub 2016 Jan 4

Needham MJ, Webb CE, Bryden DC (2017) Postoperative cognitive dysfunction and dementia: what we need to know and do. Br J Anaesth 119(Suppl_1):i115–i125. https://doi.org/10.1093/bja/aex354

NELA Project Team (2023) Eighth patient report of the national emergency laparotomy audit. Royal College of Anaesthetists (RCoA), London

Peden CJ, Aggarwal G, Aitken RJ, Anderson ID, Bang Foss N, Cooper Z, Dhesi JK, French WB, Grant MC, Hammarqvist F, Hare SP, Havens JM, Holena DN, Hübner M, Kim JS, Lees NP, Ljungqvist O, Lobo DN, Mohseni S, Ordoñez CA, Quiney N, Urman RD, Wick E, Wu CL, Young-Fadok T, Scott M (2021) Guidelines for Perioperative Care for Emergency Laparotomy Enhanced Recovery After Surgery (ERAS) society recommendations: part 1-preoperative: diagnosis, rapid assessment and optimization. World J Surg 45(5):1272–1290. https://doi.org/10.1007/s00268-021-05994-9. Epub 2021 Mar 6

Reeve KA, Schmutz Gelsomino N, Venturini M, Buddeberg F, Zozman M, Stocker R, Kedda MA, Meier P, Möller M, Wildhaber SP, Dodsworth BT (2025) Prospective external validation of the automated PIPRA multivariable prediction model for postoperative delirium on real-world data from a consecutive cohort of non-cardiac surgery inpatients. BMJ Health Care Inform 32(1):e101291. https://doi.org/10.1136/bmjhci-2024-101291

Sadeghirad B, Dodsworth BT, Schmutz Gelsomino N, Goettel N, Spence J, Buchan TA, Crandon HN, Baneshi MR, Pol RA, Brattinga B, Park UJ, Terashima M, Banning LBD, Van Leeuwen BL, Neerland BE, Chuan A, Martinez FT, Van Vugt JLA, Rampersaud YR, Hatakeyama S, Di Stasio E, Milisen K, Van Grootven B, van der Laan L, Thomson Mangnall L, Goodlin SJ, Lungeanu D, Denhaerynck K, Dhakharia V, Sampson EL, Zywiel MG, Falco L, Nguyen AV, Moss SJ, Krewulak KD, Jaworska N, Plotnikoff K, Kotteduwa-Jayawarden S, Sandarage R, Busse JW, Mbuagbaw L (2023) Perioperative factors associated with postoperative delirium in patients undergoing noncardiac surgery: an individual patient data meta-analysis. JAMA Netw Open 6(10):e2337239. https://doi.org/10.1001/jamanetworkopen.2023.37239

Scott MJ, Aggarwal G, Aitken RJ, Anderson ID, Balfour A, Foss NB, Cooper Z, Dhesi JK, French WB, Grant MC, Hammarqvist F, Hare SP, Havens JM, Holena DN, Hübner M, Johnston C, Kim JS, Lees NP, Ljungqvist O, Lobo DN, Mohseni S, Ordoñez CA, Quiney N, Sharoky C, Urman RD, Wick E, Wu CL, Young-Fadok T, Peden CJ (2023) Consensus Guidelines for Perioperative Care for Emergency Laparotomy Enhanced Recovery After Surgery (ERAS®) society recommendations part 2-emergency laparotomy: intra- and postoperative care. World J Surg 47(8):1850–1880. https://doi.org/10.1007/s00268-023-07020-6. Epub 2023 Jun 5

White S, Griffiths R, Baxter M, Beanland T, Cross J, Dhesi J, Docherty AB, Foo I, Jolly G, Jones J, Moppett IK, Plunkett E, Sachdev K (2019) Guidelines for the peri-operative care of people with dementia: guidelines from the Association of Anaesthetists. Anaesthesia 74(3):357–372. https://doi.org/10.1111/anae.14530. Epub 2019 Jan 11

Zhao L, Guo Y, Zhou X, Mao W, Li L (2024a) Preoperative cognitive training improves postoperative cognitive function: a meta-analysis and systematic review of randomized controlled trials. Front Neurol 14:1293153. https://doi.org/10.3389/fneur.2023.1293153

Zhao L, Guo Y, Zhou X, Mao W, Zhu H, Chen L, Liu X, Zhang L, Xie Y, Li L (2024b) The research progress of perioperative non-pharmacological interventions on postoperative cognitive dysfunction: a narrative review. Front Neurol 15:1369821. https://doi.org/10.3389/fneur.2024.1369821

Nursing Strategies for Older Perioperative Patients

10

Yu-Jing Ong

Take-Home Messages

- Comprehensive preoperative nursing assessment is the cornerstone of holistic perioperative care for older adults.
- Optimal nursing care for perioperative older adults must be tailored to individual needs.
- Every nurse plays a vital role in caring for perioperative older adults in any setting or encounter.
- Robust perioperative planning and coordination facilitate smooth transition of care across the care continuum.

10.1 Introduction

Our aging population is predicted to have one in two adults in Singapore above 65 years old by 2030 (Kow 2019). This demographic shift imposes a heavy burden on society and the healthcare system. Older adult often seeks to prolong life and longevity with a good quality of life, resulting in a parallel increase in surgical interventions (Kow 2019). Despite advancements in healthcare technology, older adults remain more vulnerable to tolerate the stresses of surgery compared to younger patients, who typically have higher reserve. Challenges in older adults arise not only caused by physiological changes of aging affecting visual, auditory, sensory, and

Y.-J. Ong (✉)
Department of APN and Specialty Nurse, Khoo Teck Puat Hospital, Singapore, Singapore
e-mail: ong.yu.jing@ktph.com.sg

K.-Y. Tan et al. (eds.), *Mastering Geriatric Surgery*,
https://doi.org/10.1007/978-981-95-0665-1_10

cognitive stimuli, but also from preexisting chronic medical conditions (Doerflinger 2009). A multidisciplinary approach is essential, in managing this geriatric surgical population, with nurses playing a pivotal role in caring for older surgical patients as they rotate shifts across the continuum. Nurses are the key drivers in developing and implementing individualized perioperative care plans for older surgical adults.

In this chapter, we will focus on nursing strategies in caring for older surgical patients perioperatively focusing on preoperative, intraoperative, and postoperative phases.

10.2 Preoperative Nursing Strategies

Older adults frequently present unique challenges perioperatively unlike younger patients. At baseline, they may be physiologically, psychologically, and physically compromised, which increases the risk for postoperative complications (Wolfe et al. 2020). The cornerstone in providing holistic perioperative care to older surgical patients begins with a comprehensive preoperative assessment. This thorough assessment is a baseline for identifying potential risks. By evaluating these risks, the nurse can anticipate potential issues and work with the patient and family to establish an individualized care plan.

10.2.1 Comprehensive Geriatric Assessment

Comprehensive geriatric assessment (CGA) is a tool commonly used in geriatric settings and is increasingly applied in perioperative assessment. The CGA consists of a head-to-toe assessment, encompassing cognition, functional status, psychosocial factors, and medication review. (Somnuke et al. 2024). CGA generates a list of potential issues and identifies the needs of older adults, enabling nurses to intervene and reduce the occurrence of postoperative problems as detailed in Table 10.1 (Somnuke et al. 2024).

10.2.1.1 Demographic Data

A key element of CGA is obtaining the older adult's demographic data and home situation. This information provides a context about older adults, including their preferred language, family, and living environment. In Singapore, where the majority of older adults speak dialect, the ability to communicate in their preferred language or with the assistance of a translator allows a better understanding of their condition. An overview of an older person's family and living situation facilitates early discharge planning. For example, an 82-year-old chronic smoker who is independent and lives in a landed property with his room on the third floor. Nursing considerations for this older adult might include smoking cessation at least 2 weeks before surgery, achieved by gradually reducing the number of cigarettes smoked daily. Engaging a physiotherapist for stair climbing guidance or the use of walking aids could also be beneficial. Alternatively, an early discussion with the family

Table 10.1 Nursing strategies mapped to components of CGA

Item evaluated	Details	Recommended nursing strategies
Demographic	Demographic data includes age, preferred language, previous occupation, housing, social history	Use of preferred language
Cognition	Abbreviated Mental Test (AMT) of ten questions serves as a screening tool for potential cognitive impairment	Recognize potential cognitive impairment with early involvement of geriatrician and/or occupational therapist for cognitive engagement.
Depression	Geriatric Depression Scale (GDS) of 7-item screening apparatus for major depressive in older people	Provide early access to appropriate healthcare professionals such as psychiatrist, social worker or geriatrician
Fall	Fall risk assessment such as Morse Fall Scale to stratify fall risk	Initiate fall precaution education and universal fall precaution. Early referral to physiotherapist/ occupational therapist. Encourage early ambulation with aids if needed
Functional status	Barthel Index for Activities of Daily Living (ADL) assessing the capacity to perform ADLs such as personal hygiene, transferring ranging from independent to dependent with assistance	Set goal to return back to baseline with prehabilitation to rehabilitation plan set in placed
Nutrition	Nutritional assessment is used to identify need for early dietitian referral for optimization	Initiation of early referral to dietitian and provide a meal plan with or without oral nutritional supplement
Polypharmacy	Number of medications with ≥ 5 medications suggest polypharmacy	Perform medication reconstitution, work with pharmacist and doctors to reduce pill burden
Pain	Pain assessment using numerical rating scale or visual analogue scale denoting the mild to severe pain	Educate on pain scale and medication usage postoperative as part of pre-operative education

about a temporary change of room to the first floor during the immediate postoperatively phase could be considered. As every older adult's background is unique, early discussion with family can shorten the length of stay and address any potential discharge issues.

10.2.1.2 Assessment of Cognition

Prevalence of cognitive impairment and dementia is increasingly common in older adults, particularly in Asia (Teh et al. 2021). Abbreviated mental test (AMT) is a simple and helpful screening tool for detecting cognitive impairment perioperatively (Sahadevan et al. 2000). Older adults who screen positive may undergo further evaluation and timely involvement of the geriatrician. Notifying surgeons of any cognitive impairment helps in assessing decision-making capacity and facilitates shared discussion with family regarding surgical plans. Cognitive impairment and dementia are also associated with an elevated risk for postoperative delirium. In addition to administering the AMT, nurses should engage with families to provide education on delirium and its prevention postoperatively. Families can assist by bringing familiar items such as photos, pillows, or spectacles to create a comforting environment to minimize the occurrence of delirium.

10.2.1.3 Assessment of Fall and Functional Status

An estimated 30% of older adults above the age of 65 living in the community fall annually, leading to injuries such as fractures, or head injury (Mohanty et al. 2016). This gives rise to the emphasis on fall assessment and implementation of interventions targeted at decreasing fall risk. Morse Fall Risk assessment is a commonly used tool for evaluating fall risk and guiding perioperative intervention (see Table 10.2). For example, in an older adult with diabetes and hypertension, preventing hypotensive or hypoglycemia episodes is crucial to avoiding dizziness that may lead to falls. As part of perioperative planning, targets of blood pressure or glucose level range can be set higher, deliberately resuming hypoglycemic agents (OHGAs) and antihypertensive gradually after surgery. Nurses can also refer older adults to allied health professionals such as physiotherapist and occupational therapist for assistance with mobility aids or cognitive enhancement (Wolfe et al. 2020). Routine

Table 10.2 Implications to nursing care based on Morse Fall Risk assessment

Item	Scale	Score	Perioperative nursing implication
History of fall (within past 6 months)	No	0	• Identify cause of fall and implement prevention measure postoperatively • Keeping vision or hearing within reach perioperatively
	Yes	25	
Secondary diagnosis	No	0	• Avoid too tight control of chronic disease • Set target range of chronic disease monitoring of higher level postoperatively • Review possible complication of secondary diagnosis
	Yes	15	
Walking aid	No/bedrest/ nurse assist	0	• Ensure walking aids placed within reach for accessibility • Early referral to physiotherapist for prescription of aids if needed
	Crutches/cane/ walker	15	
	Furniture cruising	30	
Intravenous therapy	No	0	• Review of need for intravenous therapy postoperatively
	Yes	20	
Gait	Normal	0	• Early referral to occupational therapist for transferring if needed
	Weak/impaired	30	
Mental status	Oriented	0	• Appropriate measures for delirium
	Confused	15	
Total	No-low risk for fall	0–<25	• Universal fall precautions
	Moderate risk for fall	25–45	
	High risk for fall	<45	

fall preventive measures should be maintained in hospitals, including ensuring all bedside rails are up, placing older adults near to nursing counter, and using visible tags to indicate higher fall risk (Watson et al. 2016).

Commonly functional status is one of the key indicators of postoperative mortality. Baseline functional status in older adults includes basic activities of daily living (BADLs) such as bathing, personal hygiene, and ambulation as well as instrumental activities of daily living (IADLs) such as meal preparation, taking transport, use of telephone, and handling of finances or medications (Eamer et al. 2018). Being aware of older adults' premorbid function, nurses can discuss with older adults and family on prehabilitation. Studies have shown that surgical patients who had prehabilitation are more likely to achieve full functional recovery post-surgery (Chia et al. 2015). Nurses should collaborate with physiotherapists to set prehabilitation goals tailored to the older adult's needs. For example, an older adult requiring one-man assistance should focus on maintaining functional abilities and preventing further decline. For patients with limited time before surgery, an institutional-based exercise program may be considered. Alternatively, home-based prehabilitation can be implemented with exercises, such as using a wheelchair for support during ambulation, and home visits by physiotherapists to focus on strength-building exercises. Figure 10.1 illustrates an older adult walking around the park support of a wheelchair before surgery.

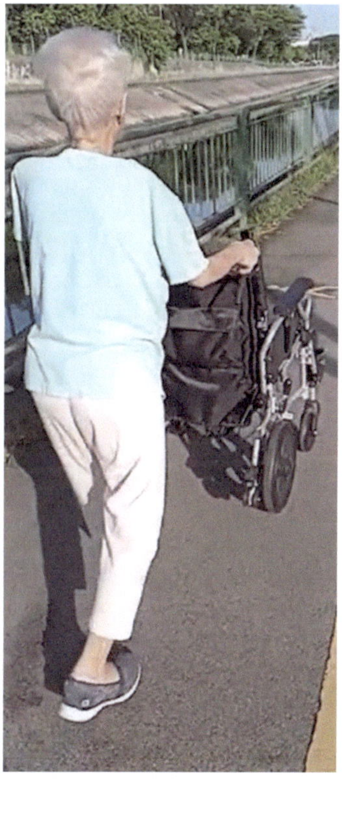

Fig. 10.1 Shows older adult walking around the park by pushing the wheelchair before surgery

10.2.2 Risk Assessment

Aging changes create unique needs in the geriatric population, making them more susceptible to postoperative complications, loss of independence, prolonged recovery, and mortality. Risk stratification is crucial for older adults to determine if the benefits of surgery outweigh the risks, facilitating shared decision-making (Eamer et al. 2018). Nurses should use various clinical predictors to anticipate and minimize risks through perioperative planning.

10.2.2.1 Reviewing of Charlson Comorbidity Index

Charlson Comorbidity Index helps nurses assess the level of complexity of the older person's condition. It is an important instrument for risk stratification, allocation of resources, development of personalized care plans, and forecasting potential complications (Charlson et al. 2022). However, it does not cover all significant, less common comorbidities. By triaging high-risk older surgical patients, nurses can mitigate the risk of complications with preventive measures. For older adults with high CCI scores, nurses can coordinate with the intensive care unit to arrange elective bookings for critical care. Placing older adults in high-acuity units or closer to the nursing counter for increased monitoring should also be considered.

10.2.2.2 Frailty Assessment

Frailty is a syndrome of diminished physiological reserve and weakened ability to adapt to stressors such as surgery or disease-related. Studies have shown that frailty is related to poor health outcomes comprised functional decline, falls, frequent hospitalization, or mortality (Wolfe et al. 2020). This emphasizes the need for nurses to be trained in frailty assessment to classify older adults into robust, pre-frail, or frail before surgery (Somnuke et al. 2024). Early detection of frailty allows for proactive strategies to mitigate and prevent adverse events. For prefrail and frail older adults, nurses advocate for prehabilitation, focusing on both physical and nutritional aspects. This includes collaborating with allied healthcare professionals—physiotherapist and dietitian to curate personalized prehabilitation plans. Examples include the prescription of high-intensity exercises or "Tai Chi" exercises for muscle strengthening, or recommending a diet with an add-on egg or nutritional supplement to improve protein intake.

10.2.3 Medication Management

Polypharmacy is a common problem in older adults due to multimorbidity, increasing the risk of frailty, falls, and mortality from side effects and drug–drug interactions (Blesynska et al. 2020). This can lead to poor medication compliance. A study in Northern Ireland found that 22.7% of prescriptions for patients over 65 years old were potentially inappropriate (Ryan et al. 2009). This emphasized the importance of nurses' roles in medication reconstitution and management and discontinuation of nonessential to lessen pill burden (Cheng et al. 2023).

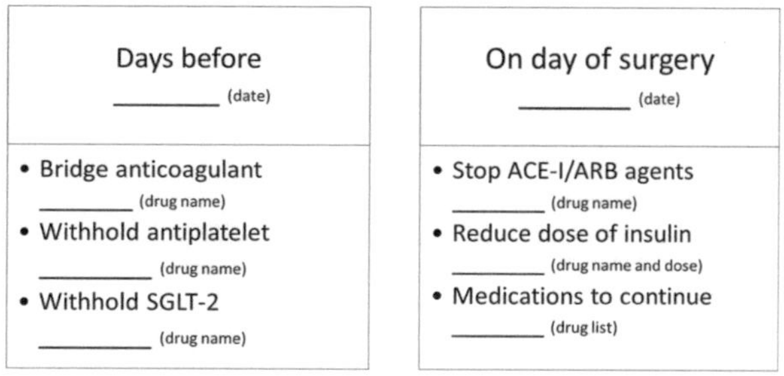

Fig. 10.2 Illustrates a sample preoperative instructional medication guide

Before surgery, older adults require review by both anesthesia and nursing staff at the pre-anesthetist clinic. Nurses reinforce the preoperative medication discontinuation using a preoperative instructional medication guide (Fig. 10.2) to enhance medication safety. For instance, older adults with diabetes on sodium-glucose co-transporter-2 (SGLT-2) like empagliflozin should stop them at least 3 days before surgery to avoid euglycemic diabetes ketoacidosis. Similarly, older adults with hypertension taking angiotensin-converting enzyme inhibitor (ACE-I) or angiotensin receptor blocking (ARB) agents like enalapril or losartan should stop them on the day of surgery to avoid severe circulatory side effects intraoperatively.

10.2.4 Ideas, Concerns, and Expectations

Given the elevated risk for mortality and morbidity in older adults, it is essential to explore their ideas, concerns, and expectations. Before initiating this conversation, nurses should ensure they allocate ample time for discussion, put away their phones, and create a conducive environment to promote a safe space. Consider the case of Mr. Toh, a 70-year-old man who was previously independent and used a walking stick. He has been diagnosed with gastric cancer, planning for gastrectomy. He is married, has no children, and is the sole caregiver for his spouse, who has hemiplegia from a stroke. Many thoughts and uncertainties might be weighing on his mind. By setting aside time with Mr. Toh, the nurses were able to elicit his ideas, concerns, and expectations, as shown in Fig. 10.3. Although he is medically guided, his health is not his top priority. His apprehension about surgery is the care of his wife. After listening to Mr. Toh, nurses work with him to list his concerns and provide psychosocial support. Additionally, nurses should communicate the concerns of older adults to the surgical team to provide appropriate recommendations. For example, nurses could confer with Mr. Toh to see if any family members can provide care for his wife or if respite services are feasible. However, nurses must be aware that each older adult has unique social situations and personalities. Not all suggested solutions may be accepted by older adults; therefore, keeping open communication with them is essential.

On the other hand, for older surgical patients at higher risk of mortality, it is important to discuss their preferences for resuscitation and advanced care planning. A 2010 study showed that more than 50% of patients over 60 years old lack

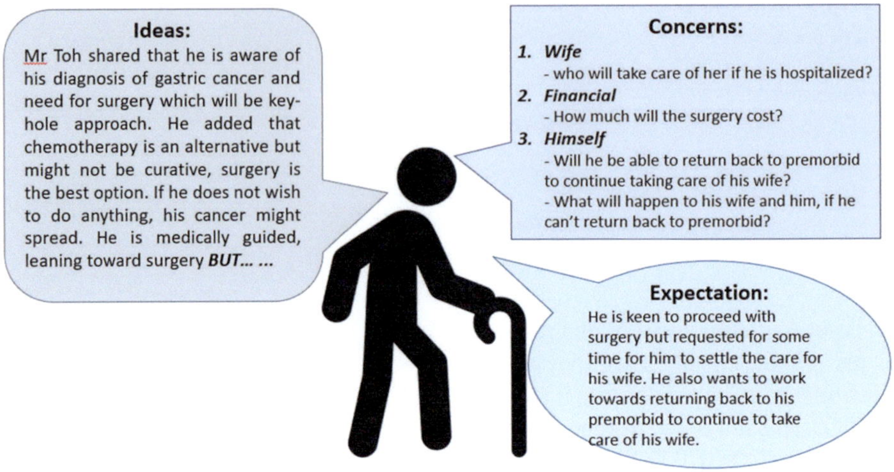

Fig. 10.3 Illustrates Mr. Toh's ideas, concerns, and expectations

decision-making capacity in the final stage of life (Silveira et al. 2010). Having an advance directive facilitates the identification of a main healthcare proxy and allows the healthcare team to plan the surgical approach. By understanding the preferences, goals, and expectations, nurses and older surgical patients can collaborate to set postoperative goals.

10.2.5 Anticipatory Risk and Mitigating Measures

Comprehensive preoperative assessments and risk evaluations can reveal potential issues or complications. Nurses should document these anticipated risks and potential complications. Developing and implementing perioperative mitigation strategies can reduce the likelihood of these identified risks occurring. Based on the potential risks, nurses should provide personalized education to patients and their families, not only to prepare them psychologically but also to establish shared goals. This also provides an opportunity to discuss discharge care planning, ensuring a smooth transition home after surgery. Table 10.3 further illustrates the mitigating measures, goals, and education targeting the anticipated risks for older adults.

Table 10.3 Mitigating measures, goals, and education targeting anticipated risks for older persons undergoing surgery

Anticipatory risk/ issue	Mitigating measures	Target/goal	Education
Risk for hypo/ hyperactive delirium	• Initiate delirium bundle • Assess for delirium timely • Refer occupational therapist for cognitive engagement	Avoid hypo/hyper delirium	• Reorientation • Bring items familiar to older adults such as spectacles or hearing aids
Risk for hypo/ hypertension	• Monitor blood pressure trend and postural blood pressure • Resume antihypertensive gradually post-operatively • Monitor for signs and symptoms of hypo/ hypotension	Set target for systolic blood pressure according to baseline	• Monitoring of blood pressure at home before surgery
Risk for hypo/ hyperglycemia	• Monitor blood glucose level especially when nil by mouth • Keep an intravenous dextrose containing therapy if on nil by mouth • Resume OHGAs gradually postoperatively • Monitor for signs and symptoms of hypo/ hyperglycemia	Keep blood glucose level between 5 and 11 mmol/L	• Monitoring of blood glucose at home • Advise on possible short-term insulin if glucose level not well control
Risk for fluid overload	• Monitor intake and output • Keep on fluid restriction accordingly • Monitor renal function if required	Aim for fluid balance	• Fluid restriction status if any
Risk for pulmonary complication • pneumonia • atelectasis	• Deep breathing exercises • Engage physiotherapist • Sit out of bed • Early ambulation	Deep breathing exercise at least 5–10 reps hourly Sit out of bed during meal time	• Teach deep breathing exercises and splinting techniques • Smoking cessation as required
Risk for malnutrition	• Availability of denture • Early resumption of diet • Supplement if needed	Start oral feeds as early as postoperative day 1	• Bring denture • Use of supplementation as indicated

(continued)

Table 10.3 (continued)

Anticipatory risk/ issue	Mitigating measures	Target/goal	Education
Risk for urinary complications • Urinary tract infection • Urinary retention	• Early Trial of Catheter (TOC) and post void residual monitoring • Resume medications for benign prostatic hyperplasia in male older adults before TOC • Monitor urine output	Keep urine output of 20–30 mL/h successful TOC post-surgery by postoperative day 2	• Expectation of lines and tubes postoperatively • May require reinsertion if fail TOC
Risk for venous thromboembolism	• Apply mechanical compression devices or thromboembolism socking • Early ambulation • Use of prophylactic subcutaneous heparin or enoxaparin	No incidence of venous thromboembolism	• Early ambulation • Use of mechanical compression devices or thromboembolism socking
Risk for functional decline	• Engage physiotherapist • Prehabilitation to rehabilitation • Sit out of bed • Early ambulation	Sit out of bed during meal time Ambulate at least 1–2 times a day Return back to premorbid	• Expectation of early ambulation
Risk for social isolation	• Engage befriender • Initiate social support such as day care center, senior activity center • Review depression scale	Engagement in activities in the day, while in hospital	• Discuss regarding engaging befriender and home situation
Discharge issue	• Identify discharge issues • Consider step-down facilities • Refer medical social worker if needed • Discuss at multidisciplinary team meeting	Identified discharge disposition	• Discuss about care option after surgery • Explain available community resources

10.3 Intraoperative Nursing Strategies

Intraoperative care for older adults presents significant difficulties due to their vulnerability to hemodynamic instability and postoperative complications. Furthermore, older adults often experience fear and anxiety before entering the operating theatre to older adults. Nurses working in the intraoperative setting play a crucial role in alleviating this anxiety and providing comfort. Introducing staff briefly, giving simple instructions in older adults' preferred language, and offering reassurance can reduce anxiety levels. Allowing an older adult to keep their visual or auditory devices such as spectacles, or hearing aids until just before induction to minimize disorientation.

10.3.1 Transfer

Maintaining communication with older adults, and encouraging their participation in care helps preserve their dignity (Doerflinger 2009). When possible, empowering them to transfer themselves from a wheelchair to trolley or operating theatre enhances older adult's independence and dignity. However, nurses at the reception area must assess their function and gait, and label any walking devices to prevent loss during transfer. Walking aids should be kept available or within sight, without compromising the sterility of the operating theatre.

10.3.2 Positioning

After transferring the older adult to the operating table, the nurse ensures proper body alignment and support. Good positioning is essential to prevent pressure on their skin or back. Use of support padding or pressure-relieving materials to protect bony prominences or pressure points, especially during long surgeries. For instance, heel protectors should be used for older adults undergoing abdominal surgery. Placing a pillow beneath the knees avoids postoperative stiffness, which may limit early mobilization whenever possible (Doerflinger 2009). Immobilization during surgery puts older adults at an increased risk for deep vein thrombosis (DVT). Nurses can apply thromboembolism socking or compression devices during surgery and continue their use immediately afterward unless contraindicated. Figure 10.4 demonstrates the use of thromboembolism socking and compression devices to reduce DVT and heel protectors to pressure injuries to heels.

10.3.3 Avoidance of Hypothermia

Older adults have impaired thermoregulation that can be further compromised in the cold environment of operating theatre. Circulating nurse can intervene by minimizing exposure of body areas and maintain patient's warmth with heating devices or

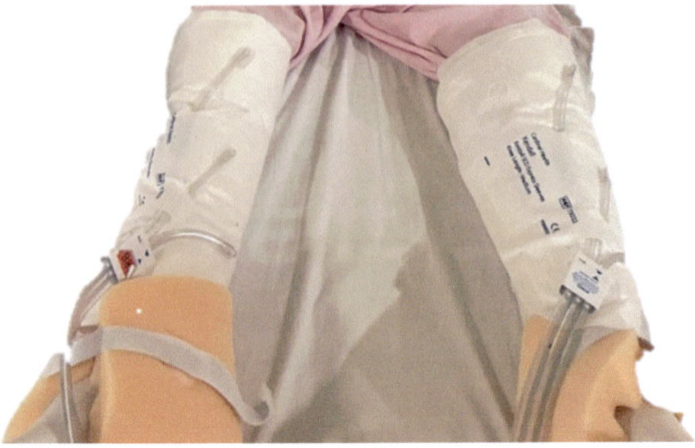

Fig. 10.4 Illustrates the use of devices for support of lower limbs

temperature-regulating blankets. Warm intravenous fluid should be readily available and older adult's temperature should be monitored, maintained above 35 °C unless contraindicated (Doerflinger 2009).

10.4 Postoperative Nursing Strategies

Immediately postoperatively, nurses in the recovery continue to monitor older adults' vital signs as they are more susceptible to hemodynamic derangement. When transferring care from the intraoperative phase to the intensive care unit or surgical ward, clear and concise communication during the handover is essential. The anticipated list of risks and targets set for older adults should be handed over to the receiving nursing team. This closes any gaps and minimizes lapses in care rendered to older adults who are more vulnerable to complications.

10.4.1 Hemodynamic Monitoring

Preoperatively, targets had been set in place for older adults. In the ward, nurses who recognize derangement in vital signs should immediately escalate the issue to the surgical team. In older adults who have had a hypotensive episode with a systolic blood pressure <80 mmHg, a small-volume fluid bolus should be considered to avoid fluid overload. Nurses are skilled in administrating bedside intervention such as hypoglycemia protocol, for older adults who are hypoglycemic. In older adults with chronic obstructive pulmonary disease and hypoxia, supplementing oxygen at no more than 2 L/min should be considered.

10.4.2 Optimizing Pain Control

Pain is subjective. Nurses should not have the misconception that older adults have a higher threshold than younger patients. Nurses should work with older adults and anesthesiologists to create a multimodal, individualized pain control plan. In older adults, especially those with cognitive impairment, pain should be assessed more frequently. The scheduling of analgesia administration and the vigilant adjustment of pain medication dosages should be considered (Doerflinger 2009). Occasionally, nurses work with therapists to time the serving of analgesia before rehabilitation to improve participation and function. Ongoing education on pain management, including medication side effects, and nonpharmacological approaches—relaxation, music therapy, or splinting technique for coughing—is implemented by ward nurses. Hence, a tailored pain management plan is needed for older adults, just as for any postoperative patient.

10.4.3 Respiratory Care

Respiratory-related complications such as pneumonia, atelectasis, and respiratory failure are common in older adults. Physiological changes associated with aging increase the risk of mortality after surgery. Close attention should be paid to the recognition of pulmonary complications, signs, and symptoms of dysphagia to optimize pulmonary status (Doerflinger 2009). Nurses reinforce coughing and deep breathing exercises and the use of incentive spirometry. Nurses ensure that older adults sit out of bed and ambulate at ward level to promote lung expansion.

10.4.4 Urinary Retention and Urinary Tract Infection (UTI)

Older adults are at risk for iatrogenic infections such as urinary tract infections (UTIs). The focus should be paid to the prevention of UTI. Nursing efforts include good hand hygiene, sterile insertion techniques, and a daily review for early removal of the catheter (Wolfe et al. 2020). However, in older males with benign prostate hyperplasia (BPH), consider removing the urinary catheter after resuming medications for BPH to avoid urinary retention. Close monitoring for lower abdominal distension and checking of post-void residual urine after TOC is essential for prompt reinsertion of urinary catheter if required.

10.4.5 Wound and Drain Care

Surgical wound infection is common, particularly in emergency surgery. Older adults who are malnourished are prone to poor wound healing. Nurses regularly review the wound, recognizing signs and symptoms of wound infection such as redness, warmth, swelling, and purulent discharge, and discuss with surgeons the need for antibiotics (Stephenson et al. 2020). Maintaining sterile techniques during wound dressing is of utmost importance in nursing intervention, along with ongoing education and caregiver training on wound care.

Post-surgery, drains, tubes, or lines are common devices seen in patients. Nurses must constantly monitor these devices and meticulously track their output for color and volume. Any significant change in output, especially if inconsistent with older adults' condition, should be immediately reported to the surgeon. However, this is particularly critical for older adults, who may not exhibit typical signs of infection and are at increased risk of developing severe complications, including septic shock. Therefore, prompt escalation of care is essential for all patients with these devices, but especially vital for this vulnerable geriatric population.

10.4.6 Ambulation

Emerging research has demonstrated the benefits of early mobilization for postsurgical patients such as quicker return to function (Tazreean et al. 2022). Patients can begin sitting up in bed or at the edge of the bed as early as the day of surgery (Fig. 10.5). However, common myths among older adults such as concerns about wound dehiscence and the need for prolonged bed rest must be addressed through ongoing education. Nurses should be mindful of each older adult's premorbid and ensure their walking devices are readily accessible. Establishing a routine of sitting out of bed during mealtime reduces the risk of lung collapse and aspiration

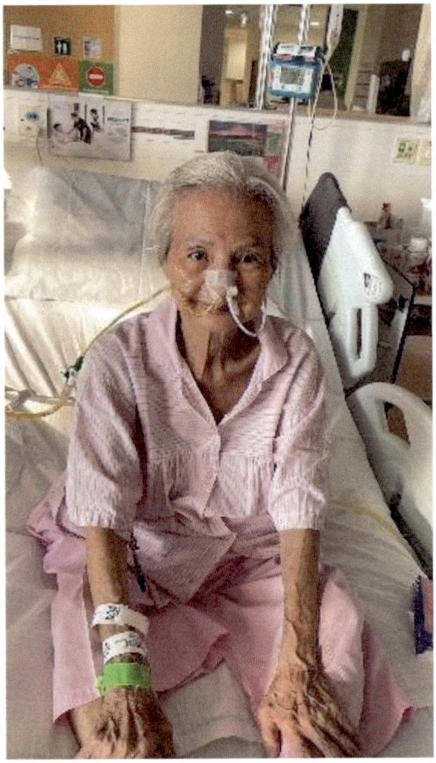

Fig. 10.5 Older adult sat up in bed after surgery

pneumonia. Nurses motivate older adults to walk to the toilet with appropriate assistance for toileting or personal hygiene. Avoiding bed sponging can also reduce pressure injury from prolonged bed rest. However, nurses need to be vigilant in recognizing alarming situations such as hemodynamic instability, low hemoglobin levels, or active bleeding.

10.4.7 Cognitive Function

Delirium is one of the most common postoperative complications in older adults and is associated with poor surgical outcomes, prolonged hospitalization, and functional decline (Wolfe et al. 2020). Fortunately, approximately 30% of older adults with delirium are preventable. This requires a conscious effort to implement delirium bundles or nonpharmacological measures to avoid the development of delirium. Strategies include early mobility, avoiding urinary retention or constipation, minimal use of restraints, and encouraging daytime activities like coloring or painting. The involvement of family members in creating a calm environment is also crucial (Mohanty et al. 2016). Figures 10.6 and 10.7 further illustrate delirium prevention strategies.

Delirium preventive strategies	
	Education on delirium
	Reorientation
	Sit out of bed
	Early mobilization
	Assistive aids such as visual; hearing or walking aids at bedside
	Adequate hydration
	Optimize pain control
	Adequate oxygen supplementation
	Avoid urinary retention or constipation
	Review of lines and tube daily for early removal
	Avoid restrainers
	Good sleep hygiene
	Minimize night activities
	Involvement of family members to be at bedside
	Engage occupational therapist for cognitive engagement

Fig. 10.6 Delirium prevention strategies

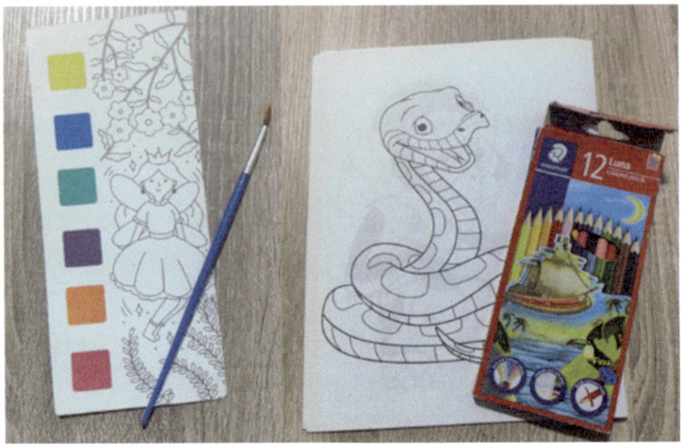

Fig. 10.7 Coloring activities to engage older adults

10.4.8 Engagement of Caregivers

Early involvement of the caregiver promotes recovery and facilitates discharge that also provides support to the healthcare team. For instance, for older adults with cognitive impairment, having a family member at the bedside can help create a calm environment. Engaging caregivers early in training of specific care needs is essential, particularly for older adults who have undergone procedures like stoma creation after colorectal surgery. Nurses should provide step-by-step instructions and demonstrations to ensure the caregiver's competency. As older adults often have poor hand dexterity, caregiver involvement can provide necessary support. However, while training caregivers, nurses should engage older adults to instill independence in self-care to avoid over-reliance on caregivers and potential caregiver stress.

Just as older adults need encouragement during the perioperative period, so do their loved ones. Provision of psychosocial support and reassurance is an essential act of nursing care. At Khoo Teck Puat Hospital, specialty nurses use their creativity and develop a caregiver competency certification as a form of encouragement. Figure 10.8 shows specialty nurses issuing a certificate to Mrs. Lee.

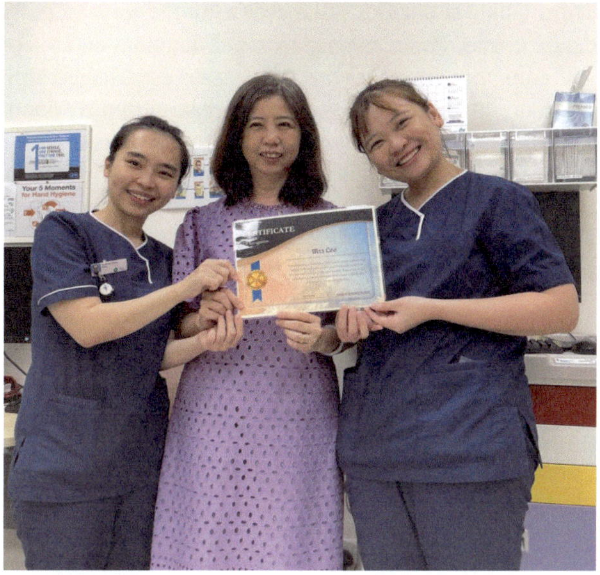

Fig. 10.8 Specialty nurses issuing certificate to Mdm Boon GB who is a caregiver for her husband

10.5 Discharge Care Planning

Intensive discharge care planning begins early in the preoperative phase, assessing older adults' social support systems and identifying discharge placement. Older adults are more prone to hospital-acquired infection. Early discharge, whenever possible, should be facilitated. Postoperatively, a joint effort involving surgeon, geriatrician, and allied healthcare professionals in the discussion of discharge care plans for older adults is essential (Mohanty et al. 2016). Nurses raise concerns about older adults and derive a discharge plan after multidisciplinary discussion. Nurses affirm the discharge process by offering suitable community resources, such as community hospital, day rehabilitation center, and timely referrals to avoid delay in transfer. Furnishing the discharge with sufficient analgesia, education on postoperative care, ambulation instructions such as avoiding heavy lifting for 6 weeks, prescription of aids, and provision of relevant follow-up appointment, if applicable, is also crucial.

10.6 Case

Mdm Chan, a 77-year-old woman, with head of pancreas lesion, was admitted for Whipple's surgery. Her medical history includes diabetes, hypertension, and hyperlipidemia. Before admission, she was independent in her activities of daily living with one person supervising her. A preoperative assessment was conducted by a surgical specialty nurse, revealing a modified Barthel index of 80/100. A frailty assessment was performed, indicating a prefrail status. During a discussion with

Mdm Chan about her perspective on surgery and any concerns, she expressed a desire to avoid being a burden to her daughter and to continue her hobbies of sewing and going out after surgery. A goal was established with her to return to her premorbid functional status. Anticipated risk and corresponding mitigating measures are documented in Table 10.4. Prehabilitation was coordinated for her at an outpatient rehabilitation clinic, supplemented with daily walking in a nearby park (Fig. 10.1).

During pre-anesthetist consultation, anesthesia nurses provided Mdm Chan and her daughter with preoperative medication instructions. In the operating theatre reception area, nurses applied thromboembolism socking before Mdm Chan enters

Table 10.4 illustrates Mdm Chan's anticipatory risk and mitigating measures

Anticipatory risk/issue	Mitigating measures	Target/goal	Education
Risk for hypo/hyperactive delirium	• Initiate delirium bundle	Avoid hypo/hyper delirium	• Reorientation • Bring Mdm Chan's phone
Risk for hypo/hypertension	• Monitor blood pressure trend and postural blood pressure • Resume anti-hypertensive gradually postoperatively • Monitor for sign and symptoms of hypo/hypertension	Set target for systolic blood pressure between 90 and 140 mmHg	• Monitoring of blood pressure at home before surgery
Risk for hypo/hyperglycemia	• Monitor blood glucose level • Keep on intravenous dextrose containing therapy when nil by mouth • Resume OHGAs gradually postoperatively • Monitor for sign and symptoms of hypo/hyperglycemia • Start caregiver training on insulin injection techniques	Keep blood glucose level between 5 and 11 mmol/L	• Monitoring of blood glucose at home • Advise on need for insulin regimen postsurgery due to nature of surgery.
Risk for functional decline	• Engage physiotherapist • Prehabilitation to rehabilitation • Sit out of bed • Early ambulation	Sit out of bed during meal time Ambulate at least once a day	• Enrolled into prehabilitation programme • Sit out of bed • Expectation of early ambulation
Discharge issue	• Consider community hospital • Installation of grab bars at home	Discharge to community hospital → Home	• Discuss about care option after surgery

operating room. Intraoperatively, her vital signs were closely monitored and she was given warmed intravenous fluids maintaining her temperature between 35 and 36 °C.

Postoperatively, given her high Charlson comorbidity index score of 7, an intensive care bed was arranged for high-acuity monitoring. Nurses provided a handover, outlining anticipated risks and initiating preventive intervention. Despite having multiple lines attached, Mdm Chan remained motivated and participated in rehabilitation with the therapist and nurse. Figure 10.9 shows Mdm Chan sitting out in the intensive care unit after surgery. Her supportive family was actively involved in her care during her hospital stay, and she did not exhibit any sign of postoperative delirium. Her daughter coordinated with the surgical ward nurses to arrange a short family gathering to celebrate Mother's Day. As planned preoperatively, a referral and arrangements were made for Mdm Chan to transition to the community hospital. Her care was seamlessly transferred, with clear documentation of her required care needs. Mdm Chan is now being followed up by surgical advanced practice nurse in conjunction with surgeons. She has recovered well and returned to her premorbid functional status, including going out for hair styling; further advancing her sewing skills and enjoying her meals outdoors with her family (Fig. 10.10).

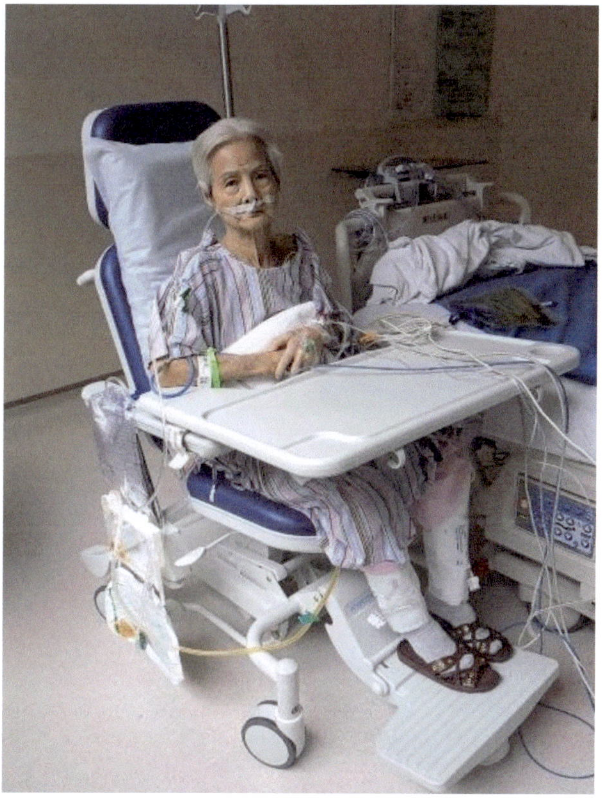

Fig. 10.9 Mdm Chan sitting out to chair in the intensive care unit

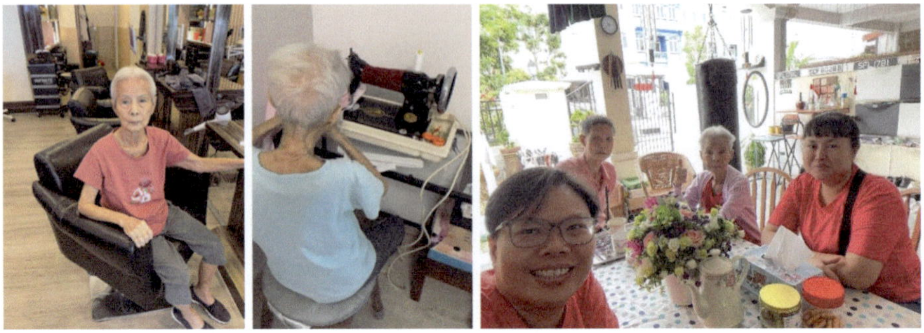

Fig. 10.10 Mdm Chan going for her hair styling, doing her sewing craft, and having her tea with her family

10.7 Conclusion

The paradigm shift toward older surgical patients requires holistic nursing care for this delicate population. Preoperative evaluation should extend beyond the surgeon's consultation. There is a need to perform a comprehensive perioperative assessment specific to the needs of older adults. Careful risk stratification and planning allow time to mitigate identified risks. Postoperatively, prompt recognition of early signs of complications, or deterioration is essential to facilitate timely escalation of care. Preventive measures to decrease complications should be integrated into routine practice. Robust perioperative planning and coordination facilitate a smooth transition of care across settings, with the return home, which are of paramount importance for optimal outcomes.

Acknowledgments A special thanks to the dedicated team of nurses at Khoo Teck Puat Hospital—ANC Lynn Tan, SSN Chong Joon Lan, SSN Tan Boon Theng, and SSN Rachel Soh—for their tireless efforts and unwavering support of perioperative older adults. Grateful appreciation to Mdm Boon GB, Mdm Chan WE, and her daughter, Ms. Lam MF, for their openness and generosity in sharing their photos and story.

References

Blesynska E, Wierucki L, Zdrojewski T, Renke M (2020) Pharmacological interactions in the elderly. Medicina (Kaunas) 56(7):320

Charlson ME, Carrozzino D, Guidi J, Patierno C (2022) Charlson comorbidity index: a critical review of clinimetric properties. Psychother Psychosom Med 91(1):8–35

Cheng C, Yu H, Wang Q (2023) Nurses' experiences concerning older adults with polypharmacy: a meta-synthesis of qualitative findings. Healthcare (Basel) 11(3):334

Chia CLK, Mantoo SK, Tan KY (2015) Start to finish trans-institutional transdisplinary care: a novel approach improves colorectal surgical results in frail elderly patients. Color Dis 18(1):43–50

Doerflinger DMC (2009) Older adult surgical patients: presentation and challenge. AORN J 90(2):223–240

Eamer G, Al-Amoodi MJH, Holroyd-Leduc J, Rolfson DB, Warkentin LM, Khadaroo RG (2018) Review of risk assessment tools to predict morbidity and mortality in elderly surgical patients. Am J Surg 216(3):585–594

Kow AWC (2019) Prehabilitation and its role in geriatric surgery. Commentary 48(11):386–392

Mohanty S, Rosenthal RA, Russell MM, Neuman MD, Ko CY, Esnaola NF (2016) Optimal perioperative management of the geriatric patient: a best practices guideline from the American College of Surgeons National Surgical Quality Improvement Program (NSQIP) and the American Geriatric Society. J Am Coll Surg 222(5):930–947

Ryan C, O'Mahony D, Kennedy J, Weedle P, Byrne S (2009) Potentially inappropriate prescribing in an Irish elderly population in primary care. Br J Clin Pharmacol 68:936–947

Sahadevan S, Lim PPJ, Tan NJL, Chan SP (2000) Diagnostic performance of two mental status tests in the older Chinese: influence of education and age on cut-off values. Int J Geriatr Psychiatry 15(3):234–241

Silveira MJ, Kim SJ, Langa KM (2010) Advance directives and outcomes of surrogate decision making before death. N Engl J Med 362:1211–1218

Somnuke P, Pongraweewan O, Siriussawakul A (2024) Optimizing perioperative care for elderly surgical patients: a review of strategies and evidence-based practices. Siriraj Med J 76(7):465–472

Stephenson C, Mohabbat A, Raslau D, Gilman E, Wight E, Kashiwagi D (2020) Management of common postoperative complications. Mayo Clin Proc 95(11):2540–2554

Tazreean R, Nelson G, Twomey R (2022) Early mobilization in enhanced recovery after surgery pathways: current evidence and recent advancements. J Comp Eff Res 11(2):121–129

Teh WL, Abdin E, Vaingankar JA, Shafie S, Jeyagurunathan A, Yunjie S, Subramaniam M (2021) Prevalence, lifestyle correlates, and psychosocial functioning among multi-ethnic older adults with mild cognitive impairment in Singapore: preliminary findings from a 10/66 population study. Yale J Biol Med 94(1):73–83

Watson BJ, Salmoni AW, Zecevic AA (2016) The use of the Morse Fall Scale in an acute care hospital. Clin Nurs Stud 4(2):32–40

Wolfe JD, Wolfe NK, Rich MW (2020) Perioperative care of the geriatric patient for noncardiac surgery. Clin Cardiol 43:127–136

Minimally Invasive Surgery in the Older Population: Challenges and Opportunities

11

Yao-Zong Lee, Hui-Yu Tham, Yen-Chen Shao, and Daniel Jin-Keat Lee

11.1 Introduction: The Evolution of Minimally Invasive Surgery

The field of abdominal surgery has made significant progress over the last few decades. Along with the advent of new imaging and surgical technologies, there is also a concomitant demand for safer, less morbid procedures with faster recovery times. Minimally invasive surgical (MIS) approaches have thus been popularized, quickly gaining immense traction to become the standard of care in many countries around the globe throughout the years.

The historical concept of MIS traces back to a journey of evolution and innovation, with initial attempts at endoscopy. In the 1800s, Philipp Bozzini invented the "Lichtleiter", a light conductor used for examining the inner cavities of the human body. By the late nineteenth century, rudimentary light scopes were widely used for diagnosis, with major advancements in endoscopy during the 1960s to 1980s. The rapidity of this development would then have ripple effects that ultimately influence the transition from diagnostic to minimally invasive surgical therapeutics. German gynecologist Kurt Semm (1927–2003) was the pioneer who truly established

Y.-Z. Lee (✉)
Colorectal Surgery, Khoo Teck Puat Hospital, Singapore, Singapore
e-mail: lee.yao.zong@ktph.com.sg

H.-Y. Tham
National Healthcare Group General Surgery Residency, Singapore, Singapore
e-mail: huiyu.tham@mohh.com.sg

Y.-C. Shao
Colorectal Surgery, China Medical University Hsinchu Hospital, Zhubei City, Taiwan

D. J.-K. Lee
General and Colorectal Surgery, Khoo Teck Puat Hospital, Singapore, Singapore
e-mail: daniel.lee@geriatricsurgery.org.sg

K.-Y. Tan et al. (eds.), *Mastering Geriatric Surgery*,
https://doi.org/10.1007/978-981-95-0665-1_11

advanced operative laparoscopy, having performed the first laparoscopic appendicectomy in 1981 (Semm 1988).

Interestingly, his operation was initially voraciously attacked by the surgical fraternity, with many criticizing his "*laparoscopic*" technique as both dangerous and unethical (Litynski 1998a). Many surgeons were then of the opinion that modern anesthetics were able to support major surgeries via laparotomies, and there was no need to replace established operative methods with technically more challenging ones. However, Semm's persistence and dedication went on further to overcome challenges and skeptics, subsequently inspiring Erich Mühe and other surgeons around the world to perform a vast array of procedures via minimally invasive means (Litynski 1998b). Laparoscopic cholecystectomy soon became the gold standard, and within a short period of time, the pendulum has now shifted to laparoscopy as the preferred approach for the majority of diseases. Single-incision laparoscopy surgery (SILS) and natural orifice specimen extraction (NOSE) surgery are even further steps to minimize surgical trauma. In recent years, there has also been a growing interest in the use of robotic platforms to realize the full potential of MIS with improved accuracy and consistency.

As the world sees the evolution of abdominal surgery from antiquity to the sophisticated techniques used in the twentieth century, many are also starting to **recognize the value of MIS for a fast-growing subgroup of patients—the *older persons***. The term "elderly" has been widely accepted as a chronological age of 65 or older. Based on this definition, the WHO estimates the proportion of older persons worldwide to reach 38% by 2050 (Rudnicka et al. 2020). Aging can impact on many physiological systems, with elderly patients having a higher incidence of postoperative complications, increased re-hospitalization rates, and longer hospital stays. Elderly individuals also experience changes in cytokine expression, leading to a pro-inflammatory state, which increases the likelihood of postoperative complications such as pneumonia, stroke, and cardiac complications. This state also contributes to fatigue, muscle loss, and postoperative pain with a resultant delay in function and independence (Rea et al. 2018). As the proportion of elderly patients in the population increases, the medical system will face new challenges. It is inevitable that these forecasted population shifts will have significant repercussions on surgical practice globally. As we jump on the bandwagon of MIS, **therein lies an exciting opportunity for anesthetists, surgeons, and physicians to collaborate** towards a shared goal of less surgical trauma and faster recovery for older persons.

11.1.1 Reduction in Surgical Stress

Open surgery has long been perceived to be associated with a shorter operative time, with improved surgical exposure and tactile sensation, thereby achieving better operative precision. While open surgery mitigates some of the challenges faced with pneumoperitoneum during minimally invasive surgeries, larger surgical incisions result in increased tissue damage, inciting a greater inflammatory cascade (Zhao and Gu 2022), hence prolonging the recovery time. Therefore, with smaller surgical incisions observed in minimally invasive surgeries, blood loss, catecholamine surge, and overall stress response with the release of inflammatory mediators are significantly less pronounced compared to bigger laparotomy wounds. The reduced tissue handling and tissue damage during minimally invasive surgeries translate to a reduction in surgical stress and are crucial in promoting recovery, especially in older patients in the immediate postoperative period.

11.1.2 Lower Risk of Postoperative Morbidities

Since the introduction of minimally invasive surgeries, various retrospective studies and randomized controlled trials have been conducted to evaluate the efficacy of laparoscopic surgeries in older persons, especially in appendicectomy, cholecystectomy, pelvic surgeries, liver resections, and colorectal surgeries. Compared to open appendicectomy, laparoscopic appendicectomy in the older persons has similarly been supported by various large observational studies and has found to be associated with reduced postoperative morbidity and reduced length of stay even in the elderly cohort (Kim et al. 2011). Similarly, in comparison to open cholecystectomy, observational series have demonstrated that laparoscopic cholecystectomy has more advantages over open cholecystectomy, especially in elderly patients with a lower incidence of postoperative complications and overall reduced length of stay (Massie et al. 1993). Minimally invasive surgery is also significantly associated with reduced odds of surgical site infections (Gandaglia et al. 2014).

In gynecological and pelvic surgeries, minimally invasive approaches have progressively become the mainstay of approach as it forms an integral component of enhanced recovery after surgery (ERAS) (Uccella et al. 2016; Leitao Jr et al. 2022). As compared to open surgeries where patients experience significant postoperative morbidity, large-center studies have demonstrated that minimally invasive approaches have been superior without increased risk of mortality and morbidity. Additionally, oncological outcomes and disease-free survival have not been compromised with minimally invasive techniques when compared to conventional open approaches (Leitao Jr et al. 2022).

11.1.3 Enhanced Functional Outcomes with Early Recovery and Independence

The role of minimally invasive surgery in colorectal cancer has been well established over the past few years with short-term benefits, without significant differences in oncological and long-term outcomes (Fujii et al. 2016). The Clinical Outcomes of Surgical Therapy (COST) Study Group trial in 2004 demonstrated superior perioperative outcomes in laparoscopic approaches compared to open surgery, with reduced length of stay (Nelson et al. 2004). In addition, the recent landmark Colon cancer Laparoscopic or Open Resection (COLOR) trial (Deijen et al. 2017) further demonstrated similar rates of disease-free survival, overall survival, and recurrences in both minimally invasive and open surgery groups. As such, laparoscopy is fast replacing traditional open colonic surgeries owing to favorable short-term outcomes such as reduced blood loss, less pain, quicker return to bowel function, and improved recovery time without compromising oncology. More recently, a retrospective comparison analysis conducted on octogenarians undergoing colorectal surgeries also showed significantly reduced hospitalization costs and length of stay with laparoscopic surgery as compared to open surgery with comparable postoperative outcomes and mortality rates (Chok et al. 2023).

The decreased pain and faster recuperation with lesser downtime in a minimally invasive approach make it highly attractive for many elder patients, **who see earlier return to function, independence, and quality of life as key priorities** when making critical treatment decisions.

MIS offers significant benefits such as
(a) ***reduction in surgical stress:*** *less blood loss, shorter recovery times, reduced post-operative pain.*
(b) ***Reduction in surgical stress****: Lower risk of post-operative complications compared to open surgery.*
(c) *Role in* ***preserving functional independence*** *in frail patients.*

11.2 Challenges of MIS Adoption in Older Persons

11.2.1 Complex Physiological Characteristics of Older Persons

Laparoscopic/robotic surgery in elderly patients pose a unique set of challenges in the perioperative period secondary to the effects of pneumoperitoneum. Carbon dioxide pneumoperitoneum may result in acid–base and blood gas disturbances as well as significant alterations to patients' pulmonary and/or cardiovascular physiology. In some elderly patients with poorer respiratory and/cardiovascular reserves, pneumoperitoneum further reduces pulmonary functional residual capacity and lung compliance and increases peak airway pressures and absorption of intraperitoneal carbon dioxide, resulting in hypercarbia and acidemia. Additionally, with pneumoperitoneum, preload reduces, resulting in decreased cardiac output, while afterload and cardiac contractility increase, bringing about an increased cardiovascular stress (Fig. 11.1) (Safran and Orlando 3rd 1994).

In addition, MIS can also involve longer operative duration compared to open surgery, thereby increasing the risks of complications in this group of patients. Clearly, the vulnerabilities of geriatric patients can be further accentuated in MIS, making the choice of surgical approach for this group of patients a complex and oftentimes a daunting task for both anesthetists and surgeons.

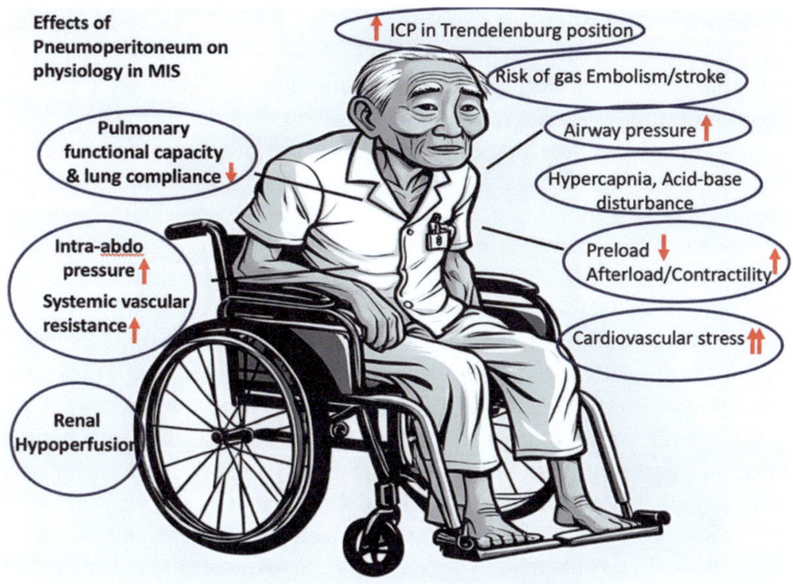

Fig. 11.1 Effects of pneumoperitoneum on the elderly physiology in MIS

11.2.2 Need for Robust Preoperative Optimization and Postoperative Rehabilitation

Older surgical patients will often require a higher acuity care than younger patients during the perioperative period. They are often more prone to developing postoperative delirium, functional decline, and loss of independence postoperatively. Henceforth, in order to provide optimal care for the older surgical patients, the uptake of MIS alone is not enough. Surgeons must never work in silos, but rather, the goal should be a tailored, comprehensive geriatric evaluation by different stakeholders at various checkpoints, starting preoperatively. A dedicated collaborative transdisciplinary Geriatric Surgery Service has been shown to improve postoperative outcomes in elderly colorectal surgery patients compared to standard management (Tan et al. 2011). Collaborative care processes among surgeons, anesthetists, geriatricians, and allied health members with a patient-centered culture are crucial in ensuring consistent successful outcomes for elderly frail patients. Unfortunately, **such a practice may not always be possible in a context of a busy surgical practice**. Certainly, as we embrace advanced MIS techniques with fervor and passion, optimizing outcomes in the frail elderly patients goes far beyond the operating room. There needs to be a **concerted, consistent surgeon-led effort** to facilitate collaboration and trust and ensure buy-in from various stakeholders in a start-to-finish endeavor for a successful surgical outcome.

11.2.3 Mounting Learning Curves in MIS

It is clear that surgical innovations are central to progress and have led to exponential growth and improvements in many facets of surgical care. However, the adoption of new techniques first comes with the need to overcome its learning curve without compromising on patient safety. Apart from being proficient with traditional open surgical techniques, the new generation of surgeons will also need to be well inversed in MIS. However, mastering laparoscopic surgery involves a steeper learning curve, making it a challenging task to train surgical residents. For example, there can be reduced tactile and depth perception in laparoscopic surgery, making it difficult to navigate and manipulate tissues. The fulcrum effect, in which the movement of the instrument's handles results in the opposite movement of the instrument tip, requires good hand–eye coordination coupled with spatial awareness. **The challenges mentioned underscore the importance of adaptability and continuous upskilling in this dynamic field of surgery.** Similarly, with the increasing adoption of robotic surgery, institutions intending to adopt this technology will need to devise strategies to support the process of skill acquisition in a safe and efficient way. Providing opportunities for fellowships and robotic surgical stimulation, along with a structured training program complemented by proctorship, are some of the ways institutions can consider to help their surgeons acquire new skills in their practice. Various statistical methods, such as the more commonly described cumulative sum (CUSUM) analysis can also be an effective tool for learning curve assessments (Lin et al. 2023).

In summary, the minimally invasive approach has revolutionized surgical care and has proven to be a game changer over traditional open surgery, especially for frail elderly patients. However, new techniques will undoubtedly face multiple roadblocks to its adoption, either due to cultural or organizational factors. To overcome such barriers, hospital systems will need to focus on strategies such as providing comprehensive training opportunities and support, **fostering partnership between surgeons and hospital leadership** to address the financial concerns about costs and reimbursements that may impede adoption.

In elderly patients undergoing MIS, it is imperative to recognize the unique physiological changes of ageing and their impact on anesthetic management. There needs to be a robust and collaborative multidisciplinary team work in ensuring overall quality care for geriatric patients.

Effective hospital leadership and a strong support system are crucial in creating an environment of innovation and surgical upskilling.

11.3 Opportunities for Novel Minimally Invasive Surgical Techniques in Colorectal Surgery in Older Persons

11.3.1 Natural Orifice Specimen Extraction

Natural orifice specimen extraction, NOSE, is an advanced minimally invasive technique. It allows surgeons to extract surgical specimens from hollow organs that communicate with outside, such as the vagina or the gastrointestinal tract. The specimen could be extracted without creating an outer incision, therefore reducing surgical trauma, pain, and infection rate (Fig. 11.2) (Chin et al. 2021; Izquierdo et al. 2018). NOSE has comparable long-term oncological outcomes when compared to

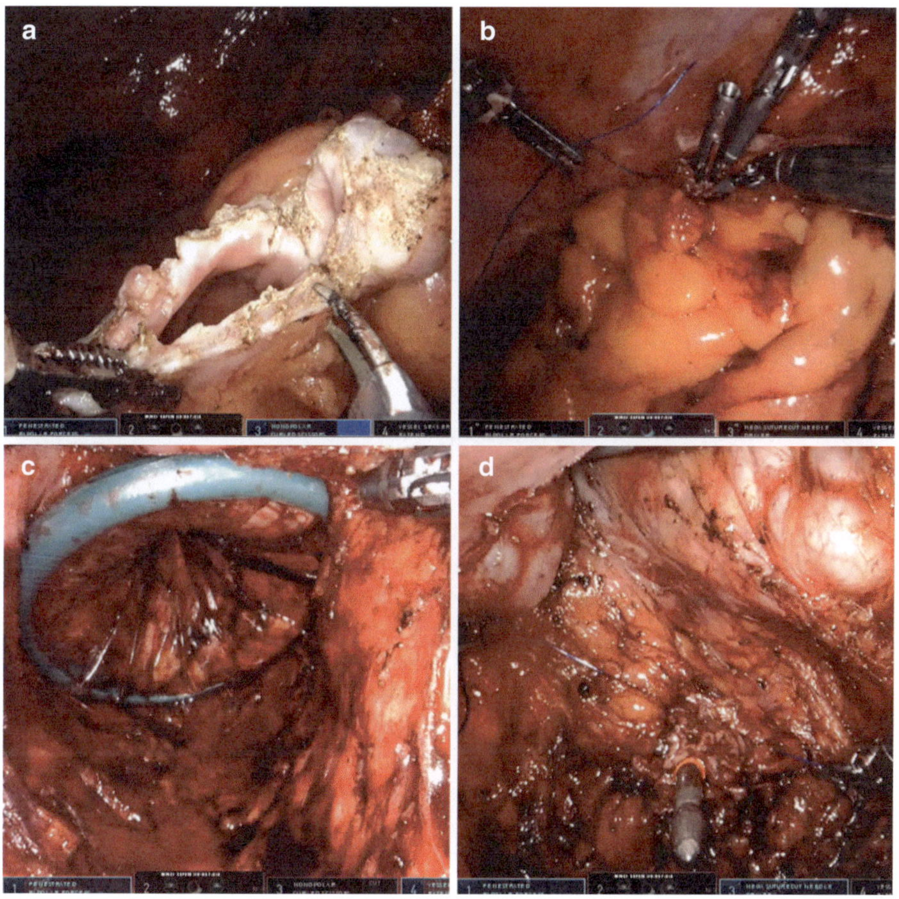

Fig. 11.2 Natural orifice specimen extraction. (**a**) Division of proximal cut end (**b**) Purse-string suture of proximal cut end (**c**) Wound protector placed to faciliate extraction of specimen through natural orifice (**d**) Purse-string suture of distal cut end followed by insertion of circular stapler

conventional laparoscopic surgery. NOSE was widespread adopted in many fields; the specimen can be extracted via colon, anus, vagina, and stomach (Izquierdo et al. 2018). For example, the gallbladder can be extracted from the stomach after laparoscopic cholecystectomy. One can also deliver the colon specimen from anus or vagina.

NOSE in colorectal surgery has been proven to have many benefits in meta-analysis; it is associated with shorter hospital stay, less wound pain, faster first flatus passage, fewer wound complications, less postoperative inflammatory response, and less incisional hernia rates, compared to transabdominal wall wound specimen retrieval (Liu et al. 2025). **By eliminating the need for a large abdominal wound to extract the specimen, this significantly reduces the risk of developing an incisional hernia. This is particularly advantageous for a frail elderly patient with limited tolerance for abdominal wall trauma.** In our colorectal department, the most commonly selected routes for specimen retrieval are rectum and vagina (in female patients). After completing the dissection and dividing the bowel segment, an incision was made in the upper rectum or posterior wall of vagina. A wound protector would then be inserted, and the specimen was retrieved through the natural orifice. We can also transect at the descending colon and then retrieve the specimen from the descending colon opening by using colonoscopy. However, in order to preserve the integrity of the specimen so as to achieve a better oncological outcome, not all patients with malignancy are suitable for NOSE. There are some limitations of NOSE, which are contraindicated in patients with a body mass index (BMI) more than 30 kg/m^2, a T3 or T4 staging tumor, bulky tumor, and/or mesentery size.

11.3.2 Intracorporeal Anastomosis

Anastomosis is one of the most difficult procedures in MIS. Despite the ability to perform dissection, transection, and ligation laparoscopically, intracorporeal anastomosis remains technically challenging. Bouras et al. reported a series with 82 patients who underwent total intracorporeal anastomosis after laparoscopic distal gastrectomy and Roux-en-Y reconstruction. Compared to extracorporeal anastomosis (ECA), intracorporeal anastomosis (ICA) is technically feasible and safe, without obvious poor outcomes. In esophagojejunostomy after total gastrectomy, intracorporeal anastomosis is associated with less blood loss, earlier time to first oral intake, and shorter hospital stay, and compared to extracorporeal anastomosis, there was no statistically significant difference in safety (Bouras et al. 2011). As far as we know, intracorporeal anastomosis is widely accepted in gastrojejunostomy, jejunojejunostomy, and choledochojejunostomy in our institute. In the lower gastrointestinal tract surgery, intracorporeal compared to extracorporeal anastomosis in right colectomy is associated with less hernia rate, short incision site length, less bowel length sacrifice, faster gastrointestinal recovery, and shorter hospital stay in many meta-analyses (Bou Saleh et al. 2020). Similar findings were also found in left colectomy; intracorporeal anastomosis is associated with less overall morbidity, less SSI, shorter incision length, and faster postoperative gastrointestinal recovery compared to extracorporeal anastomosis (Fig. 11.3) (Vaghiri et al. 2023). Additionally, in ECA, the site of specimen extraction is often limited by the location of anastomosis (Fig. 11.4). On the contrary, ICA gives the surgeon the freedom to choose the extraction site. In our experience, specimen extraction via a Pfannenstiel incision reduces wound pain, lowers the risk of infection, and decreases the likelihood of future hernias. Our findings are also compatible with many studies (Benlice et al. 2016; Benlice et al. 2019).

11.3.3 Robotic Surgery for Colorectal Cancer

Although robotic surgery has gained acceptance in many fields, sufficient evidence to support its superiority over laparoscopic surgery is still lacking. Lu et al. concluded that robotic distal gastrectomy is not inferior to laparoscopic approach in a phase 2 trial (Lu et al. 2024). The overall incidence of postoperative complications

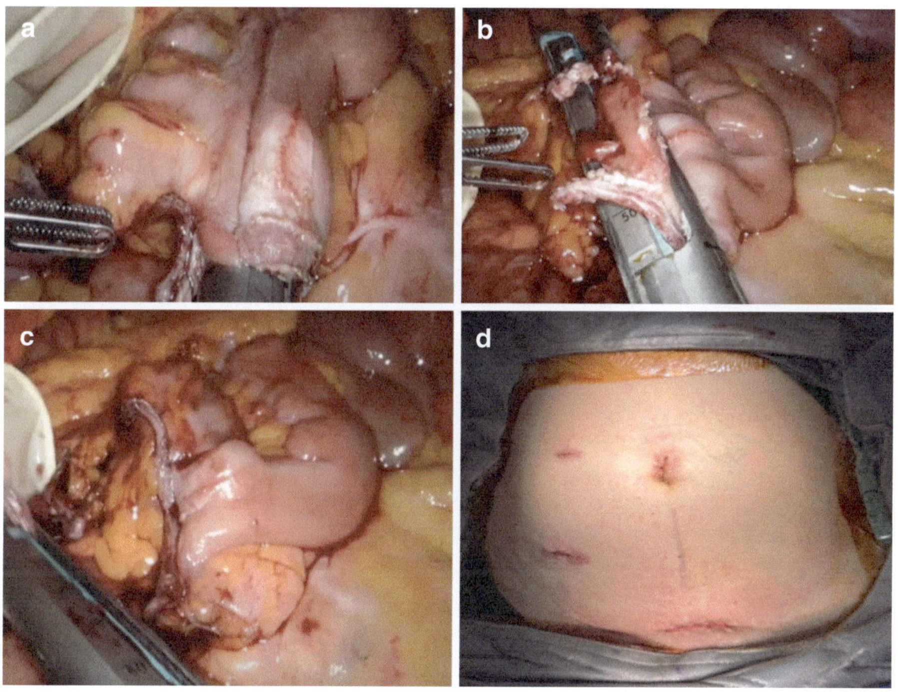

Fig. 11.3 Surgical conduct for intracorporeal anastomosis (ICA). (**a**) Side-to-side antiperistaltic intracorporeal anastomosis performed in a right hemicolectomy, (**b**) Closure of enterotomies done intracorporeally, (**c**) Tension-free anastomosis achieved **intracorporeally** with **minimal bowel manipulation**, (**d**) ICA allows for **off-midline** extraction of specimen, with benefits of reduced pain, faster recovery, and lower risks of incisional hernia

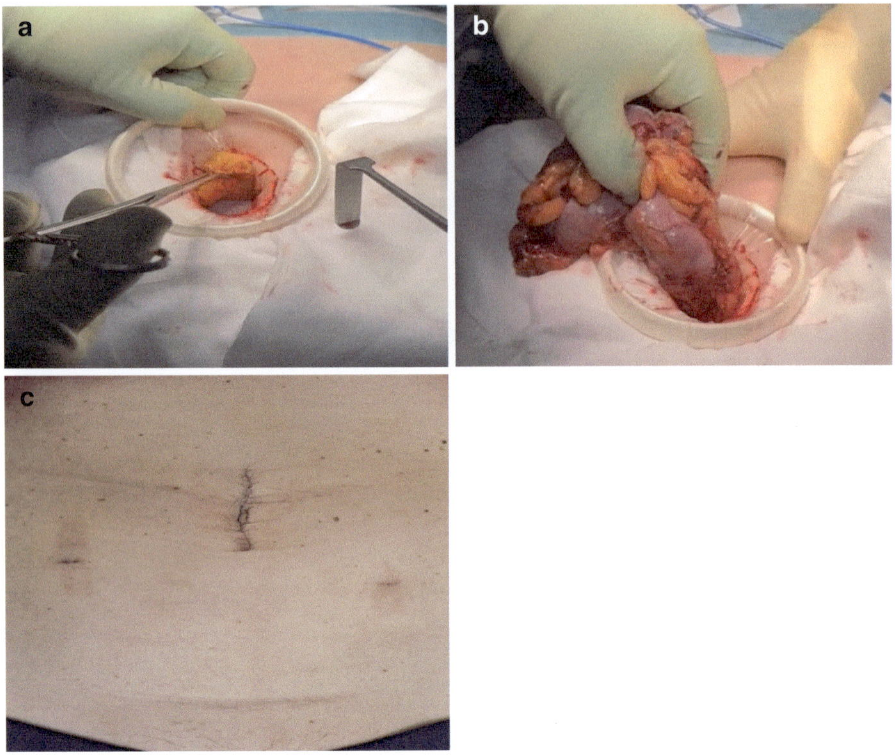

Fig. 11.4 Surgical conduct for extracorporeal anastomosis (ECA). (**a**) **Larger midline incision** is required in extracorporeal anastomosis to facilitate bowel exteriorization, (**b**) There is also **more bowel manipulation** and **traction on the mesentery** as the specimen is being exteriorized, (**c**) Postoperative laparoscopic right hemicolectomy (extracorporeal anastomosis). Specimen extracted via midline incision

shows no significant difference between robotic and laparoscopic gastrectomy in a phase 3 randomized controlled trial (Ojima et al. 2021).

There are currently few randomized controlled trials (RCTs) comparing robotic and laparoscopic surgeries for rectal cancer; two RCTs from Korea found no significance in the circumferential margin between the robotic and laparoscopic approaches for rectal cancer, which is one of the most important factor by doing malignant rectal surgery (Kim et al. 2018; Park et al. 2023). However, the patients were collected in the early 2010s. In the recent study from China, Feng et al. found that for middle and low rectal cancer, robotic surgery provides better CRM, less surgical trauma, and better postoperative recovery compared to conventional laparoscopic surgery (Feng et al. 2022). Although robotic colorectal surgery does not seem to provide statistically significant benefits compared to laparoscopic surgery, we still believe it has several advantages. Compared to the traditional laparoscopic approach, the more stable view and the increased wrist mobility allow for more efficient suturing during surgery, saving time and reducing the fatigue of the surgeon. Robotic-assisted surgery offers enhanced precision and ergonomics in handling complex anatomy and offers great utility in patients with narrow pelvises or prior surgical adhesions. Unfortunately, cost and robotic access still remain as significant barriers for many healthcare systems. As such, robotic surgery may well coexist as a complementary tool to laparoscopic surgery presently, gradually taking over more complex cases as costs decrease and utilization spreads.

11.4 Future Opportunities

The evidence for MIS is unequivocal for its feasibility and oncologic safety. As it gains widespread acceptance within the surgical community in recent years, its utilization is also rapidly growing, especially in the realm of ***elective*** **geriatric surgery**. Interestingly, there **still appears to be a dearth of available literature on MIS emergency surgery in the older persons.** According to large retrospective studies in the surgical literature, laparoscopic appendicectomy, cholecystectomy, and even laparoscopic repair of perforated viscus (gastric and duodenal ulcers) are generally well-accepted emergency surgical procedures. However, the utilization of the MIS approach in such scenarios, even within the same institutions, can still be variable and influenced by insufficient surgical expertise. Similarly, while other surgical procedures such as laparoscopic repair for incarcerated hernias, bowel resection, and laparoscopic Hartmann's are also becoming more frequent, they are still not being routinely suggested in the current literature. This underutilization of MIS in emergency surgery in older persons can be attributed to several reasons, for instance, more complex and sicker frail elderly patients in the acute setting, lack of a dedicated emergency surgical team with homogeneous surgical skills, inadequate experience, and diagnostic dilemma. A recent survey by Ceresoli et al. revealed that only 28.7% of surgeons declared the use of laparoscopy in more than 50% of the time in primary emergencies (Ceresoli et al. 2022). **These findings underscore a missed opportunity to potentially lower costs and improve outcomes in geriatric emergency surgery patients.** There need to be a greater focus and intent on training a group of dedicated emergency surgeons who are well versed in laparoscopy and minimally invasive surgeries.

In addition, Artificial Intelligence (AI) is also poised to further transform patient care by enhancing surgical decision-making before, after, and even intraoperatively by integrating information from many sources. For instance, the Supporting SURgery with Geriatric Co-Management and AI (SURGE-Ahead) initiative supports geriatric co-management by integrating evidence-based recommendations and continuity of care decisions into a digital platform for personalized surgical planning (Leinert et al. 2023). AI can also facilitate postoperative care by analyzing patient data to predict complications and guide follow-up care.

11.5 Closing

As the global population ages, the number of geriatric patients requiring surgical interventions would indubitably increase. From the advent of laparoscopy to robotic surgery, this technological leap has significantly expanded the scope and capability of minimally invasive surgery. Compared to traditional open surgery, MIS has now been shown to be an equally feasible, if not more efficient, way of achieving safe and improved surgical outcomes for geriatric patients. Today, MIS stands at the critical intersection of technology and patient, playing a pivotal role in guiding surgical planning and conduct through the complexities of geriatric surgery. The upcoming generation of residents and surgeons will have a vast array of tools and advanced techniques in their surgical armamentarium to minimize surgical morbidity and restore function for the aged. Nevertheless, despite having the best intents, surgeons and patients can infrequently still have differing viewpoints and perspectives on whether a surgical intervention will or will not improve patients' quality of life. Ultimately, a patient-centered care model, encouraging active collaboration and shared decision-making between patients and clinicians, **remains the cornerstone and bedrock of good-quality healthcare.**

The field of minimally invasive surgery is still evolving with further opportunities such as NOSE, robotic surgery.

Minimally invasive techniques in Geriatric Emergency Surgery and the integration of AI in perioperative care are potential areas of growth as we strive to optimize surgical outcomes for the frail and elderly.

References

Benlice C, Stocchi L, Costedio MM, Gorgun E, Kessler H (2016) Impact of the specific extraction-site location on the risk of incisional hernia after laparoscopic colorectal resection. Dis Colon Rectum 59(8):743–750. https://doi.org/10.1097/DCR.0000000000000632

Benlice C, Stocchi L, Sapci I et al (2019) Impact of the extraction-site location on wound infections after laparoscopic colorectal resection. Am J Surg 217(3):502–506. https://doi.org/10.1016/j.amjsurg.2018.10.034

Bou Saleh N, Voron T, De'Angelis N et al (2020) Intracorporeal versus extracorporeal anastomosis in laparoscopic right hemicolectomy: results from the CLIMHET study group. Tech Coloproctol 24(6):585–592. https://doi.org/10.1007/s10151-020-02202-z

Bouras G, Lee SW, Nomura E, Tokuhara T, Nitta T, Yoshinaka R, Tsunemi S, Tanigawa N (2011) Surgical outcomes from laparoscopic distal gastrectomy and Roux-en-Y reconstruction: evolution in a totally intracorporeal technique. Surg Laparosc Endosc Percutan Tech 21(1):37–41. https://doi.org/10.1097/SLE.0b013e3182073fdb

Ceresoli M, Pisano M, Abu-Zidan F et al (2022) Minimally invasive surgery in emergency surgery: a WSES survey. World J Emerg Surg 17:18

Chin YH, Decruz GM, Ng CH et al (2021) Colorectal resection via natural orifice specimen extraction versus conventional laparoscopic extraction: a meta-analysis with meta-regression. Tech Coloproctol 25(1):35–48. https://doi.org/10.1007/s10151-020-02330-6

Chok AY, Tan IE, Zhao Y et al (2023) Clinical outcomes and cost comparison of laparoscopic versus open surgery in elderly colorectal cancer patients over 80 years. Int J Color Dis 38(1):160. https://doi.org/10.1007/s00384-023-04459-w

Deijen CL, Vasmel JE, de Lange-de Klerk ESM, Cuesta MA, Coene PLO, Lange JF, Meijerink WJHJ, Jakimowicz JJ, Jeekel J, Kazemier G, Janssen IMC, Påhlman L, Haglind E, Bonjer HJ, COLOR (COlon cancer Laparoscopic or Open Resection) Study Group (2017) Ten-year outcomes of a randomised trial of laparoscopic versus open surgery for colon cancer. Surg Endosc 31(6):2607–2615. https://doi.org/10.1007/s00464-016-5270-6

Feng Q, Yuan W, Li T et al (2022) Robotic versus laparoscopic surgery for middle and low rectal cancer (REAL): short-term outcomes of a multicentre randomised controlled trial. Lancet Gastroenterol Hepatol 7(11):991–1004. https://doi.org/10.1016/S2468-1253(22)00248-5

Fujii S, Tsukamoto M, Fukushima Y, Shimada R, Okamoto K, Tsuchiya T, Nozawa K, Matsuda K, Hashiguchi Y (2016) Systematic review of laparoscopic vs open surgery for colorectal cancer in elderly patients. World J Gastrointest Oncol 8(7):573–582

Gandaglia G, Ghani KR, Sood A et al (2014) Effect of minimally invasive surgery on the risk for surgical site infections: results from the National Surgical Quality Improvement Program (NSQIP) database. JAMA Surg 149(10):1039–1044. https://doi.org/10.1001/jamasurg.2014.292

Izquierdo KM, Unal E, Marks JH (2018) Natural orifice specimen extraction in colorectal surgery: patient selection and perspectives. Clin Exp Gastroenterol 11:265–279. https://doi.org/10.2147/CEG.S135331

Kim MJ, Fleming FJ, Gunzler DD, Messing S, Salloum RM, Monson JR (2011) Laparoscopic appendectomy is safe and efficacious for the elderly: an analysis using the National Surgical Quality Improvement Project database. Surg Endosc 25(6):1802–1807. https://doi.org/10.1007/s00464-010-1467-2

Kim MJ, Park SC, Park JW et al (2018) Robot-assisted versus laparoscopic surgery for rectal cancer: a phase II open label prospective randomized controlled trial. Ann Surg 267(2):243–251. https://doi.org/10.1097/SLA.0000000000002321

Leinert C, Fotteler M, Kocar TD, Dallmeier D, Kestler HA, Wolf D, Gebhard F, Uihlein A, Steger F, Kilian R, Mueller-Stierlin AS, Michalski CW, Mihaljevic A, Bolenz C, Zengerling F, Leinert E, Schütze S, Hoffmann TK, Onder G, Andersen-Ranberg K, O'Neill D, Wehling M, Schobel J, Swoboda W, Denkinger M, SURGE-Ahead Study Group (2023) Supporting SURgery with GEriatric co-management and AI (SURGE-ahead): a study protocol for the development of a digital geriatrician. PLoS One 18(6):e0287230. https://doi.org/10.1371/journal.pone.0287230

Leitao MM Jr, Zhou QC, Brandt B et al (2022) The MEMORY Study: MulticentEr study of Minimally invasive surgery versus Open Radical hYsterectomy in the management of early-stage cervical cancer: survival outcomes. Gynecol Oncol 166(3):417–424. https://doi.org/10.1016/j.ygyno.2022.07.002

Lin PL, Zheng F, Shin M, Liu X, Oh D, D'Attilio D (2023) CUSUM learning curves: what they can and can't tell us. Surg Endosc 37(10):7991–7999. https://doi.org/10.1007/s00464-023-10252-1

Litynski GS (1998a) Kurt Semm and the fight against skepticism: endoscopic hemostasis, laparoscopic appendectomy, and Semm's impact on the "laparoscopic revolution". JSLS 2:309–313

Litynski GS (1998b) Erich Mühe and the rejection of laparoscopic cholecystectomy (1985): a surgeon ahead of his time. JSLS 2:341–346

Liu X, Yuan X, Ye P, Yang J, Li K (2025) Comparison of postoperative inflammatory response between natural orifice specimen extraction surgery and conventional laparoscopy in the treatment of colorectal cancer: a meta-analysis and systematic review. Int J Surg 111(1):1244–1254. https://doi.org/10.1097/JS9.0000000000001912

Lu J, Xu BB, Zheng HL et al (2024) Robotic versus laparoscopic distal gastrectomy for resectable gastric cancer: a randomized phase 2 trial. Nat Commun 15(1):4668. https://doi.org/10.1038/s41467-024-49013-6

Massie MT, Massie LB, Marrangoni AG, D'Amico FJ, Sell HW Jr (1993) Advantages of laparoscopic cholecystectomy in the elderly and in patients with high ASA classifications. J Laparoendosc Surg 3(5):467–476. https://doi.org/10.1089/lps.1993.3.467

Nelson H, Sargent DJ, Wieand HS et al (2004) A comparison of laparoscopically assisted and open colectomy for colon cancer. N Engl J Med 350:2050–2059. https://doi.org/10.1056/NEJMoa032651

Ojima T, Nakamura M, Hayata K et al (2021) Short-term outcomes of robotic gastrectomy vs laparoscopic gastrectomy for patients with gastric cancer: a randomized clinical trial. JAMA Surg 156(10):954–963. https://doi.org/10.1001/jamasurg.2021.3182

Park JS, Lee SM, Choi GS et al (2023) Comparison of laparoscopic versus robot-assisted surgery for rectal cancers: the COLRAR randomized controlled trial. Ann Surg 278(1):31. https://doi.org/10.1097/SLA.0000000000005788

Rea IM, Gibson DS, McGilligan V, McNerlan SE, Alexander HD, Ross OA (2018) Age and age-related diseases: role of inflammation triggers and cytokines. Front Immunol 9:586. https://doi.org/10.3389/fimmu.2018.00586

Rudnicka E, Napierała P, Podfigurna A, Męczekalski B, Smolarczyk R, Grymowicz M (2020) The World Health Organization (WHO) approach to healthy ageing. Maturitas 139:6–11. https://doi.org/10.1016/j.maturitas.2020.05.018

Safran DB, Orlando R 3rd (1994) Physiologic effects of pneumoperitoneum. Am J Surg 167(2):281–286

Semm K (1988) Pelviscopic appendectomy (in German). Dtsch Med Wochenschr 113:3–5

Tan KY, Tan P, Tan L (2011) A collaborative transdisciplinary "geriatric surgery service" ensures consistent successful outcomes in elderly colorectal surgery patients. World J Surg 35(7):1608–1614. https://doi.org/10.1007/s00268-011-1112-9

Uccella S, Bonzini M, Palomba S et al (2016) Laparoscopic vs. open treatment of endometrial cancer in the elderly and very elderly: an age-stratified multicenter study on 1606 women. Gynecol Oncol 141(2):211–217. https://doi.org/10.1016/j.ygyno.2016.02.029

Vaghiri S, Prassas D, Krieg S, Knoefel WT, Krieg A (2023) Intracorporeal versus extracorporeal colo-colic anastomosis in minimally-invasive left colectomy: a systematic review and meta-analysis. J Gastrointest Surg 27(12):3024. https://doi.org/10.1007/s11605-023-05827-1

Zhao Z, Gu J (2022) Open surgery in the era of minimally invasive surgery. Chin J Cancer Res 34(1):63–65. https://doi.org/10.21147/j.issn.1000-9604.2022.01.06

12 Strategies for Older Women Undergoing Breast Surgery

Rachel Xue-Ning Lee and Clement Luck-Khng Chia

12.1 Introduction

The global trend of population ageing is irreversible. In 2021, one in ten people worldwide were aged 65 years and above. According to the World Social Report 2023 (United Nations Department of Economic and Social Affairs 2023), it is projected that by 2050, this age group will account for one in six people globally. Breast cancer is the most common malignancy in females worldwide; its incidence correlates with increasing age (World Cancer Research Fund International 2024). In 2020, approximately 48% of the 2.26 million new cases of breast cancer diagnoses worldwide were in older women aged 65 years and above (Cancer Research UK 2015; Brendler-Spaeth et al. 2020). In the USA, a study conducted in 2015 has estimated that the number of invasive breast cancer cases will double by 2030, of which older women aged 70–84 were expected to make up a larger rising proportion of diagnoses, increasing from 24% in 2011 to 35% (Breast Cancer Research Foundation 2021). As life expectancy increases and the population ages, understanding the specific considerations for breast cancer in older women becomes increasingly important.

R. X.-N. Lee
Nottingham Breast Cancer Research Centre, University of Nottingham, Nottingham, UK

Royal Derby Hospital, University Hospitals of Derby and Burton NHS Foundation Trust, Derby, UK

C. L.-K. Chia (✉)
Khoo Teck Puat Hospital, NHG Health, Singapore, Singapore

Lee Kong Chian School of Medicine, Nanyang Technological University, Singapore, Singapore

Yong Loo Lin School of Medicine, National University of Singapore, Singapore, Singapore
e-mail: chia.clement.lk@ktph.com.sg

K.-Y. Tan et al. (eds.), *Mastering Geriatric Surgery*,
https://doi.org/10.1007/978-981-95-0665-1_12

This chapter will explore an older patient's breast cancer journey from the time of screening for breast cancer, treatment options, psychosocial support, prognosis and follow-up care. There are important considerations for personalising the care of breast cancer in older women, which can be categorised into patient-, physician- and system-associated factors, as seen in Fig. 12.1. There is a complex interplay between these factors throughout an older patient's breast cancer journey.

12.2 Breast Cancer Screening

One of the primary considerations for breast cancer in older women is screening. In the United Kingdom (UK), women aged 50–70 are offered mammograms every 3 years as part of the population screening programme (National Institute for Health and Care Excellence 2022). While mammography remains the gold standard for breast cancer screening, there is ongoing debate regarding the age at which screening should be stopped in older women. The Ministry of Health of Singapore (Ministry of Health Singapore 2010) and German Guideline Program in Oncology (Wöckel et al. 2018) recommended stopping screening at age 70. Some guidelines, including those of American Cancer Society, American College of Radiology and Brazilian Society for Breast Disease, recommended that the age to end screening

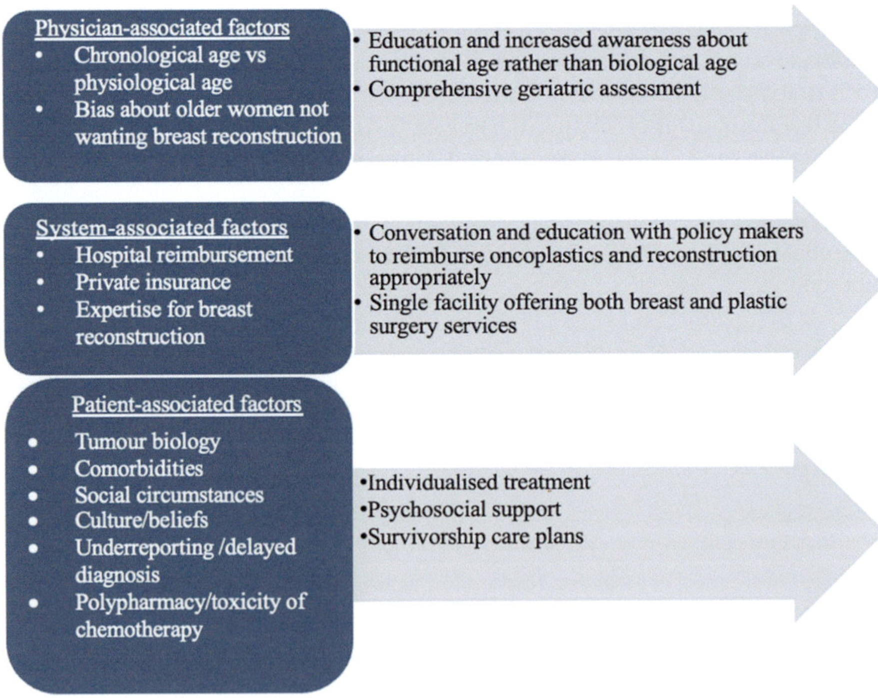

Fig. 12.1 Considerations for breast cancer in older women

should be determined based on the patient's health status and to consider stopping screening for women whose life expectancy is lower than 5–7 years or 10 years. Some guidelines recommend continuing regular mammography screening for women aged 65 and older, while others suggest individualised screening based on a woman's overall health and life expectancy. We believe that rather than looking at age as an absolute 'number', the functional and personal health status of the patient should be considered before recommending whether to screen the patient for breast cancer, as seen in Fig. 12.2.

12.3 Breast Cancer Treatment Options

The management of breast cancer in older women requires a comprehensive understanding of tumour biology, patient characteristics and treatment tolerability. Surgery, radiation therapy, chemotherapy, hormone therapy and targeted therapies constitute the mainstay of treatment, but their utilisation may vary based on factors such as tumour subtype, stage and patient comorbidities.

Older women diagnosed with breast cancer exhibit a wide range of diversity, encompassing variations in physiological status, personal priorities and social dynamics. Consequently, they encounter distinct challenges throughout each phase of their breast cancer treatment and may undergo different treatment modalities.

12.3.1 Surgery

Surgery is a key element of treatment for early breast cancer, with significant benefit in terms of local control and survival. We have summarised the surgical options available for older patients with breast cancer in Table 12.1. A few guidelines

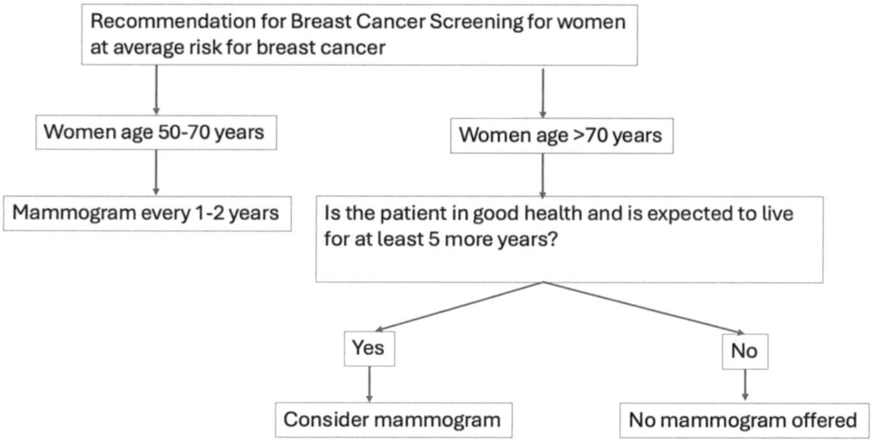

Fig. 12.2 Breast cancer screening algorithm

Table 12.1 Summary of surgical options for older patients with breast cancer

Surgical options for older patients with breast cancer
• Breast surgery – Breast-conserving surgery – Mastectomy – Breast reconstruction • Axillary surgery – Axillary lymph node dissection – Sentinel lymph node biopsy – Targeted axillary dissection – Omission of axillary surgery

(National Institute for Health and Care Excellence 2016; Biganzoli et al. 2021) have stated that patients should be offered the same breast cancer treatment options irrespective of age but with careful consideration of individual preferences and coexisting comorbidities. However, surgery has higher morbidity rates and significant rates of functional decline post-surgery (Morgan et al. 2020). In some older women who declined surgery as the primary treatment for cancer and breast reconstruction, old age (Schonberg et al. 2014; Morgan et al. 2015) and concerns about surgery impacting their independence (Lu et al. 2010; Burton et al. 2015) were cited as reasons.

Considering that older women have coexisting health and social care needs, introducing a comprehensive geriatric assessment (CGA) into breast clinics may assist surgeons in assessing older women's fitness for treatment and appropriateness of treatment (Parks et al. 2012). This will help surgeons develop a personalised approach to assessing older women's suitability for different types of breast cancer treatment, breast reconstruction options and maximising their quality of life.

Over the last three decades, there has been a considerable evolution of the role of axillary surgery in the management of breast cancer, moving away from axillary lymph node dissection to sentinel lymph node biopsy, to perhaps omission of axillary surgery in selected patients (Boughey et al. 2013; Kuehn et al. 2013; Donker et al. 2014; Jung et al. 2022). The 'Choosing Wisely' initiative launched by the American Board of Internal Medicine Foundation recommended the omission of sentinel node biopsy in women aged 70 years and above, with early-stage hormone receptor-positive, HER2-negative invasive breast cancer, who are clinically node-negative women (Grossi et al. 2023). In recent years, targeted axillary dissection emerged in an attempt to further reduce the false-negative rate of sentinel lymph node dissection in patients who underwent neoadjuvant chemotherapy. This trend towards de-escalation of axillary surgery has been supported by many studies that demonstrated a reduction in patient morbidity without compromising oncologic outcomes (Classe et al. 2019; Piltin et al. 2020; Wong et al. 2021). Similarly, in the older population, the PRIME II trial (Kunkler et al. 2023) concluded that although the omission of radiotherapy after breast-conserving surgery in women aged 65 years and above with hormone receptor-positive early breast cancer receiving adjuvant endocrine therapy was associated with an increased risk of local recurrence (9.5% vs 0.9%), it had no detrimental effect on distant recurrence or overall survival. Given that lymphoedema and limited shoulder ability after breast cancer surgery present a significant concern for survivors (Fu and Rosedale 2009), it is even more challenging to older women as these restrict their ability to carry out their daily activities and independence (Fenlon et al. 2013); as such, the move towards de-escalating axilla surgery should be even more strongly considered in this group of patients. We have included a summary of axillary management algorithm in older patients, as seen in Fig. 12.3.

12.3.2 Breast Reconstruction

Despite the demonstrable benefits of post-mastectomy immediate breast reconstruction, the uptake of PMIBR remains lower in older women. The UK's National Audit of Breast Cancer in Older Patients 2021 annual report (NABCOP 2021) clearly demonstrated that women aged 70 and over were less likely to receive PMIBR and standardised breast cancer treatment in comparison to younger women. The reasons behind this disparity in the uptake of PMIBR in older women can be divided into three categories: surgeon, system and patient factors, as seen in Table 12.2 (Lee et al. 2022).

12.3.2.1 Surgeon Factors

Patients' decisions are strongly influenced by surgeons. A study reported that 'surgeon strong recommendation' was reported by approximately 92% of women as a reason for undergoing post-mastectomy breast reconstruction (Ishak et al. 2018). Surgeons may have an increasingly significant role in the treatment decisions for older women, who were described to depend heavily on healthcare professionals' advice, believing that treatment should be determined by surgeons with specialised knowledge and expertise (Burton et al. 2015).

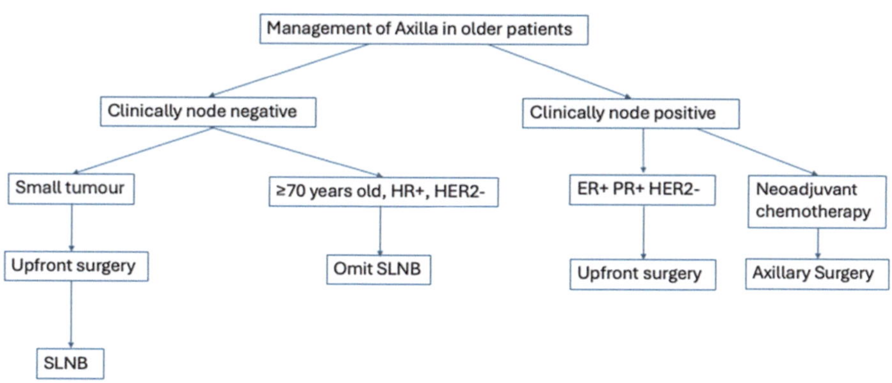

Fig. 12.3 Summary of axillary management in older patients

Table 12.2 Factors affecting the uptake of PMIBR in older women

Surgeon factors	System factors	Patient factors
• Surgeon's recommendations	• Insurance status • Hospital type and location	• Age • Comorbidities • Socioeconomic status • Ethnicity

12.3.2.2 System Factors

A recent study highlighted how system-associated factors like outdated reimbursement policies have adversely influenced best clinical practices for breast cancer care (Cardoso et al. 2019). Healthcare funders have often mistaken oncoplastic and reconstructive breast surgery for cosmetic surgery, categorising them as non-essential. Consequently, reimbursement policies fail to reflect the true costs of these complex surgeries. This discrepancy results in hospitals incurring an economic loss for each operation, which restricts the volume of surgeries performed and the availability of breast reconstruction services.

Access to breast reconstruction may be influenced by various factors including the healthcare system of the country of residence, personal income and the availability of health insurance. Higher income and private insurance coverage often facilitate the access to post-mastectomy breast reconstruction. Studies have shown that African American (AA) women with higher income are more likely to undergo PMBR.

In the UK, where there is universal access to the National Health Service (NHS), there exists significant regional variation in PMBR uptake depending on patients' residential addresses, a phenomenon known as the "postcode lottery". This indicates that women may face unequal access to various types of breast reconstruction procedures (Jeevan et al. 2010). As not all hospitals provide oncoplastic or plastic surgery services, patients may need to travel considerable distances to access specific hospitals that offer breast reconstruction procedures. Given that older women may face unique challenges such as caregiving responsibilities, financial constraints and limited social support networks, travelling long distances to a different hospital for a second operation such as delayed reconstruction may not be feasible.

12.3.2.3 Patient Factors

Traditionally, increased patient morbidity has been cited as a barrier to offering breast reconstruction (Spyrou et al. 1998). The presence of comorbidities and the change in perception of body image with ageing may also explain why some older women are less likely to receive IBR compared to younger women. Studies have also reported a significantly lower uptake of PMBR in some ethnic groups such as African American, Hispanic and Asian women (Yang et al. 2013; Butler et al. 2016).

12.3.3 Hormonal Therapy

Surgical interventions encompass a spectrum of approaches, ranging from simple local excision to various forms of wider excision like segmental resection, quadrantectomy and mastectomy. Surgery seems to offer better local control of breast cancer (Chan et al. 2023); however, primary endocrine therapy is still an appropriate option for women with ER-positive tumours who are unfit for surgery or do not consent for surgery (Hind et al. 2007).

Older women with breast cancer are usually diagnosed with more favourable tumour biology compared to younger women. In general, breast cancer in older patients is a more indolent disease, with favourable features including lower histologic grade, lower proliferative indices, less peritumoral vascular invasion and more well-differentiated tumours as compared to younger patients (Wildiers et al. 2007; Le Saux et al. 2015). Considering that nearly a third of all breast cancer cases occur in older women (aged 70 years and above), with most cases being oestrogen receptor-positive (ER+), this allows us to focus on unique clinical considerations for screening, detection and treatment regimens for older women who develop ER+ breast cancers specifically. Table 12.3 outlines several factors to consider when addressing hormonal therapy in older patients. Older women may be more susceptible to treatment-related toxicities and less tolerant to aggressive interventions, necessitating a judicious approach to treatment decision-making. Moreover, considerations regarding functional status, cognitive function and social support networks should inform treatment recommendations to optimise outcomes and minimise treatment-related morbidity.

12.3.4 Chemotherapy

While numerous studies have assessed the impact of ageing on cancer, few have focused on therapeutic decision-making among older adults. In early-stage breast cancer, the decision-making process for chemotherapy in older women is complex (Puts et al. 2015). Some studies have indicated that older women derive comparable benefits from adjuvant chemotherapy compared to their younger counterparts (Carlson et al. 2008; Tew et al. 2014). However, due to the under-representation of

Table 12.3 Summary of considerations for approach to hormonal therapy in older patients

Considerations for older patients on hormonal therapy
1. Side effects of medications
• Bone health/risk of osteoporosis
– Yearly bone mineral density test
• Joint aches and pain associated with aromatase inhibitors
2. Risks of toxicity
• Comorbidities
• Polypharmacy
3. Patient preferences and adherence to treatment

older adults in clinical trials, which has led to under- and overtreatment of breast cancer (Bertagnolli and Singh 2021), more efforts are needed to understand the safety and efficacy of chemotherapy in this population (Hurria et al. 2015).

Few studies that have examined decisions regarding chemotherapy in older women with early-stage breast cancer have suggested that treatment decision-making in older breast cancer patients is often influenced by various factors. These factors may include tumour characteristics, the balance between treatment benefits and risks, logistical considerations such as transportation and patient's comorbidities (Schonberg et al. 2014). A qualitative study looked at older women's information-gathering processes and contextual considerations related to their decision-making (Karuturi et al. 2022). Quality-of-life trade-offs, family roles, spirituality and anecdotal stories from others influenced their consideration for adjuvant chemotherapy. Fostering active engagement and open communication between clinicians, older women and their support networks may contribute to higher quality decision-making in the context of adjuvant chemotherapy among older women with breast cancer. From a clinical perspective, CGA can be used to determine the factors affecting survival and quality of life in breast cancer patients and can therefore be used to aid treatment decision-making (Reid-Agboola et al. 2023).

12.4 Psychosocial Support

Breast cancer diagnosis and treatment can have significant psychosocial implications for older women. According to a systematic review (Angarita et al. 2020), older women experienced unique barriers to breast cancer treatment due to physiological and psychosocial reasons. Older women who had pre-existing medical conditions influenced the treatments they could tolerate. Several psychosocial factors influenced older women's breast cancer treatment experience. Older women who needed assistance from others to travel to hospital appointments experienced psychological distress as they saw themselves as a burden to their support system (Pieters et al. 2011), complicating their ability to attend multiple hospital appointments. In contrast, those who received help from their families for transportation had a more seamless breast cancer treatment experience (Lu et al. 2010). Another social barrier is some older women have a caregiving role. Having to attend multiple hospital appointments while caring for their partners proves challenging, leading them to ignore their symptoms and health problems (29). However, for others, the prospect of being able to continue caregiving for their frail partners may motivate them to accept treatment (Lu et al. 2010). Given this variability, it is imperative that the clinician considers each older woman's unique social circumstances before recommending a personalised treatment plan.

Psychological complications of breast cancer diagnosis and treatment in older women may include concerns about body image, sexuality, relationships and end-of-life planning. Body image is important for older women. In some women, their main concern after surgery was disfigurement (Husain et al. 2008). It was reported that some women felt less of a woman because they had lost their breast, and some consider cosmetic disfigurement the worse part of their breast cancer treatment experience, regardless of whether they are married or widowed (Husain et al. 2008). Therefore, comprehensive care for older women with breast cancer should include psychosocial support services such as counselling, support groups and assistance with practical issues like transportation and financial planning.

12.5 Prognosis

Breast cancer incidence dramatically increases with age and will rise with the expanding population of older adults and increasing life expectancy. As older adults make up a larger proportion of new breast cancer diagnoses, it is important to understand the age-related disparities in breast cancer.

In general, breast cancer in older patients is a more indolent disease and displays less aggressive biological features including lower histologic grade, lower proliferative indices, less peritumoral vascular invasion and more well-differentiated tumours as compared to younger patients (Wildiers et al. 2007; Le Saux et al. 2015). Even if older women referred to surgery had larger tumour size and greater lymph node involvement (Wildiers et al. 2009), they have a more favourable biologic tumour profile overall; as the human epidermal receptor 2 (HER2) positivity decreases with age, ER positivity increases with age (Anderson et al. 2011). The proportion of ER-positive cancer increases from 56% among women aged 30–34 years to 85% among women aged 80–84 years (Anderson et al. 2011).

Improvements in breast cancer screening and advances in treatments (Walton et al. 2011) have improved breast cancer mortality rates over time. However, survival among women diagnosed in older age has not substantially improved. Many studies have revealed that breast cancer-related mortality increases with patient's age, regardless of the disease stage (Bastiaannet et al. 2010; Rosso et al. 2010; Smith et al. 2011). A few reasons that could contribute toward the worse prognosis seen in older women with breast cancer compared to their younger counterparts include decreased tolerability of treatment, comorbidities and potential overtreatment which adversely affects the morbidity and mortality of older patients. This age-related disparity in prognosis has largely been attributed to advanced disease at presentation related to delays in time to diagnosis.

12.6 Follow-Up Care

The survival rates for breast cancer patients are steadily increasing, exceeding 80% at 10 years for early-stage breast cancers (Shapiro 2018; Siegel et al. 2022), due to advances in early diagnosis and multimodal effective therapeutic strategies. As breast cancer is being considered a chronic condition rather than a life-threatening condition, this now presents new challenges for healthcare professionals. They must be able to manage the long-term side effects of treatments and also manage pre-existing health issues which may be exacerbated by their treatment (Bodai and Tuso 2015). Studies have revealed that up to 50% of breast cancer survivors live with at least one distressing long-term physical symptom (Ferreira et al. 2019), 30% face emotional distress (Charles et al. 2022) and 20% struggle to rejoin workforce (Dumas et al. 2020).

After completing their breast cancer treatment, older women require ongoing survivorship care and monitoring. Survivorship care plans (SCPs) are sometimes called a follow-up care plan upon a patient's discharge from cancer treatment to the community (Hewitt et al. 2005). The objective of SCPs is to enhance the coordination and continuity of patient care by providing adequate information about cancer treatment and follow-up care from cancer specialist teams to primary care providers (Hewitt et al. 2005; Cancer Care Ontario 2019). SCPs are highly endorsed by cancer survivors (Palmer et al. 2015; Husain et al. 2019; Nekhlyudov et al. 2019), evidenced by literature reviews supporting the utilisation of SCPs in improving disease management. Older women may benefit from having regular follow-up visits with healthcare providers to monitor for recurrence or late effects of treatment and being taught strategies for managing long-term side effects. They may also benefit from lifestyle recommendations such as good dietary habits, physical activity and smoking cessation to prevent further preventable disease.

In conclusion, older women with breast cancer have unique challenges at various stages of their breast cancer journey. There is a complex interplay between the patient, surgeon and system factors throughout an older patient's breast cancer journey that may affect an older woman's treatment choice and experience. Older women may benefit from more proactive treatment discussions with the wider multidisciplinary team involved in a breast cancer patient's care to address their specific needs.

References

Anderson WF, Katki HA, Rosenberg PS (2011) Incidence of breast cancer in the United States: current and future trends. J Natl Cancer Inst 103(18):1397–1402. https://doi.org/10.1093/jnci/djr257

Angarita FA et al (2020) Older women's experience with breast cancer treatment: a systematic review of qualitative literature. Breast (Edinburgh, Scotland) 54:293–302. https://doi.org/10.1016/j.breast.2020.11.009

Bastiaannet E et al (2010) Breast cancer in elderly compared to younger patients in The Netherlands: stage at diagnosis, treatment and survival in 127,805 unselected patients. Breast Cancer Res Treat 124(3):801–807. https://doi.org/10.1007/s10549-010-0898-8

Bertagnolli MM, Singh H (2021) Treatment of older adults with cancer - addressing gaps in evidence. N Engl J Med 385(12):1062–1065. https://doi.org/10.1056/NEJMp2106089

Biganzoli L et al (2021) Updated recommendations regarding the management of older patients with breast cancer: a joint paper from the European Society of Breast Cancer Specialists (EUSOMA) and the International Society of Geriatric Oncology (SIOG). Lancet Oncol 22(7):e327–e340. https://doi.org/10.1016/S1470-2045(20)30741-5

Bodai BI, Tuso P (2015) Breast cancer survivorship: a comprehensive review of long-term medical issues and lifestyle recommendations. Perm J 19(2):48–79. https://doi.org/10.7812/TPP/14-241

Boughey JC et al (2013) Sentinel lymph node surgery after neoadjuvant chemotherapy in patients with node-positive breast cancer: the ACOSOG Z1071 (Alliance) clinical trial. JAMA 310(14):1455–1461. https://doi.org/10.1001/jama.2013.278932

Breast Cancer Research Foundation (2021) Breast cancer in the elderly: treating this growing patient population. https://www.bcrf.org/blog/breast-cancer-elderly-treating-growing-patient-population/. Accessed 15 July 2024

Brendler-Spaeth CI et al (2020) Autologous breast reconstruction in older women: a retrospective single-centre analysis of complications and uptake of secondary reconstructive procedures. J Plast Reconstr Aesthet Surg 73(5):856–864. https://doi.org/10.1016/j.bjps.2019.11.039

Burton M et al (2015) The information and decision support needs of older women (>75 yrs) facing treatment choices for breast cancer: a qualitative study. Psycho-Oncology 24(8):878–884. https://doi.org/10.1002/pon.3735

Butler P et al (2016) Racial and age disparities persist in immediate breast reconstruction: an updated analysis of 48,564 patients from the 2005 to 2011 American College of Surgeons National Surgery Quality Improvement Program data sets. Am J Surg 212(1):96–101. https://doi.org/10.1016/j.amjsurg.2015.08.025

Cancer Care Ontario (2019) Follow-up model of care for cancer survivors. https://www.cancercareontario.ca/sites/ccocancercare/files/assets/FollowUpModelsOfCareRecommendations.pdf

Cancer Research UK (2015) Breast cancer incidence (invasive) statistics. Cancer Research UK. https://www.cancerresearchuk.org/health-professional/cancer-statistics/statistics-by-cancer-type/breast-cancer/incidence-invasive. Accessed 15 July 2024

Cardoso F et al (2019) Early breast cancer: ESMO Clinical Practice Guidelines for diagnosis, treatment and follow-up†. Ann Oncol 30(8):1194–1220. https://doi.org/10.1093/annonc/mdz173

Carlson RW et al (2008) NCCN task force report: breast cancer in the older woman. J Natl Compr Cancer Netw 6 Suppl 4:S1–S25; quiz S26–27

Chan KS et al (2023) Revisiting primary endocrine therapy versus surgery in older women with breast cancer: meta-analysis. Br J Surg 110(4):420–431. https://doi.org/10.1093/bjs/znac435

Charles C et al (2022) Characterization of depressive symptoms trajectories after breast cancer diagnosis in women in France. JAMA Netw Open 5(4):e225118. https://doi.org/10.1001/jamanetworkopen.2022.5118

Classe J-M et al (2019) Sentinel lymph node biopsy without axillary lymphadenectomy after neoadjuvant chemotherapy is accurate and safe for selected patients: the GANEA 2 study. Breast Cancer Res Treat 173(2):343–352. https://doi.org/10.1007/s10549-018-5004-7

Donker M et al (2014) Radiotherapy or surgery of the axilla after a positive sentinel node in breast cancer (EORTC 10981-22023 AMAROS): a randomised, multicentre, open-label, phase 3 non-inferiority trial. Lancet Oncol 15(12):1303–1310. https://doi.org/10.1016/S1470-2045(14)70460-7

Dumas A et al (2020) Impact of breast cancer treatment on employment: results of a multicenter prospective cohort study (CANTO). J Clin Oncol Off J Am Soc Clin Oncol 38(7):734–743. https://doi.org/10.1200/JCO.19.01726

Fenlon D et al (2013) Living into old age with the consequences of breast cancer. Eur J Oncol Nurs 17(3):311–316. https://doi.org/10.1016/j.ejon.2012.08.004

Ferreira AR et al (2019) Differential impact of endocrine therapy and chemotherapy on quality of life of breast cancer survivors: a prospective patient-reported outcomes analysis. Ann Oncol 30(11):1784–1795. https://doi.org/10.1093/annonc/mdz298

Fu MR, Rosedale M (2009) Breast cancer survivors' experiences of lymphedema-related symptoms. J Pain Symptom Manage 38(6):849–859. https://doi.org/10.1016/j.jpainsymman.2009.04.030

Grossi S, Le J, Armani A (2023) Omitting axillary staging in selected patients: rationale of choosing wisely in breast cancer treatment. Surgery 174(2):413–415. https://doi.org/10.1016/j.surg.2023.03.023

Hewitt M, Greenfield S, Stovall E (2005) From cancer patient to cancer survivor: lost in transition. National Academies Press, Washington, D.C. https://doi.org/10.17226/11468

Hind D, Wyld L, Reed MW (2007) Surgery, with or without tamoxifen, vs tamoxifen alone for older women with operable breast cancer: Cochrane review. Br J Cancer 96(7):1025–1029. https://doi.org/10.1038/sj.bjc.6603600

Hurria A et al (2015) Improving the evidence base for treating older adults with cancer: American Society of Clinical Oncology statement. J Clin Oncol Off J Am Soc Clin Oncol 33(32):3826–3833. https://doi.org/10.1200/JCO.2015.63.0319

Husain LS et al (2008) Choices in cancer treatment: a qualitative study of the older women's (>70 years) perspective. Psycho-Oncology 17(4):410–416. https://doi.org/10.1002/pon.1242

Husain M et al (2019) An overview of the unique challenges facing African-American breast cancer survivors. Support Care Cancer 27(3):729–743. https://doi.org/10.1007/s00520-018-4545-y

Ishak A, Yahya MM, Halim AS (2018) Breast reconstruction after mastectomy: a survey of surgeons' and patients' perceptions. Clin Breast Cancer 18(5):e1011–e1021. https://doi.org/10.1016/j.clbc.2018.04.012

Jeevan R et al (2010) Regional variation in use of immediate breast reconstruction after mastectomy for breast cancer in England. Eur J Surg Oncol 36(8):750–755. https://doi.org/10.1016/j.ejso.2010.06.008

Jung JG et al (2022) No axillary surgical treatment for lymph node-negative patients after ultrasonography [NAUTILUS]: protocol of a prospective randomized clinical trial. BMC Cancer 22(1):189. https://doi.org/10.1186/s12885-022-09273-1

Karuturi MS et al (2022) Exploring and supporting older women's chemotherapy decision-making in early-stage breast cancer. J Geriatr Oncol 13(2):170–175. https://doi.org/10.1016/j.jgo.2021.11.018

Kuehn T et al (2013) Sentinel-lymph-node biopsy in patients with breast cancer before and after neoadjuvant chemotherapy (SENTINA): a prospective, multicentre cohort study. Lancet Oncol 14(7):609–618. https://doi.org/10.1016/S1470-2045(13)70166-9

Kunkler IH et al (2023) Breast-conserving surgery with or without irradiation in early breast cancer. N Engl J Med 388:585–594. https://doi.org/10.1056/NEJMoa2207586

Le Saux O et al (2015) Optimal management of breast cancer in the elderly patient: current perspectives. Clin Interv Aging 10:157–174. https://doi.org/10.2147/CIA.S50670

Lee RXN et al (2022) Immediate breast reconstruction uptake in older women with primary breast cancer: systematic review. Br J Surg 109(11):1063–1072. https://doi.org/10.1093/bjs/znac251

Lu M-H, Lin H-R, Lee M-D (2010) The experiences among older Taiwanese women facing a new diagnosis of breast cancer. Cancer Nurs 33(5):398. https://doi.org/10.1097/NCC.0b013e3181d72c45

Ministry of Health Singapore (2010) Cancer screening MOH clinical practice guidelines. https://www.moh.gov.sg/docs/librariesprovider4/guidelines/cpg_cancer-screening.pdf. Accessed 15 July 2024

Morgan JL et al (2015) The balance of clinician and patient input into treatment decision-making in older women with operable breast cancer. Psycho-Oncology 24(12):1761–1766. https://doi.org/10.1002/pon.3853

Morgan JL et al (2020) Breast cancer surgery in older women: outcomes of the Bridging Age Gap in Breast Cancer study. Br J Surg 107(11):1468–1479. https://doi.org/10.1002/bjs.11617

NABCOP (2021) NABCOP 2021 annual report. National Audit of Breast Cancer in Older Patients. https://www.nabcop.org.uk/reports/nabcop-2021-annual-report/. Accessed 15 July 2024

National Institute for Health and Care Excellence (2016) Breast cancer. NICE. https://www.nice.org.uk/guidance/qs12. Accessed 15 July 2024

National Institute for Health and Care Excellence (2022) The NHS breast screening programme | Background information | Breast screening | CKS | NICE. https://cks.nice.org.uk/topics/breast-screening/background-information/the-nhs-breast-screening-programme/. Accessed 15 July 2024

Nekhlyudov L et al (2019) Developing a quality of cancer survivorship care framework: implications for clinical care, research, and policy. J Natl Cancer Inst 111(11):1120–1130. https://doi.org/10.1093/jnci/djz089

Palmer SC et al (2015) Outcomes and satisfaction after delivery of a breast cancer survivorship care plan: results of a multicenter trial. J Oncol Pract 11(2):e222–e229. https://doi.org/10.1200/JOP.2014.001404

Parks RM et al (2012) Comprehensive geriatric assessment for older women with early breast cancer - a systematic review of literature. World J Surg Oncol 10:88. https://doi.org/10.1186/1477-7819-10-88

Pieters HC et al (2011) Older women's reflections on accessing care across their breast cancer trajectory: navigating beyond the triple barriers. Oncol Nurs Forum 38(2):175–184. https://doi.org/10.1188/11.ONF.175-184

Piltin MA et al (2020) Oncologic outcomes of sentinel lymph node surgery after neoadjuvant chemotherapy for node-positive breast cancer. Ann Surg Oncol 27(12):4795–4801. https://doi.org/10.1245/s10434-020-08900-0

Puts MTE et al (2015) A systematic review of factors influencing older adults' decision to accept or decline cancer treatment. Cancer Treat Rev 41(2):197–215. https://doi.org/10.1016/j.ctrv.2014.12.010

Reid-Agboola C et al (2023) Comprehensive geriatric assessment for older women with early-stage (non-metastatic) breast cancer-an updated systematic review of the literature. Curr Oncol 30(9):8294–8309. https://doi.org/10.3390/curroncol30090602

Rosso S et al (2010) Up-to-date estimates of breast cancer survival for the years 2000-2004 in 11 European countries: the role of screening and a comparison with data from the United States. Eur J Cancer 46(18):3351–3357. https://doi.org/10.1016/j.ejca.2010.09.019

Schonberg MA et al (2014) Older women's experience with breast cancer treatment decisions. Breast Cancer Res Treat 145(1):211–223. https://doi.org/10.1007/s10549-014-2921-y

Shapiro CL (2018) Cancer survivorship. N Engl J Med 379(25):2438–2450. https://doi.org/10.1056/NEJMra1712502

Siegel RL et al (2022) Cancer statistics, 2022 - Siegel – 2022. CA Cancer J Clin 72(1):7–33. https://doi.org/10.3322/caac.21708

Smith BD et al (2011) Improvement in breast cancer outcomes over time: are older women missing out? J Clin Oncol Off J Am Soc Clin Oncol 29(35):4647–4653. https://doi.org/10.1200/JCO.2011.35.8408

Spyrou GE et al (1998) A survey of general surgeons' attitudes towards breast reconstruction after mastectomy. Ann R Coll Surg Engl 80(3):178–183

Tew WP et al (2014) Breast and ovarian cancer in the older woman. J Clin Oncol Off J Am Soc Clin Oncol 32(24):2553–2561. https://doi.org/10.1200/JCO.2014.55.3073

United Nations Department of Economic and Social Affairs (2023) World social report 2023: leaving no one behind in an ageing world. United Nations (World Social Report). https://doi.org/10.18356/9789210019682

Walton L, Ommen K, Audisio RA (2011) Breast reconstruction in elderly women breast cancer: a review. Cancer Treat Rev 37(5):353–357. https://doi.org/10.1016/j.ctrv.2011.02.001

Wildiers H et al (2007) Management of breast cancer in elderly individuals: recommendations of the International Society of Geriatric Oncology. Lancet Oncol 8(12):1101–1115. https://doi.org/10.1016/S1470-2045(07)70378-9

Wildiers H et al (2009) Relationship between age and axillary lymph node involvement in women with breast cancer. J Clin Oncol Off J Am Soc Clin Oncol 27(18):2931–2937. https://doi.org/10.1200/JCO.2008.16.7619

Wöckel A et al (2018) The screening, diagnosis, treatment, and follow-up of breast cancer. Dtsch Arztebl Int 115(18):316–323. https://doi.org/10.3238/arztebl.2018.0316

Wong SM et al (2021) Oncologic safety of sentinel lymph node biopsy alone after neoadjuvant chemotherapy for breast cancer. Ann Surg Oncol 28(5):2621–2629. https://doi.org/10.1245/s10434-020-09211-0

World Cancer Research Fund International (2024) Breast cancer. WCRF International. https://www.wcrf.org/diet-activity-and-cancer/cancer-types/breast-cancer/. Accessed 15 July 2024

Yang RL et al (2013) Racial disparities in immediate breast reconstruction after mastectomy: impact of state and federal health policy changes. Ann Surg Oncol 20(2):399–406. https://doi.org/10.1245/s10434-012-2607-9

Strategies for Older Person Undergoing Colorectal Surgery

13

Kai-Siang Chan, Shen-Leong Oh, and Daniel Jin-Keat Lee

Highlights

1. Older patients undergoing colorectal surgery face distinct challenges that influence both short- and long-term outcomes. Frailty, sarcopenia, and comorbidities contribute to higher surgical risks and recovery complexities.
2. A transdisciplinary, individualized perioperative approach is essential, integrating prehabilitation, risk stratification, and patient-centered decision-making to optimize surgical outcomes.
3. Surgical strategies must be tailored to patient risk profiles, incorporating minimally invasive techniques, staged procedures in high-risk or emergency cases, and surgical palliation to prioritize symptom control and functional preservation.
4. Evidence guiding rectal cancer management often excludes older adults, leaving the impact of surgery and treatment toxicity underexplored. A multimodal strategy is crucial, balancing oncological control with functional outcomes and quality of life.

K.-S. Chan
National Healthcare Group General Surgery Residency, Singapore, Singapore
e-mail: KCHAN023@e.ntu.edu.sg

S.-L. Oh
Colorectal Surgery, Khoo Teck Puat Hospital, Singapore, Singapore
e-mail: oh.shen.leong@ktph.com.sg

D. J.-K. Lee (✉)
General and Colorectal Surgery, Khoo Teck Puat Hospital, Singapore, Singapore
e-mail: Daniel.lee@geriatricsurgery.org.sg

K.-Y. Tan et al. (eds.), *Mastering Geriatric Surgery*,
https://doi.org/10.1007/978-981-95-0665-1_13

13.1 Case Study

Meet Mr. T, an 80-year-old widower who is as resilient as he is reserved. Living a quiet, mostly inactive life, he carries a challenging medical history to match. Parkinson's disease keeps his gait unsteady; a past brush with ischemic heart disease left him with an ejection fraction of 40%; and chronic medical conditions such as hypertension and diabetes have led to kidney impairment, edging him close to requiring dialysis. But in a typical fashion, Mr. T did not like to "make a fuss" and kept quiet even when he noticed unsettling changes in his bowel habits and rectal bleeding. It took him months before mentioning it to anyone. After all, as he put it, "There's always a bit of something to worry about at my age."

Initial investigations revealed a circumferential malignant tumor in the rectosigmoid region, too bulky to let the scope pass. Surgery would be necessary, but given his age and health, the journey from here was not going to be straightforward. The prehabilitation team recommended he start some strength-building exercise before the surgery, but with his shaky balance, these exercises turned into something of an obstacle course. Nevertheless, Mr. T took it in stride, and surgery was scheduled. Then, as if on cue, his story took a twist: Mr. T came down with a Covid-19 pneumonia, needing hospital admission and oxygen therapy—a tough setback for someone already short on physical reserves. This left him even more frail, with added functional decline.

In many ways, Mr. T's case is emblematic of the reality we face with older patients in colorectal surgery. Health conditions layer upon each other, mobility is limited, and unexpected detours—like infections—can quickly change the picture. Beyond the medical complexities, social and psychological factors also weigh heavily; patients like Mr. T may have limited support networks, and the stress of surgery can impact mental health, adding to the challenge of preserving their independence.

While every patient's story is unique, scenarios like Mr. T's are, in fact, quite typical in our work with older adults. They remind us just how complex and nuanced surgical planning can be when balancing immediate surgical needs with the broader goal of preserving the function and quality of life. While the story of Mr. T is a case of newly diagnosed rectosigmoid tumor, this chapter will discuss about the challenges faced with surgical intervention in the older population, as well as key considerations in the surgical planning for colorectal surgery in general.

13.2 Challenges Encountered in Older Patients Undergoing Colorectal Surgery

The global situation is facing a silver tsunami, with about one in six people who will be ≥60 years old by 2030, and people aged ≥80 years are expected to triple by 2050 to reach 426 million (World Health Organization 2024). With an increase in age, there is an associated physiological decline and increase in comorbidities (Mohan et al. 2020). Moreover, syndromes such as frailty and sarcopenia have been shown to be more prevalent in the older population, with an estimated incidence of 24% and 10–27% reported worldwide (O'Caoimh et al. 2021; Petermann-Rocha et al.

2022). Frailty is defined as a clinically recognizable state of increased vulnerability resulting from aging-associated decline in reserve and function (Xue 2011), while sarcopenia is defined as progressive and generalized loss of skeletal muscle mass and strength (Cruz-Jentoft et al. 2018), of which, each has been shown to be independently associated with worse postoperative outcomes, higher short-term mortality, and even inferior long-term survival (Reisinger et al. 2015; Chen et al. 2022).

Apart from these medical problems faced in the older population, there are psychosocial factors which are less explored on. These include cognitive decline, poor medical literacy, differences in health beliefs, social isolation with a lack of adequate social support, and financial difficulties, ultimately impacting health-seeking behaviors (Wallace et al. 2014; Hämmig 2019; Guessous et al. 2010). For instance, in the context of colorectal cancer, Berkowitz et al. reported that there was a concerning 25% and 17% of adults ≥65 years old who have not heard of fecal occult blood test (FOBT) or colonoscopy, respectively, for screening for colorectal cancer (Berkowitz et al. 2008). This may delay the diagnosis of colorectal cancer, result in more advanced disease on presentation, and increase the technical difficulty of surgery (Alexiusdottir et al. 2012; Langenfeld et al. 2024); this is associated with increased operating time, need for more extended resections (e.g. pelvic exenteration), higher chance of open surgery (Gefen et al. 2023), and the resulting increased anesthetic risks and postoperative morbidity, or even mortality (Moghadamyeghaneh et al. 2016a). This concept of delayed presentation resulting in worse outcomes similarly applies for benign colorectal pathologies, such as in the instance of acute diverticulitis, where patients with uncomplicated acute diverticulitis are managed nonoperatively with antibiotics (Sartelli et al. 2020). The risk of progression to complicated diverticulitis including perforation has been shown to be higher in those with delayed presentation and initial treatment (Balk et al. 2022).

Figure 13.1 summarizes the pressing issues encountered in the perioperative management of older patients undergoing colorectal surgery.

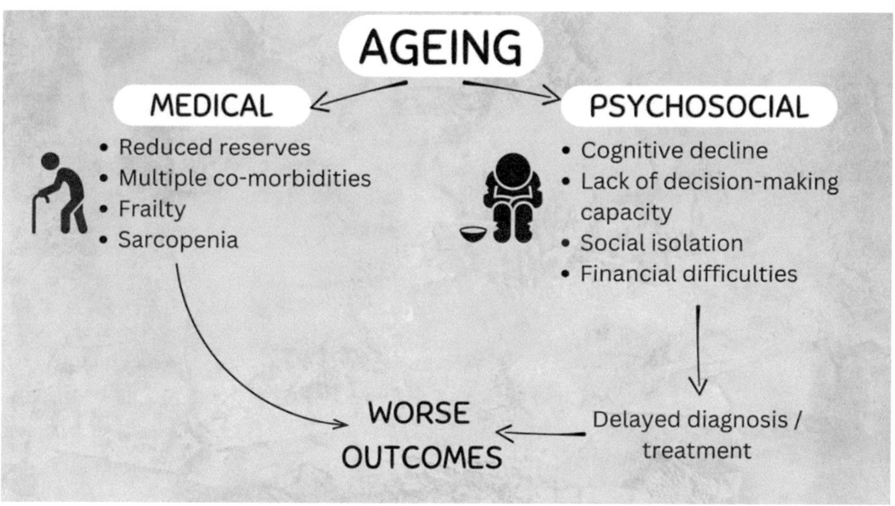

Fig. 13.1 Challenges faced in the management of older patients in colorectal surgery

13.3 Special Considerations for Decision-Making for Surgery in the Geriatric Population

Given the special issues faced in the older population as highlighted above, older adults undergoing major surgery often face higher risks of postoperative complications, functional decline, and mortality. Outcomes relevant to them, such as the quality of life, physical function, and independent living are more important than disease-specific endpoints. Hence, there needs to be a structured, yet patient-centric, approach in the perioperative management of older patients undergoing colorectal surgery. Recommendations have been made by the American Society of Colon and Rectal Surgeons (ASCRS) Clinical Practice Guidelines (CPG) in 2022 with supporting evidence on the perioperative management of older and/or frail patients undergoing colorectal surgery (Saur et al. 2022).

Family members should be actively engaged throughout the perioperative management in older patients, especially for those without decision-making capacity (Repetto et al. 2009). A qualitative study by Dijkman et al. showed that the inclusion of family members in the deliberation process and discussion of treatment options allowed patients to make better informed decisions, with observed positive outcomes on the entire care trajectory for colorectal cancer (Dijkman et al. 2022). Family conferences should be conducted to explain the disease pathology, various management options, and their respective risks. This is largely guided by patient factors, disease factors, and surgery factors, which are summarized in Table 13.1.

Decision-making for surgery in older patients is challenging; the primary surgeon should oversee this and jointly make a decision for, or against, surgery after the above considerations.

Table 13.1 Various factors which play important roles in the discussion for surgery in older patients

Patient factors	• Age • Severity of underlying comorbidities • Premorbid functional status • Existing perceived quality of life and anticipated quality of life postoperatively
Disease factors	• Severity of disease, e.g., impending demise from septic shock • Benign vs malignant pathology—Implication on long-term survival
Surgery factors	• Minimally invasive vs open approach • Single vs staged surgery • Extent of surgery, e.g., need for extensive resection vs "damage control" such as diverting stoma

13.4 Perioperative Optimization in Older Patients

One of the key challenges with surgery for older patients is the higher incidence of frailty and sarcopenia and lower physiological reserves. Perioperative optimization may be broadly categorized into preoperative and postoperative phases. Figure 13.2 shows the algorithm and possible interventions during each phase to optimize care.

There are a few studies which showed that multimodal prehabilitation, inclusive of physiotherapy, nutritional supplementation, and psychological support, has been shown to improve postoperative outcomes, though evidence is weak (Garoufalia et al. 2024; Molenaar et al. 2023). Duration of prehabilitation ranged from 2 to 4 weeks (Garoufalia et al. 2024). To facilitate the multidisciplinary management of these patients, it is more ideal for these patients to be placed inside a perioperative pathway. For instance, our institution introduced a colorectal pathway for all older patients undergoing elective colorectal surgery which is managed by a geriatric surgical service (GSS)—inclusive of a team of surgeons, geriatricians, specialized nurse clinicians, physiotherapists, dieticians, anesthetists, and cardiologists—since 2007 (Tan et al. 2011). We recently reported good and sustainable results 10 years following its implementation, attributed by accumulation of experience with the same GSS team, regular quarterly reviews, and provision of an individualized approach for various goals (e.g., prehabilitation and nutritional goals) (Chan et al. 2024).

However, preoperative optimization is only possible for patients planned for elective surgery. Patients who present urgently with an acute abdomen due to various pathologies such as ischemic bowel, obstructed colon cancer, or perforated diverticulitis with hemodynamic instability do not have the luxury of time for prehabilitation and will need urgent surgery. While preoperative optimization is not possible, there is still a window for early intervention postoperative in these group of patients, i.e., the well-established Enhanced After Recovery Surgery (ERAS) guidelines, which were first initiated by Professor Henrik Kehlet in 1997 (Kehlet 1997). Since then, revisions have been made to the ERAS guidelines—the latest recommendations were made by the American Society of Colon and Rectal Surgeons (ASCRS) Clinical Practice Guidelines (CPG) in 2022 with supporting evidence on the perioperative management of older and/or frail patients undergoing colorectal surgery (Saur et al. 2022). These include intraoperative measures to reduce the risk of surgical site infections, adoption of a multimodal opioid-sparing pain management plan, anti-emetic prophylaxis, and use of balanced crystalloids with goal-directed hemodynamic monitoring.

Postoperatively, standard ERAS interventions include the early review of the need for lines, drains, and catheters and for early removal once deemed unnecessary (Irani et al. 2023). Patients should also be started early on enteral feeding within 24 h (Stannard 2020). Especially for older patients, early postoperative mobilization is important to avoid skeletal muscle loss (for which some of them may already have); early postoperative mobilization has been shown to reduce the length of stay (Daskivich et al. 2019).

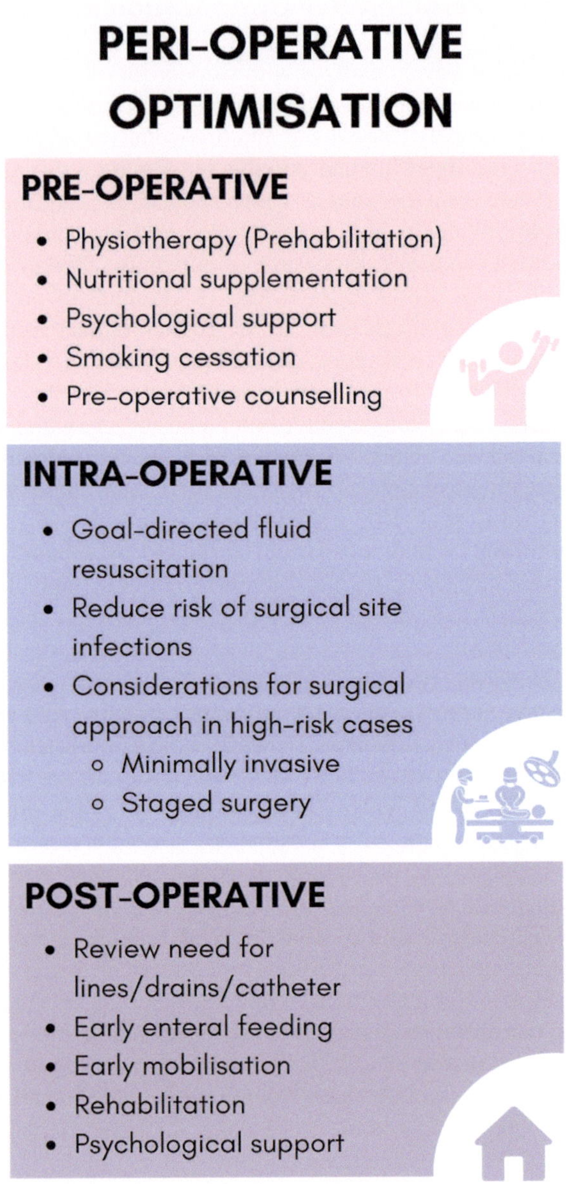

Fig. 13.2 Interventions available during each phase of the perioperative care to optimize outcomes for older patients

13.5 Minimally Invasive Surgery Versus Open Surgery

One of the ways to reduce postoperative complications is the adoption of minimally invasive surgery (MIS). MIS, which encompasses both robotic and laparoscopic techniques, has emerged as a preferred approach for colorectal procedures, particularly in geriatric patients. Benefits of MIS include shorter hospital stays and faster recovery compared to those undergoing open surgery (Horsey et al. 2022; Luo et al. 2022). The benefits of smaller wounds and less manipulation of bowel during the approach of MIS facilitate a quicker return of bowel function and reduced postoperative pain, allowing patients to resume normal activities sooner (Horsey et al. 2022; Luo et al. 2022). This faster recovery process can be especially beneficial for elderly individuals, who may experience more pronounced declines in mobility and independence after surgery. Furthermore, MIS is also linked to lower rates of postoperative complications, including wound infections, respiratory issues, and intraoperative blood loss. These reduced complication rates have a more pronounced impact on the geriatric patient population that have reduced physiological reserves and healing potential, overall mitigating further morbidity and mortality (Horsey et al. 2022).

Despite its advantages, MIS is not without its concerns. MIS requires the use of pneumoperitoneum which can lead to deleterious physiological effects, including reduced venous return, cardiac output, and pulmonary compliance. These effects are more significant, especially in the older population with underlying cardiovascular or respiratory conditions (Irani et al. 2023). Other drawbacks of MIS include the increased operative duration and the need to overcome its initial learning curve prior to reaping its benefits (Xue et al. 2023; Kayano et al. 2011). Hence, these factors need careful consideration in geriatric patients with limited physiological reserves, as prolonged anesthesia and operative stress may increase perioperative risks.

In this group of patients who are already at higher risks from the physiological derangements due to the need for pneumoperitoneum, another important consideration is whether the surgery is performed in an elective or emergency setting. Traditionally, the mainstay surgical approach to any surgical emergency is upfront laparotomy, but there is an increasing trend toward the adoption of MIS in emergency colorectal surgery for both benign and malignant conditions, with good outcomes reported (Smyth et al. 2023; Le et al. 2024; Zhang et al. 2022). However, the last guidelines by WSES on the management of perforated diverticulitis only provided weak recommendations on the use of laparoscopy compared with open sigmoidectomy (Sartelli et al. 2020); this was in 2020, and evidence has evolved since then. Special attention also needs to be paid on the underlying physiology of patients; in this context of older patients, deciding on laparoscopic surgery is even prudent as older patients exhibit delayed wound healing due to reduced cellular proliferation, impaired immune response, and decreased angiogenesis (Dube et al. 2022; Brubaker et al. 2013). This is compounded by the presence of other comorbidities such as diabetes mellitus, frailty, and sarcopenia which also impair wound healing and recovery from a major laparotomy. A recent audit on the National

Surgical Quality Improvement Program database from 2017 to 2021 on 11,976 frail patients showed that MIS was independently associated with 4.6%, 6.9%, and 4.2% reduction in 30-day mortality, severe complications, and need for prolonged length of stay >14 days, respectively (Khan et al. 2024).

In light of this, it is important to analyze whether minimally invasive surgery (MIS) is beneficial in these groups of patients who are at increased risk of complications by weighing the extent of physiologic derangement on presentation and the need for an expedient surgery. In complex situations or patients presenting with hemodynamic instability and/or severe physiologic derangement, open surgery remains the cornerstone. It provides direct access and visualization, which can be crucial for extensive resections or when dealing with complex anatomical variations (Moghadamyeghaneh et al. 2016b; Zelhart and Kaiser 2018). Despite the longer recovery times and higher postoperative pain associated with open surgery, it remains a critical option in the surgical armamentarium for cases where MIS is not feasible or safe.

13.6 Is Primary Anastomosis Always Beneficial?

The decision between primary anastomosis and stoma creation must be carefully evaluated based on patient-specific factors and disease factors (e.g., elective vs. emergency settings). The best situation for any patient would be primary anastomosis as this eliminates the need for a stoma and stoma-related complications such as skin irritation, high output, stomal prolapse, and parastomal hernias (Meisner et al. 2012). Additionally, it reduces long-term healthcare costs associated with stoma care supplies and follow-up interventions (Geisler et al. 2023). From a psychological and social perspective, avoiding a stoma can improve a patient's quality of life, reducing the stigma, social isolation, and distress often associated with an ostomy. Patients who maintain bowel continuity tend to experience fewer disruptions in daily activities and social interactions, which is particularly important in preserving the overall well-being of older adults (Neuberger et al. 2022; Ketelaers et al. 2022).

Despite its advantages, primary anastomosis carries an inherent risk of anastomotic leakage. While older age in itself may not increase the risk of anastomotic leakage (Zaimi et al. 2018), the aging population often has reduced physiological reserves, impaired wound healing, and comorbidities such as diabetes, cardiovascular disease, and malnutrition that increase the likelihood of poor anastomotic healing. This risk is more pronounced in patients who present acutely with intestinal obstruction from a tumor or perforation with peritoneal soilage (Bakker et al. 2014). In cases where anastomotic leakage occurs, the morbidity and mortality rates are substantially higher in comparison to younger patients, often leading to prolonged hospital stays, reoperations, and even sepsis-related complications (van Loon et al. 2021). For colon or rectal cancers which present acutely with obstruction, the choice of a staged procedure with colonic stenting may be considered for the left-sided tumor to bypass the acute obstruction, with an aim to perform definitive colonic resection via a MIS approach following nutritional optimization and prehabilitation

(Shang et al. 2023). Primary anastomosis should be reserved for geriatric patients with favorable risk profiles who are likely to tolerate the procedure and its recovery phase and in the elective setting.

While primary anastomosis is preferred in most situations, there are certain unique circumstances, especially in the geriatric population, where stoma creation may be preferred. In individuals with neurodegenerative diseases, mobility limitations, or pre-existing bowel dysfunction, a stoma can simplify bowel management and improve the overall quality of life (Johns et al. 2021). Patients with severe constipation, fecal incontinence, or rectal dysfunction may benefit from a stoma by achieving better control over their bowel movements, reducing the risk of soiling, and improving hygiene (van Loon et al. 2021). Additionally, a stoma can prevent low anterior resection syndrome (LARS), a distressing complication characterized by frequent bowel movements, urgency, and incontinence following low rectal anastomosis (Algie et al. 2022).

The choice between primary anastomosis and stoma creation in geriatric patients during colorectal surgery should be individualized, considering the patient's overall health status, surgical risk, and anticipated recovery. Primary anastomosis may be beneficial in avoiding stoma-related morbidities and the distress it confers; however, its complications can be lethal and must be taken into serious consideration; a stoma thus remains a valuable option in high-risk patients and select groups. This decision should be made collaboratively with a multidisciplinary team, including geriatricians, anesthesiologists, and stoma care specialists to optimize patient outcomes.

13.7 Role of Surgical Palliation

Despite every surgeon's attempt to aim for a curative resection, this is not possible for geriatric patients with advanced colorectal pathology, particularly when curative treatment is not feasible due to extensive disease burden, comorbid conditions, or poor functional status. However, surgery is still not obsolete, whereby there is a crucial role for surgical palliation. Surgeons often feel a reluctance to bring up palliative options, fearing that they may be perceived as not offering the "best" treatment, especially when curative surgery is technically possible. Addressing palliative options requires shifting the focus from "doing everything possible" to "doing what's best for this patient," taking into account their frailty, personal values, and quality of life.

The primary goal of palliative surgery in this context is to alleviate symptoms such as obstruction, bleeding, perforation, or intractable pain, thereby improving the patient's quality of life (Zattoni and Christoforidis 2020; Ahmed et al. 2021). Even though the primary focus may not be on survival, there are some studies that have shown surgical intervention in elderly colorectal cancer patients, even those aged 90 and above, which can lead to improved overall and cancer-specific survival compared to nonoperative treatments (Kim et al. 2021; Gefen et al. 2025). For geriatric patients who survive the postoperative period, the oncological prognosis is similar to that of younger patients, and the maintenance of functional status is a key goal (Zattoni and Christoforidis 2020). Hence, decision-making should be patient-centered, taking into account the patient's overall prognosis, goals of care, and preferences, while minimizing surgical morbidity and hospitalization.

A variety of surgical approaches can be employed for palliation in colorectal diseases, each tailored to the patient's condition and clinical presentation. For patients with malignant large bowel obstruction, options include diverting colostomy or ileostomy, bypass procedures, or placement of self-expanding metallic stents (SEMS) as less invasive alternatives (Ma et al. 2024).

These interventions can relieve obstruction and allow for enteral nutrition, enhancing patient comfort. In cases of intractable bleeding from colorectal malignancies that do not respond to endoscopic or medical therapy, segmental resection or, in some cases, subtotal colectomy may be considered, particularly if the bleeding is life-threatening (Ma et al. 2024).

For patients experiencing perforation or impending perforation due to malignancy or ischemic colitis, surgical intervention is often necessary to prevent sepsis and systemic complications. Diverting ostomies may be preferable in frail patients, avoiding the need for more extensive resections. Additionally, for those with severe perineal symptoms related to advanced rectal cancer, procedures such as diverting colostomy or palliative pelvic exenteration in select cases may provide symptom relief and enhance dignity in end-of-life care (Zattoni and Christoforidis 2020; Ma et al. 2024).

Ultimately, surgical palliation in geriatric colorectal patients must balance the potential benefits of symptom relief with the risks of surgical intervention. Multidisciplinary discussions involving surgeons, geriatricians, oncologists, palliative care specialists, and the patient's family are essential to ensure a comprehensive approach that aligns with the patient's goals and best interests. Nonsurgical options such as palliative radiotherapy, chemotherapy, or medical management should also be weighed as part of a holistic strategy for symptom control in patients with advanced colorectal disease.

13.8 Targeted Approach to Rectal Cancer in Older Patients

While the above subsections discussed about the perioperative considerations and surgical approaches in the management of older patients undergoing colorectal surgery in general, rectal cancer should be discussed separately, as it is a distinct disease entity within colorectal malignancies, requiring a multidisciplinary treatment approach due to its significant risk of both local recurrence after surgery and distant metastasis. Unlike colon cancer, rectal cancer management is more complex due to anatomical constraints, the need for sphincter preservation, and the potential impact on bowel, urinary, and sexual function—issues that are particularly relevant in older adults who may have pre-existing functional impairments.

Recent data suggest that colorectal cancers exhibit intrinsic biological differences based on tumor location (Salem et al. 2017). These differences have implications for treatment strategies, particularly in older patients where balancing efficacy and tolerability is crucial. Colon cancer is more likely to exhibit microsatellite instability (MSI), CpG island methylator phenotype (CIMP), and BRAF mutations, particularly in right-sided tumors, while rectal cancer typically arises through chromosomal instability and often has higher rates of TOPO1 expression and HER2/neu amplification compared to colon cancers (Ciepiela et al. 2024). Rectal cancer's higher rates of TOPO1 expression and HER2/neu amplification can make it more responsive to neoadjuvant chemoradiotherapy (CRT). Additionally, the induction of immune pathways by CRT in rectal cancer can enhance the effectiveness of immunotherapy, particularly in cases where surgery is not considered.

Fortunately, the incidence of rectal cancer is generally lower than that of colon cancer among the older adults (>80 years old) (Gefen et al. 2023), but its management often requires a combination of surgery, chemotherapy, and radiation therapy. Although extensive evidence supports current guidelines, many randomized controlled trials exclude patients older than 70 years. As a result, these guidelines often fail to address the specific challenges faced by this elderly population. In older adults, treatment decisions must consider factors such as frailty, comorbidities, and life expectancy to ensure an optimal balance between oncological control and quality of life.

13.8.1 Key Considerations in the Management of Rectal Tumors

When a rectal tumor is detected, management is guided by two main factors: (1) anatomical considerations and (2) the patient's overall health status, particularly frailty. From an anatomical perspective, the key distinction is whether the tumor is located in the upper third or the lower two-thirds of the rectum. For upper rectal tumors (Fig. 13.3), upfront surgery may be considered if the radial margin is not threatened. In contrast, tumors in the lower two-thirds often require a more cautious approach, with neoadjuvant chemoradiotherapy (CRT) being a key consideration. Therefore, detailed local imaging—such as MRI of the rectum or endorectal ultrasound—is an essential part of the preoperative workup to assess tumor staging and guide treatment planning.

In older patients with rectal cancer, prognosis and treatment decisions are equally determined by comorbidities and frailty, alongside the disease stage. As a result, geriatric assessment has become an essential component of the preoperative evaluation to guide individualized management. Given that cancer treatment in older persons differs from that of the general population—placing greater emphasis on functional outcomes, quality of life, and patient-specific goals of care—comprehensive geriatric assessment is crucial in optimizing treatment strategies and ensuring a balanced approach between oncological control and overall well-being.

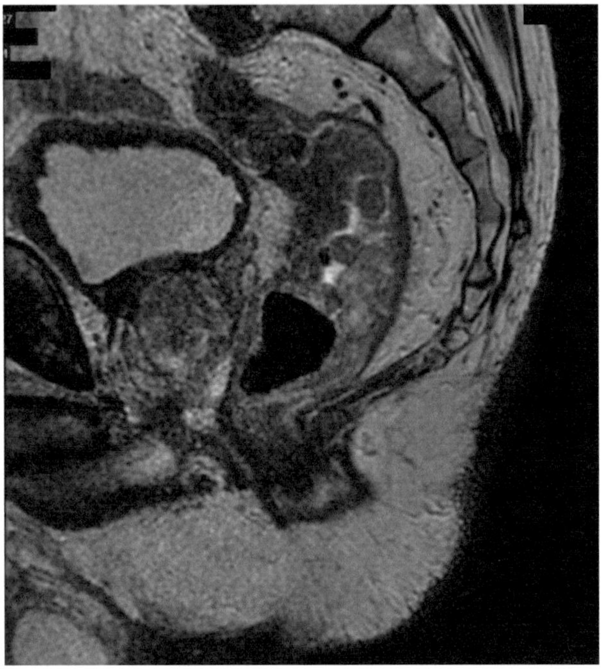

Fig. 13.3 MRI of an 82-year-old male patient showed an upper rectal tumor extending to the peritoneal reflection. Upfront surgery was performed, and postoperative histology revealed T3N0. No adjuvant treatment was required. Preoperative chemoRT might have been overtreatment, considering his age and comorbidities

The following are examples of a few recommended assessments:

1. Comprehensive geriatric assessment (CGA): The American Society of Clinical Oncology (ASCO) recommends CGA to evaluate comorbidities, functional status, cognition, psychological state, social support, nutritional status, and polypharmacy. CGA helps identify vulnerabilities and guides interventions to improve treatment tolerability and outcomes (Dale et al. 2023).
2. Nutritional status assessment: Pretreatment nutritional indicators such as body mass index (BMI), prognostic nutritional index (PNI), geriatric nutrition risk index (GNRI), and platelet–albumin ratio (PAR) are essential. These indicators independently predict the overall survival and progression-free survival in elderly rectal cancer patients, guiding early nutritional interventions (Qiu et al. 2024).
3. Chemotherapy risk assessment scale for high age (CRASH) scores: The CRASH score is designed to predict the risk of severe chemotherapy toxicity in older patients. The score categorizes patients into risk groups, helping clinicians tailor chemotherapy regimens to minimize toxicity. This is particularly useful for older adults with rectal cancer, who may have varying degrees of functional reserve and comorbidities (Extermann et al. 2012).
4. Charlson comorbidity index (CCI): CCI assesses the burden of comorbidities and predicts 6-month mortality. Higher CCI scores are associated with increased postoperative complications and mortality, aiding in risk stratification and management planning (Cooper et al. 2020).

5. Modified frailty index (mFI): This five-item score is a significant predictor of clinical outcomes in elderly rectal cancer patients. Higher mFI scores are associated with increased postoperative morbidity, prolonged recovery times, and elevated medical costs. An mFI score of ≥2 is an independent risk factor for severe postoperative complications and cancer-specific survival (CSS) (Miller et al. 2020). This tool helps stratify patients preoperatively, guiding decisions on the intensity of surgical and adjuvant treatments.
6. Sarcopenia index (SI): Sarcopenia index is a measure used to assess skeletal muscle mass, typically calculated using the skeletal muscle index (SMI) at the third lumbar vertebral (L3) level via computed tomography (CT) scans. It is defined as the total cross-sectional area of skeletal muscle at L3 divided by height squared (cm^2/m^2). Sarcopenia is an independent predictor of worse overall survival in rectal cancer patients (Zhu et al. 2022); it is associated with increased postoperative complications, prolonged hospital stays, and higher chemotherapy toxicity (Bliggenstorfer et al. 2023; Li et al. 2023). Given its impact on treatment tolerability and outcomes, preoperative identification of sarcopenia allows for targeted interventions, such as nutritional support and prehabilitation, to optimize patient fitness and improve therapeutic success.

We will not cover the stage-based management of rectal cancer, as comprehensive guidelines and major surgical textbooks already provide detailed recommendations on standard treatment protocols. Instead, the focus will be on practical considerations specific to older adults that balance oncological outcome with functional preservation and quality of life. Key considerations here would include reduction of surgical stress, patient-centered approach, and nonoperative management strategies where appropriate.

When surgery is indicated, minimally invasive surgery (MIS) techniques—such as laparoscopy- or robotic-assisted approaches—are preferred to minimize postoperative stress and facilitate faster recovery. Recent evidences have shown both laparoscopic and robotic approaches are associated with reduced postop complications, shorter length of hospital stay, and comparable or improved survival outcomes to open surgery (Horsey et al. 2022; van Harten et al. 2020). In addition, the enhanced recovery after surgery (ERAS) protocol is found to be safe and beneficial, with evidence proving that it reduces surgical complications and hospital stays, which is particularly beneficial for frail older adults (Wei et al. 2024).

As discussed earlier in this chapter, surgeons have come to recognize that traditional oncological outcomes, such as disease-free survival and overall survival, have limited relevance for the geriatric population. In older adults, the primary goal is often to preserve functional independence and ensure survival with a satisfactory quality of life (QoL).

The GOSAFE (Geriatric Oncology Surgical Assessment and Functional Recovery after Surgery) study, published in 2023 (Montroni et al. 2023), provided valuable insights into functional outcomes following colorectal cancer surgery in older adults. The study included 625 patients aged 70 years and older undergoing major elective colorectal surgery, with a significant proportion undergoing rectal cancer surgery. The findings were reassuring, demonstrating that a substantial proportion of older adults experienced good postoperative QoL and functional recovery (FR). Specifically, 60.1%–63.9% of rectal cancer patients reported equal or better QoL at 3–6 months post-surgery, and 70.6% achieved functional recovery. Notably, the study found that neither permanent nor temporary stomas were associated with poorer QoL or FR, challenging the assumption that restorative procedures inherently lead to superior outcomes. Instead, preoperative frailty, a history of delirium, and postoperative complications emerged as independent predictors of poor QoL and FR. These findings reinforce the importance of frailty screening in preoperative counselling and treatment planning, ensuring that surgical strategies align with patient-centered goals.

For older patients who are deemed fit following a comprehensive geriatric assessment (CGA), standard treatment can be pursued with careful monitoring for treatment-related toxicity. However, for those who are frail or decline surgery, alternative strategies such as external beam radiotherapy (EBRT) or chemoradiotherapy (EBCRT) with a watch-and-wait (WW) approach may be considered if a clinical complete response (cCR) (Fig. 13.4) is achieved. The NCCN guidelines endorse the WW approach for patients within a multidisciplinary team framework (Benson et al. 2022). This strategy should be carefully discussed with the patient, taking into account their preferences and overall health status. Haak et al. reported that in patients aged ≥75 years who achieved cCR, the 3-year local regrowth-free rate was 88%, with an overall survival rate of 97% (Haak et al. 2020). Additionally, data from the International Watch & Wait Database (IWWD) reinforce this approach, showing that most local recurrences occur within the first 2–3 years, emphasizing the need for intensive surveillance during this period (Fernandez et al. 2021). Beyond oncological safety, the WW approach offers significant functional benefits compared to radical surgery. Custers et al. found that patients managed nonoperatively reported better quality of life, fewer instances of major bowel dysfunction,

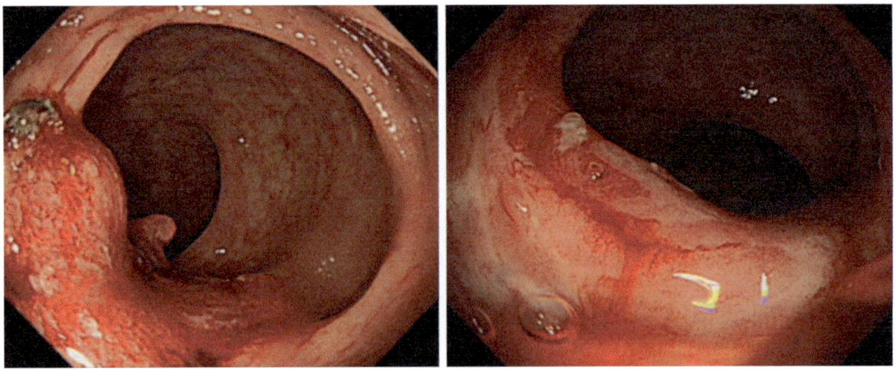

Fig. 13.4 (**a**) Endoscopic image of a 75-year-old female with Child's B liver cirrhosis showing a low rectal tumor before treatment. (**b**) Post-treatment endoscopic image showing complete response after long-course chemoRT, with no recurrence observed after 2 years on a watch-and-wait approach

and improved preservation of urinary and sexual function (Custers et al. 2023). These factors are particularly important for older adults, who often prioritize maintaining independence and functional status. Given these findings, the WW approach presents a balanced strategy for managing rectal cancer in older adults, aligning with their goals of care while ensuring oncological safety through vigilant monitoring.

In cases where there is residual disease but the patient is not fit for major surgery, local excision can be considered. This approach is less invasive and can be effective in managing small, residual tumors. The American Radium Society notes that local excision can be an option for patients with residual disease after CRT, with careful selection and follow-up (Russo et al. 2019).

Given the multimodal nature of rectal cancer treatment and its associated toxicity and morbidity, we recommend a patient-centered approach that prioritizes shared decision-making, thorough evaluation of geriatric syndromes and frailty, and a clear discussion of treatment options aligned with the patient's priorities. The decision to pursue or withhold radical surgery should consider not only perioperative risks but also life expectancy and the patient's primary goals—whether prioritizing functional independence and symptom relief or maximizing disease-free survival. For patients who are physically and cognitively fit, standard treatments used in younger populations remain appropriate. However, for those with reduced functional reserves and significant comorbidities, alternative strategies that minimize surgical trauma should be considered to optimize outcomes while maintaining the quality of life.

13.9 Conclusion

The clinical journey of patients like Mr. T exemplifies the multifaceted challenges inherent in managing older adults undergoing colorectal surgery. These patients often present with complex medical comorbidities, frailty/sarcopenia, and functional limitations that significantly influence perioperative risk and recovery trajectories. Optimal care necessitates a transdisciplinary, individualized approach that integrates comprehensive prehabilitation, meticulous risk stratification, and patient-centered decision-making to enhance surgical outcomes and preserve postoperative function.

Notably, the evidence base guiding the management of older adults, particularly in the context of rectal cancer, remains limited due to their frequent underrepresentation in clinical trials. This paucity of data complicates treatment planning and underscores the need to balance oncological efficacy with the preservation of quality of life and functional independence. Consequently, a nuanced, multimodal strategy that carefully weighs the benefits and risks of surgical and adjunctive therapies is essential.

In summary, the care of older colorectal surgery patients demands a holistic framework that addresses not only the biological aspects of disease but also the broader psychosocial factors affecting recovery and long-term well-being.

References

Ahmed O, Lee JH, Thompson CC et al (2021) AGA clinical practice update on the optimal management of the malignant alimentary tract obstruction: expert review. Clin Gastroenterol Hepatol 19(9):1780–1788

Alexiusdottir KK, Möller PH, Snaebjornsson P et al (2012) Association of symptoms of colon cancer patients with tumor location and TNM tumor stage. Scand J Gastroenterol 47(7):795–801

Algie JPA, van Kooten RT, Tollenaar R et al (2022) Stoma versus anastomosis after sphincter-sparing rectal cancer resection; the impact on health-related quality of life. Int J Color Dis 37(10):2197–2205

Bakker IS, Grossmann I, Henneman D et al (2014) Risk factors for anastomotic leakage and leak-related mortality after colonic cancer surgery in a nationwide audit. Br J Surg 101(4):424–432; discussion 432

Balk EM, Adam GP, Bhuma MR et al (2022) Diagnostic imaging and medical management of acute left-sided colonic diverticulitis: a systematic review. Ann Intern Med 175(3):379–387

Benson AB, Venook AP, Al-Hawary MM et al (2022) Rectal cancer, version 2.2022, NCCN clinical practice guidelines in oncology. J Natl Compr Cancer Netw 20(10):1139–1167

Berkowitz Z, Hawkins NA, Peipins LA et al (2008) Beliefs, risk perceptions, and gaps in knowledge as barriers to colorectal cancer screening in older adults. J Am Geriatr Soc 56(2):307–314

Bliggenstorfer JT, Hashmi A, Bingmer K et al (2023) Sarcopenia in patients with rectal adenocarcinoma: an opportunity for preoperative rehabilitation. Am Surg 89(12):5631–5637

Brubaker AL, Rendon JL, Ramirez L et al (2013) Reduced neutrophil chemotaxis and infiltration contributes to delayed resolution of cutaneous wound infection with advanced age. J Immunol 190(4):1746–1757

Chan KS, Lee DJK, Kok Y et al (2024) A 10-year review on older patients undergoing colorectal cancer surgery: surgeon-led geriatric service and good quality surgery are drivers of good outcomes. J Gastrointest Surg 28(1):40–46

Chen WZ, Shen ZL, Zhang FM et al (2022) Prognostic value of myosteatosis and sarcopenia for elderly patients with colorectal cancer: a large-scale double-center study. Surgery 172(4):1185–1193

Ciepiela I, Szczepaniak M, Ciepiela P et al (2024) Tumor location matters, next generation sequencing mutation profiling of left-sided, rectal, and right-sided colorectal tumors in 552 patients. Sci Rep 14(1):4619

Cooper L, Siam B, Sagee A et al (2020) Some nursing screening tools can be used to assess high-risk older adults who undergo colorectal surgery for cancer. Clin Interv Aging 15:1505–1511

Cruz-Jentoft AJ, Bahat G, Bauer J et al (2018) Sarcopenia: revised European consensus on definition and diagnosis. Age Ageing 48(1):16–31

Custers PA, van der Sande ME, Grotenhuis BA et al (2023) Long-term quality of life and functional outcome of patients with rectal cancer following a watch-and-wait approach. JAMA Surg 158(5):e230146

Dale W, Klepin HD, Williams GR et al (2023) Practical assessment and management of vulnerabilities in older patients receiving systemic cancer therapy: ASCO guideline update. J Clin Oncol 41(26):4293–4312

Daskivich TJ, Houman J, Lopez M et al (2019) Association of wearable activity monitors with assessment of daily ambulation and length of stay among patients undergoing major surgery. JAMA Netw Open 2(2):e187673

Dijkman BL, Paans W, Van der Wal-Huisman H et al (2022) Involvement of adult children in treatment decision-making for older patients with cancer - a qualitative study of perceptions and experiences of oncology surgeons and nurses. Support Care Cancer 30(11):9203–9210

Dube CT, Ong YHB, Wemyss K et al (2022) Age-related alterations in macrophage distribution and function are associated with delayed cutaneous wound healing. Front Immunol 13:943159

Extermann M, Boler I, Reich RR et al (2012) Predicting the risk of chemotherapy toxicity in older patients: the chemotherapy risk assessment scale for high-age patients (CRASH) score. Cancer 118(13):3377–3386

Fernandez LM, São Julião GP, Figueiredo NL et al (2021) Conditional recurrence-free survival of clinical complete responders managed by watch and wait after neoadjuvant chemoradiotherapy for rectal cancer in the International Watch & Wait Database: a retrospective, international, multicentre registry study. Lancet Oncol 22(1):43–50

Garoufalia Z, Emile SH, Meknarit S et al (2024) A systematic review and meta-analysis of high-quality randomized controlled trials on the role of prehabilitation programs in colorectal surgery. Surgery 176:1352

Gefen R, Emile SH, Garoufalia Z et al (2025) Characteristics and role of surgery in nonagenarians with colorectal cancer: SEER database analysis. Surgery 181:109161

Gefen R, Emile SH, Horesh N et al (2023) Age-related variations in colon and rectal cancer: an analysis of the national cancer database. Surgery 174(6):1315–1322

Geisler BP, Cao KN, Ryschon AM et al (2023) Cost associated with diverting ostomy after rectal cancer surgery: a transnational analysis. Surg Endosc 37(10):7759–7766

Guessous I, Dash C, Lapin P et al (2010) Colorectal cancer screening barriers and facilitators in older persons. Prev Med 50(1–2):3–10

Haak HE, Maas M, Lambregts DMJ et al (2020) Is watch and wait a safe and effective way to treat rectal cancer in older patients? Eur J Surg Oncol 46(3):358–362

Hämmig O (2019) Health risks associated with social isolation in general and in young, middle and old age. PLoS One 14(7):e0219663

van Harten MJ, Greenwood EB, Bedrikovetski S et al (2020) Minimally invasive surgery in elderly patients with rectal cancer: an analysis of the Bi-National Colorectal Cancer Audit (BCCA). Eur J Surg Oncol 46(9):1649–1655

Horsey ML, Parascandola SA, Sparks AD et al (2022) The impact of surgical approach on short- and long-term outcomes after rectal cancer resection in elderly patients: a national cancer database propensity score matched comparison of robotic, laparoscopic, and open approaches. Surg Endosc 36(2):1269–1277

Irani JL, Hedrick TL, Miller TE et al (2023) Clinical practice guidelines for enhanced recovery after colon and rectal surgery from the American Society of Colon and Rectal Surgeons and the Society of American Gastrointestinal and Endoscopic Surgeons. Surg Endosc 37(1):5–30

Johns J, Krogh K, Rodriguez GM et al (2021) Management of neurogenic bowel dysfunction in adults after spinal cord injury. Clinical practice guideline for healthcare providers. J Spinal Cord Med 44(3):442–510. https://doi.org/10.1080/10790268.2021.1883385

Kayano H, Okuda J, Tanaka K et al (2011) Evaluation of the learning curve in laparoscopic low anterior resection for rectal cancer. Surg Endosc 25(9):2972–2979

Kehlet H (1997) Multimodal approach to control postoperative pathophysiology and rehabilitation. Br J Anaesth 78(5):606–617

Ketelaers SHJ, Orsini RG, Nieuwenhuijzen GAP et al (2022) Outcomes on diverting ostomy formation and reversal after low anterior resection in the older more advanced rectal cancer patient. Eur J Surg Oncol 48(6):1414–1420

Khan MS, Meier J, Afsari M et al (2024) The effect of minimally invasive surgery on thirty-day postoperative outcomes of frail patients undergoing emergency colon resections. Surgery 180:109004

Kim S, Kim DS, Soh JS et al (2021) Clinical characteristics and prognosis of elderly patients with colorectal cancer: comparison between surgical resection and supportive care. Medicine (Baltimore) 100(7):e24609

Langenfeld SJ, Davis BR, Vogel JD et al (2024) The American Society of Colon and Rectal Surgeons clinical practice guidelines for the management of rectal cancer 2023 supplement. Dis Colon Rectum 67(1):18–31

Le NK, Cho NY, Mallick S et al (2024) Open versus minimally invasive emergent colectomy for diverticulitis. Am Surg 90(10):2560–2569

Li Q, An T, Wu J et al (2023) The impact of sarcopenia on the outcome of patients with left-sided colon and rectal cancer after curative surgery. BMC Cancer 23(1):640

van Loon YT, van Erning FN, Maas HA et al (2021) Primary anastomosis versus end-ostomy in left-sided colonic and proximal rectal cancer surgery in the elderly Dutch population: a propensity score matched analysis. Ann Surg Oncol 28(12):7450–7460

Luo W, Wu M, Chen Y (2022) Laparoscopic versus open surgery for elderly patients with colorectal cancer: a systematic review and meta-analysis of matched studies. ANZ J Surg 92(9):2003–2017

Ma B, Ren T, Cai C et al (2024) Palliative procedures for advanced obstructive colorectal cancer: a systematic review and meta-analysis. Int J Color Dis 39(1):148

Meisner S, Lehur PA, Moran B et al (2012) Peristomal skin complications are common, expensive, and difficult to manage: a population based cost modeling study. PLoS One 7(5):e37813

Miller SM, Wolf J, Katlic M et al (2020) Frailty is a better predictor than age for outcomes in geriatric patients with rectal cancer undergoing proctectomy. Surgery 168(3):504–508

Moghadamyeghaneh Z, Hanna MH, Carmichael JC et al (2016b) Comparison of open, laparoscopic, and robotic approaches for total abdominal colectomy. Surg Endosc 30(7):2792–2798

Moghadamyeghaneh Z, Hanna MH, Hwang G et al (2016a) Outcomes of colon resection in patients with metastatic colon cancer. Am J Surg 212(2):264–271

Mohan R, Huey CWT, Junnarkar S et al (2020) Prehabilitation in elderly patients scheduled for liver resection and protocol for recovery of surgery in elderly. Hepatoma Res 6:13

Molenaar CJL, Minnella EM, Coca-Martinez M et al (2023) Effect of multimodal prehabilitation on reducing postoperative complications and enhancing functional capacity following colorectal cancer surgery: the PREHAB randomized clinical trial. JAMA Surg 158(6):572–581

Montroni I, Ugolini G, Saur NM et al (2023) Predicting functional recovery and quality of life in older patients undergoing colorectal cancer surgery: real-world data from the international GOSAFE study. J Clin Oncol 41(34):5247–5262

Neuberger L, Braude P, Weeks K et al (2022) A new stoma for an older person-An association with quality of life and physical function: a systematic review. J Am Geriatr Soc 70(8):2415–2425

O'Caoimh R, Sezgin D, O'Donovan MR et al (2021) Prevalence of frailty in 62 countries across the world: a systematic review and meta-analysis of population-level studies. Age Ageing 50(1):96–104

Petermann-Rocha F, Balntzi V, Gray SR et al (2022) Global prevalence of sarcopenia and severe sarcopenia: a systematic review and meta-analysis. J Cachexia Sarcopenia Muscle 13(1):86–99

Qiu J, Yu Y, Wang Z et al (2024) Comprehensive analysis of the prognostic value of pre-treatment nutritional indicators in elderly rectal cancer patients. Sci Rep 14(1):22078

Reisinger KW, van Vugt JL, Tegels JJ et al (2015) Functional compromise reflected by sarcopenia, frailty, and nutritional depletion predicts adverse postoperative outcome after colorectal cancer surgery. Ann Surg 261(2):345–352

Repetto L, Piselli P, Raffaele M et al (2009) Communicating cancer diagnosis and prognosis: when the target is the elderly patient-a GIOGer study. Eur J Cancer 45(3):374–383

Russo S, Anker CJ, Abdel-Wahab M et al (2019) Executive summary of the American Radium Society appropriate use criteria for local excision in rectal cancer. Int J Radiat Oncol Biol Phys 105(5):977–993

Salem ME, Weinberg BA, Xiu J et al (2017) Comparative molecular analyses of left-sided colon, right-sided colon, and rectal cancers. Oncotarget 8(49):86356–86368

Sartelli M, Weber DG, Kluger Y et al (2020) 2020 update of the WSES guidelines for the management of acute colonic diverticulitis in the emergency setting. World J Emerg Surg 15(1):32

Saur NM, Davis BR, Montroni I et al (2022) The American Society of Colon and Rectal Surgeons clinical practice guidelines for the perioperative evaluation and management of frailty among older adults undergoing colorectal surgery. Dis Colon Rectum 65(4):473–488

Shang R, Han X, Zeng C et al (2023) Colonic stent as a bridge to surgery versus emergency rection for malignant left-sided colorectal obstruction: a systematic review and meta-analysis of randomized controlled trials. Medicine (Baltimore) 102(50):e36078

Smyth R, Darbyshire A, Mercer S et al (2023) Trends in emergency colorectal surgery: a 7-year retrospective single-centre cohort study. Surg Endosc 37(5):3911–3920

Stannard D (2020) Early enteral nutrition within 24 hours of lower gastrointestinal surgery versus later commencement for length of hospital stay and postoperative complications. J Perianesth Nurs 35(5):541–542
Tan KY, Tan P, Tan L (2011) A collaborative transdisciplinary "geriatric surgery service" ensures consistent successful outcomes in elderly colorectal surgery patients. World J Surg 35(7):1608–1614
Wallace D, Walker K, Kuryba A et al (2014) Identifying patients at risk of emergency admission for colorectal cancer. Br J Cancer 111(3):577–580
Wei PL, Huang YJ, Wang W et al (2024) Modified enhanced recovery after surgery protocol in octogenarians undergoing minimally invasive colorectal cancer surgery. J Am Geriatr Soc 72(9):2679–2689
World Health Organization (2024) Ageing and health 2024. https://www.who.int/news-room/fact-sheets/detail/ageing-and-health. Updated 1 Oct 2024
Xue QL (2011) The frailty syndrome: definition and natural history. Clin Geriatr Med 27(1):1–15
Xue Y, Li S, Guo S et al (2023) Evaluation of the advantages of robotic versus laparoscopic surgery in elderly patients with colorectal cancer. BMC Geriatr 23(1):105
Zaimi I, Sparreboom CL, Lingsma HF et al (2018) The effect of age on anastomotic leakage in colorectal cancer surgery: a population-based study. J Surg Oncol 118(1):113–120
Zattoni D, Christoforidis D (2020) How best to palliate and treat emergency conditions in geriatric patients with colorectal cancer. Eur J Surg Oncol 46(3):369–378
Zelhart M, Kaiser AM (2018) Robotic versus laparoscopic versus open colorectal surgery: towards defining criteria to the right choice. Surg Endosc 32(1):24–38
Zhang Y, Liu C, Nistala KRY et al (2022) Open versus laparoscopic Hartmann's procedure: a systematic review and meta-analysis. Int J Color Dis 37(12):2421–2430
Zhu Y, Guo X, Zhang Q et al (2022) Prognostic value of sarcopenia in patients with rectal cancer: a meta-analysis. PLoS One 17(6):e0270332

Strategies for Older Persons Undergoing Upper Gastrointestinal Surgery

14

Kheng-Tian Lim

> Biology is King, selection is Queen, technical manoeuvres are the Prince and Princess; occasionally the Prince or Princess tries to usurp the throne; they almost always fail to overcome the powerful forces of the King and Queen. (Cady 1997)

This chapter focuses on the strategies of older persons undergoing upper gastrointestinal cancer (UGIC) management due to their nature of higher complexity and complication risks from invasive surgical treatment in comparison to benign upper gastrointestinal disease. UGIC discussed in this chapter includes oesophageal cancer (squamous cell carcinoma and adenocarcinoma), oesophago-gastric (OG) junction cancer and gastric cancer.

K.-T. Lim (✉)
Central Queensland Hospital and Health Service, Gladstone Hospital, Gladstone, QLD, Australia

Rural Clinical School, The University of Queensland, Rockhampton, QLD, Australia
e-mail: KhengTian.Lim@health.qld.gov.au

K.-Y. Tan et al. (eds.), *Mastering Geriatric Surgery*,
https://doi.org/10.1007/978-981-95-0665-1_14

Take-Home Messages

- Apply geriatric assessment (GA) tools to select the most appropriate and safe medical and surgical intervention in older persons with UGIC diagnosis.
- Collaborate in a transdisciplinary or multidisciplinary team for holistic UGIC management in older persons with geriatric care emphasis during their continuum of cancer care from the hospital to the community.
- Implement a standardised pathway in multimodal prehabilitation programme for medical optimisation, physical exercise, nutritional support and psychological support.
- Adopt minimally invasive surgery (MIS) techniques and instruments such as endoscopy, laparoscopy, thoracoscopy or robotic-assisted surgery as appropriate. Consider initial non-operative management of UGIC crisis, allowing opportunity for perioperative optimization or prehabilitation.
- Implement Enhance Recovery After Surgery (ERAS) protocol in UGIC surgery focusing on pain control, nutrition and rehabilitation.
- Respect older persons' view and wish in shared decision-making.

14.1 Introduction

14.1.1 Older Persons and the Burden of Cancer Globally

Older persons aged 65 years or older worldwide are rising from 761 million in 2021 to 1.6 billion in 2050 (United Nations 2023). The rapid growth in older persons' population highlights the importance of promoting health, preventing and treating illness during their life expectancy. From the estimated 20 million new cancer cases in 2022, over 35 million cases are predicted in 2050 (World Health Organisation 2024).

There were over 968,000 new cases of gastric cancer in 2022 and close to 660,000 deaths, ranking as fifth cancer in both incidence and mortality worldwide. Oesophageal cancer is the 11th most diagnosed cancer and the seventh leading cause of cancer death worldwide, with an estimate of 511,000 new cases and 445,000 deaths in 2022 (Bray et al. 2024). By 2040, the estimates are 957,000 new cases (141,300 adenocarcinoma cases and 806,000 squamous cell carcinoma cases) and 880,000 deaths from oesophageal cancer (Morgan et al. 2022).

Older persons requiring cancer surgery have been associated with higher morbidity and mortality. The burden of treatment such as the invasiveness of treatment and length of hospital stay, its outcomes such as severity of functional and cognitive impairment and the likelihood of the outcomes such as death influence the attitude and preference of older persons (Fried et al. 2002).

14.1.2 Surgical Risk in Older Persons with UGIC

A Swedish single-centre study of 548 patients, with 122 (22.3%) older persons (age ≥75 years) with either oesophageal or gastric cancer who underwent oesophagectomy or gastrectomy, showed a statistically significant increase in 90-day mortality after cancer surgery in older persons compared to younger persons (Klevebro et al. 2019).

In a Dutch study, looking at the impact of age and comorbidity on the surgical resection rate and survival in 6223 patients with oesophageal and gastric cancer, it was found that surgical treatment of OG cancer was associated with better survival than no surgery. However, the postoperative mortality was increased in patients with advanced age (≥70 years) and those with one or more comorbidities (Koppert et al. 2012).

In cancer surgery, it is a standard practice that the surgeons shall provide the necessary information to the older persons and their caregivers, detailing the cancer diagnosis, outlining the treatment options, the potential benefits of each option, the likelihood of good outcome and the risks of complication related to cancer surgery (Fig. 14.1). The possibility of functional or cognitive impairment risks influencing patients' preferences and surgeons' selection should be addressed during the shared decision-making.

Modern older persons with cancer and skilled surgeons are not alone in cancer care management. Current collaborating practice in a transdisciplinary or multidisciplinary team approach involving geriatrician (GRM), anaesthetist, cardiologist, specialist nurse, pharmacist, dietician, physiotherapist, occupational therapist, medical social worker (MSW), psychologist, oncologist, surgeon and other stakeholders providing their expert input is important in the evidence-based clinical decision-making in the overall cancer care of older persons.

Redesigning the surgical decision-making for high-risk patients in a more patient-centred and team-based approaches should be done (Glance et al. 2014). The recommended treatment plan should balance the advantages and disadvantages of surgical and non-surgical approaches to disease management, taking the patient's values and goals into consideration.

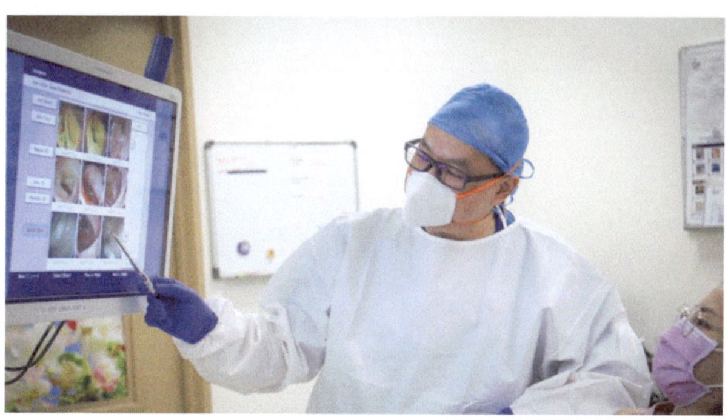

Fig. 14.1 Doctor and patient consultation during shared decision-making

14.1.3 UGIC Diagnosis and Treatment

The treatment of UGIC such as oesophageal cancer (Fig. 14.2) and gastric cancer (Fig. 14.3) is often surgically complex, challenging and even more so in the older persons with underlying functional and cognitive impairment, frailty and malnutrition.

Older persons with UGIC may present with the symptoms of progressive dysphagia, nausea, vomiting, haematemesis, melaena, syncope, anorexia, significant unexplained weight loss, fatigue, lethargy, epigastric pain, early satiety and bloated abdomen. These red-flag symptoms warrant further assessment and investigation.

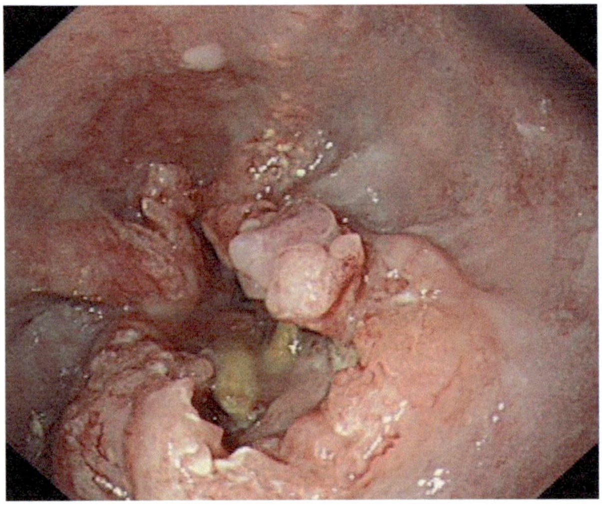

Fig. 14.2 Endoscopic view of an ulcerating partially obstructing lower oesophageal cancer

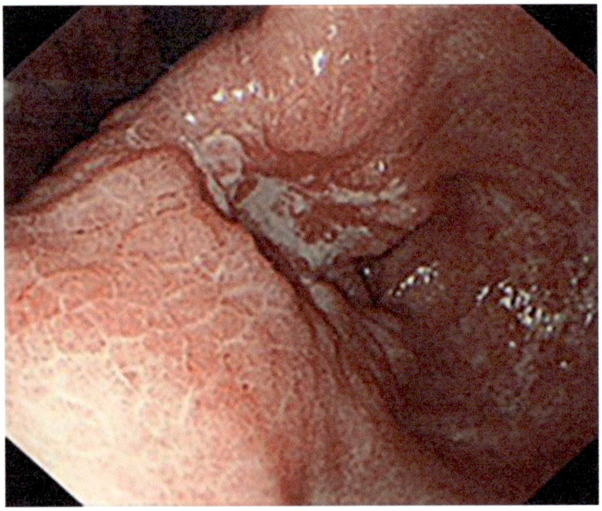

Fig. 14.3 Endoscopic view of an ulcerating gastric incisura cancer

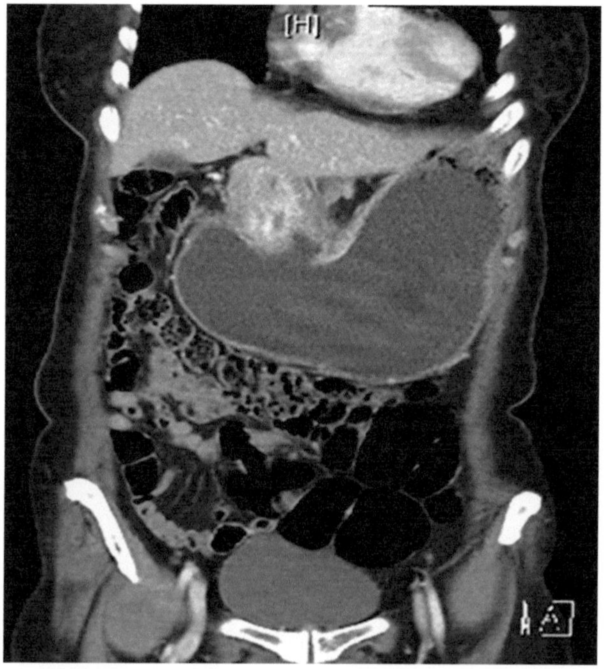

Fig. 14.4 Coronal view of a CT scan of the abdomen and pelvis showing fluid-filled distended stomach with a gastric outlet obstruction from a primary obstructing gastric pyloric cancer

The risk factors for oesophageal cancer include tobacco smoking, alcohol consumption, obesity, diet low in fresh fruits and vegetables, chronic gastro-oesophageal acid reflux, Barrett's oesophagus and male gender. While the risk factors for gastric cancer are somewhat like that for oesophageal cancer, they include the family history of gastric cancer or genetic syndromes, *Helicobacter pylori* infection, autoimmune atrophic gastritis and diet high in fatty, salty and smoked or pickled food. Some of these risk factors can be modifiable through diet and lifestyle changes. There are opportunities to raise public health awareness in these modifiable factors targeted early at a younger generation and to promote healthy lifestyles by the responsible healthcare system.

The diagnostic workup for suspected UGIC includes upper gastrointestinal endoscopy (UGIE) with biopsy, with or without endoscopic ultrasound scan and fine needle biopsy, staging computed tomography (CT) scan (Fig. 14.4) and/or positron emission tomography (PET) scan (Fig. 14.5). Laparoscopy is useful for staging gastro-oesophageal and gastric cancer. Baseline blood workup should be performed, such as haematology (full blood count, coagulation profile, blood type and screen), biochemistry (electrolytes, liver and renal profile, bone and metabolic profile and glucose) and tumour markers (such as CEA, CA19.9). The number of tests is not exhaustive, such as MSI or MMH, but HER-2 and PD-L1 molecular markers may be required.

The treatment specifics of oesophageal and gastric cancer can be referred to the National Comprehensive Cancer Network (NCCN) Clinical Practice Guidelines in

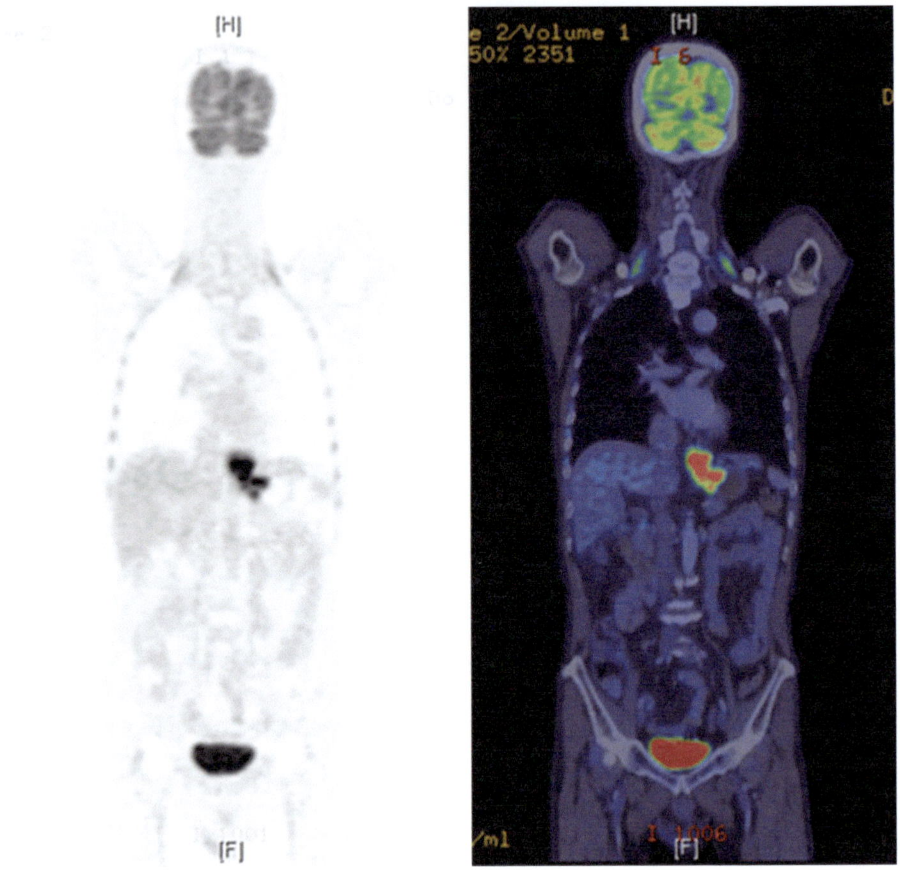

Fig. 14.5 PET scan showing FDG-avid lesion at the gastro-oesophageal junction

Oncology (NCCN Guidelines®), Esophageal and Esophagogastric Junction Cancers and Gastric Cancer Version 5.2024 (NCCN 2024a, b).

Depending on the clinicopathological and radiological stage of UGIC, the general treatment of early UGIC limited to mucosa (T1a or earlier) with good prognostic indicator may be in the form of endoscopic therapy, utilising endoscopic mucosal resection (EMR) (Fig. 14.6a–f) and endoscopic submucosal dissection (ESD) (Fig. 14.7a, b).

In brief, early UGIC without nodal disease may be offered an upfront oesophagectomy (Fig. 14.8) or gastrectomy (Fig. 14.9a, b), possibly followed by adjuvant therapy in the form of chemotherapy and/or radiotherapy, depending on the final histopathological stage. Curative-intent resectable UGIC with locally advanced or nodal disease may be offered multimodal therapy in the form of neoadjuvant chemoradiotherapy or neoadjuvant chemotherapy, followed by surgery, such as in the CROSS and FLOT trials (van Hagan et al. 2012; Al-Batran et al. 2019). Targeted therapy in HER-2-positive patients and immunotherapy in PD-L1-positive patients

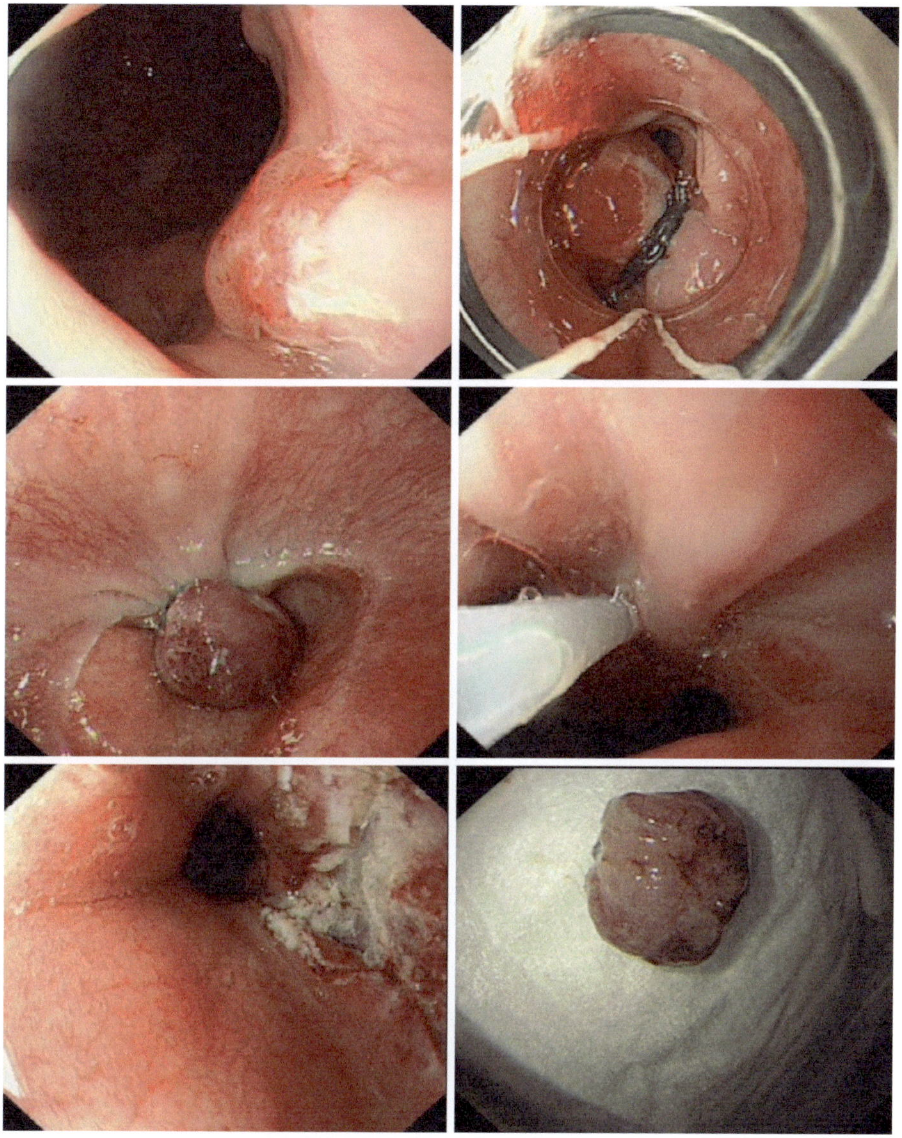

Fig. 14.6 (**a**) Endoscopic view of an early pT1a OG junction cancer. (**b**, **c**) Endoscopic band ligation to create a polyp. (**d**) Snare EMR performed. (**e**) Base of the OG junction post-EMR. (**f**) OG junction and EMR specimen, respectively

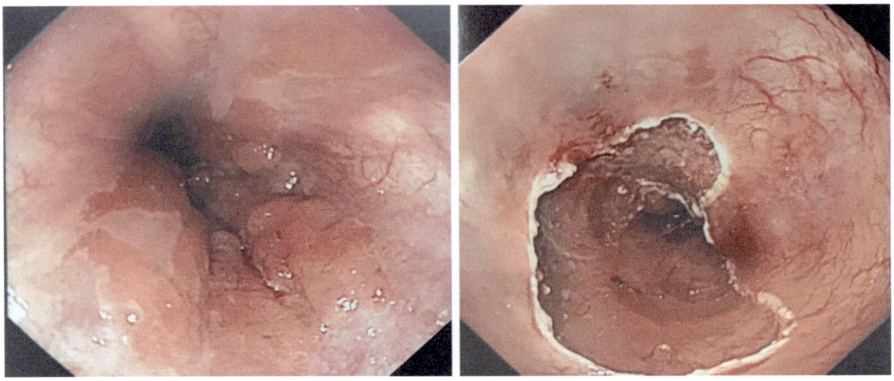

Fig. 14.7 (**a**) Endoscopic view of early lower oesophageal cancer in the background of Barrett's oesophagus. (**b**) Endoscopic view of lower oesophagus following ESD procedure

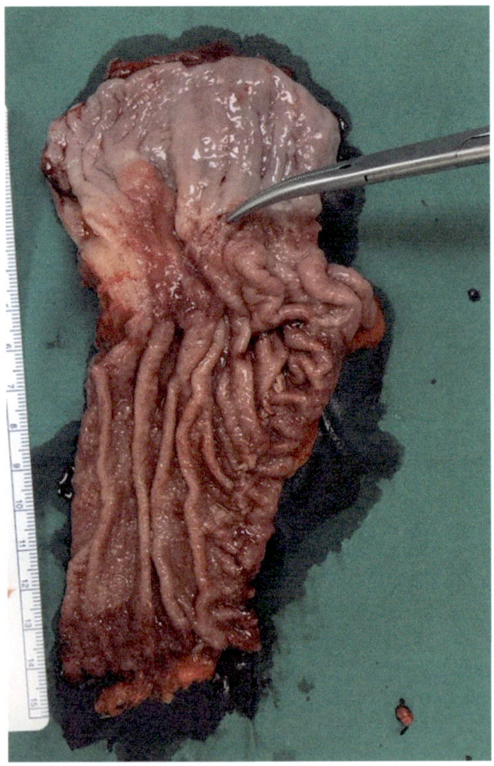

Fig. 14.8 Oesophagectomy specimen with macroscopic view of the lower third oesophageal cancer following neoadjuvant therapy

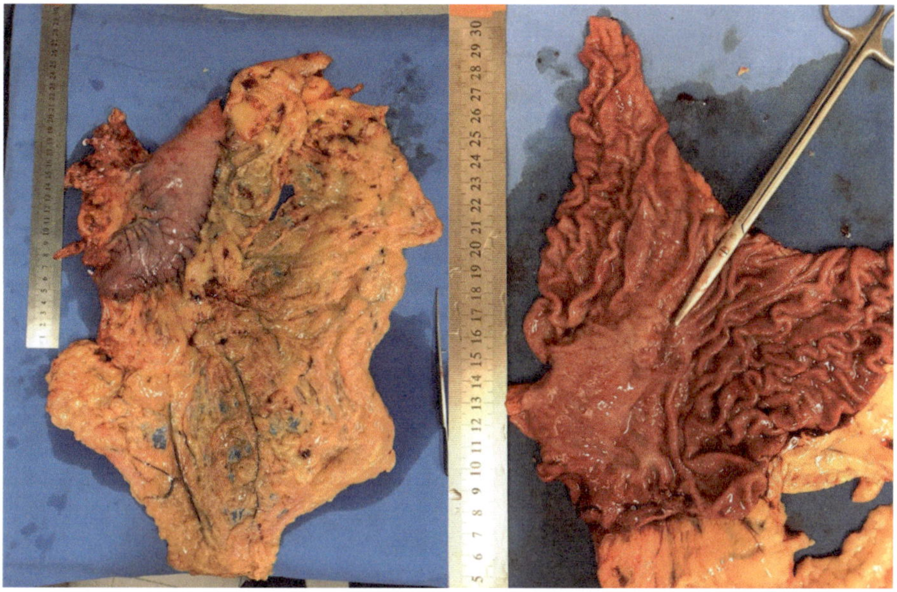

Fig. 14.9 (**a**) Specimen from a laparoscopic subtotal gastrectomy, D2 lymphadenectomy and partial omentectomy. (**b**) Macroscopic view of the resected gastric lumen showing an ulcerating gastric lesser curve cancer

with a high combined positive score may be offered in advanced or metastatic UGIC (Bang et al. 2010; Muro et al. 2016).

More importantly, the older persons' ability to withstand the rigors of multimodal therapy can be similarly challenging and risky due to their limited physiological reserves, cognitive and functional decline, frailty and malnutrition. The effects of neoadjuvant therapy may result in physiological deconditioning. Quite often, the older persons have concurrent chronic cardiovascular, respiratory, metabolic and renal disease. Despite the relative lack of elderly specific data in the management of locally advanced and metastatic oesophageal cancer in a review article citing 89 references, the fitter older person population appears to similarly benefit from multimodal therapy in early-stage and palliative therapy in metastatic disease (Bracken-Clarke et al. 2018).

14.1.4 Importance of Transdisciplinary or Multidisciplinary Team

Hence, the incorporation of a transdisciplinary or multidisciplinary team with geriatric care emphasis is ever more important, to optimize cognitive, physical and organ functions that will improve medical and surgical outcomes. To address these geriatric surgery issues, multimodal strategies are used to promote better outcomes including GA, prehabilitation (which includes medical optimisation, physical exercise, nutritional support and psychological support), MIS, ERAS and rehabilitation.

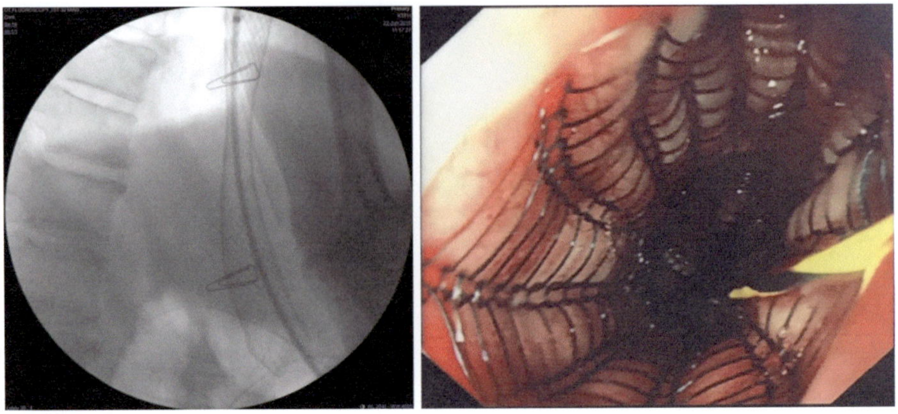

Fig. 14.10 (**a**) Fluoroscopic view of a palliative-intent oesophageal stent insertion under image intensifier guidance with paper clip markers placed around the proximal and distal ends of malignant oesophageal stricture. (**b**) Endoscopic view of a successfully and satisfactorily placed oesophageal stent

Initial non-operative management of UGIC crisis, allowing the opportunity for perioperative optimization or prehabilitation can be considered in some suitable cases.

In the late stage of UGIC, palliative non-resectable therapy in the form of oesophageal stent (Fig. 14.10a, b) or gastroduodenal stent (Fig. 14.11a–c) insertion, palliative bypass surgery may be considered along with palliative chemotherapy and/or radiotherapy and/or targeted therapy and/or immunotherapy. In a systematic review and meta-analysis of 23 studies totalling 999 patients, looking at the role of repeated normothermic intraperitoneal chemotherapy (catheter-based or pressurised aerosol) in patients with gastric cancer and peritoneal metastases, it was found that the treatment is safe and conversion surgery is possible in 16% of the patients (Guchelaar et al. 2024). However, it is unclear what percentage of older persons is included in the study. The alternative palliative-intent cytoreductive surgery (CRS) and hyperthermic intraperitoneal chemotherapy (HIPEC) would be considered too aggressive in older persons with metastatic disease.

Best supportive care should be considered in older persons not fit for such treatment above. The palliative medicine team should be consulted early, and those skilled in discussing advanced care planning with the older persons and their carers should be arranged for better coordination of end-of-life care.

The guidance of four ethical principles of beneficence, non-maleficence, autonomy and justice should be adhered to during the counselling process, regardless of whether the intent is for curative or palliative management. The professional and therapeutic relationship built on competent and compassionate care by the clinician should meet the expectation and benefits of the patient without adding unnecessary harm (Varkey 2021).

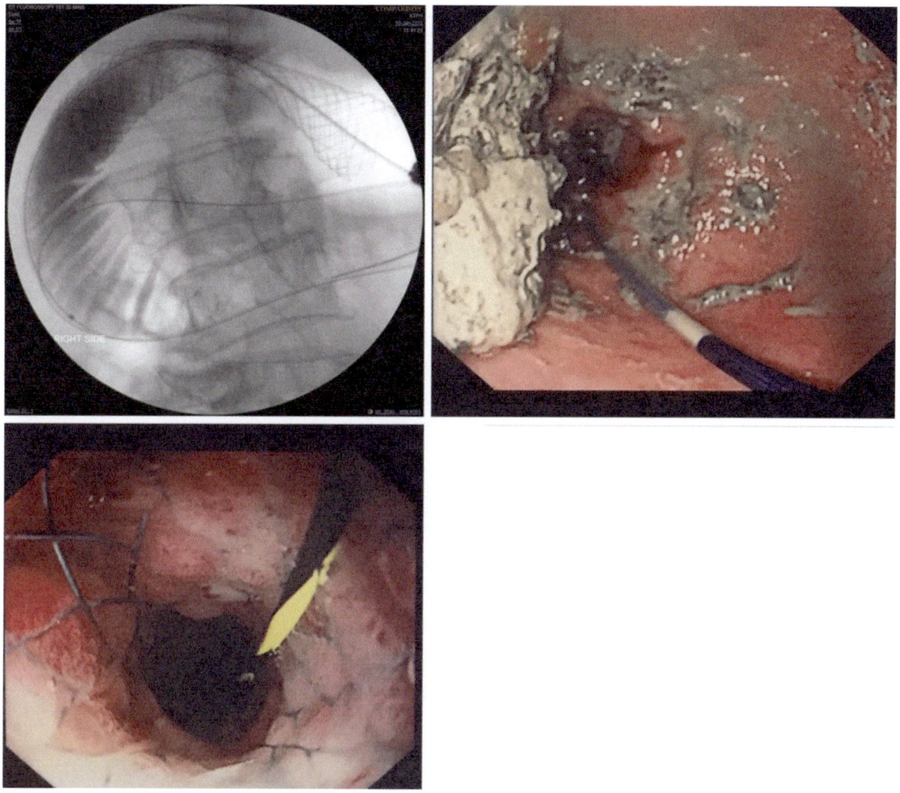

Fig. 14.11 (**a**) Fluoroscopic view of a palliative-intent gastroduodenal stent insertion with central 'waisting' and some flow of contrast from the gastric side into the duodenum. (**b**) Endoscopic view of a malignant gastric pylorus stricture causing gastric outlet obstruction. (**c**) Endoscopic view of the lumen of malignant gastric pylorus stricture following a gastroduodenal stent insertion

14.2 Geriatric Assessment (GA)

GA is an assessment in the domains of functional status, objective physical performance, falls, cognitive function, mood, nutritional status, comorbidity, polypharmacy and social support (Rostoft et al. 2021). There are many assessment tools available in each domain with the aim of evaluating and optimising diagnostic and treatment plans, improving prognostication and risk stratification. For example, the GA screening tools include Vulnerable Elderly Survey, Triage Risk Screening Tool, Geriatric-8, Groningen Frailty Index, Comprehensive Geriatric Assessment (CGA), Clinical Frailty Scale (also known as Rockwood Frailty Scale), Baldacci Score and Fried Frailty Scale. Each of these GA tools has different levels of sensitivity and specificity in predicting frailty in older persons with cancer (Kenig et al. 2015).

14.2.1 Vulnerability of Older Persons with UGIC

Older persons with UGIC are a vulnerable group of patients, especially with reduced physiological reserves, medical comorbidity, frailty and cognitive impairment. In one review article citing 113 references, physical fitness was found as an independent risk factor, and its effect on other risk factors is a significant indicator of developing pulmonary and cardiac complications after oesophagectomy (Feeney et al. 2010). An intervention that would improve physical activity and fitness may positively influence these complications.

Frailty is a complex state of diminished physiologic reserve that results in decreased resiliency, adaptive capacity, and increased vulnerability to stressors. A review article citing 132 references concluded that frailty in particularly older persons with cancer is a predictor of postoperative complications, chemotherapy intolerance, disease progression and death (Ethun et al. 2017).

Postoperative delirium is common in older persons undergoing surgery. In a Japanese cohort study of 255 patients utilising CGA, the combined use of Mini-Mental State Examination (MMSE) and Eastern Cooperative Oncology Group Performance Status (ECOG-PS) can easily predict postoperative delirium in older persons with gastric cancer undergoing gastrectomy (Itami et al. 2024). In this study, the CGA consisted of five assessments: the Barthel Index and Instrumental Activities of Daily Living scale (IADL) was used to assess physical function, while the MMSE, the Geriatric Depression Scale 15 (GDS-15) and the Vitality Index (VI) were used to assess the mental function.

14.2.2 Why Use GA in UGIC?

The European Society for Medical Oncology (ESMO) recommends the use of GA before initiating treatment in older persons with gastric cancer (Smyth et al. 2016). Older persons have been shown to have the same benefits from radical treatment and palliative chemotherapy as younger patients. With the use of GA, an individualised approach to treatment decisions can achieve improved outcomes in this cohort (Joharatnam-Hogan et al. 2020).

In an American database study from M. D. Anderson Cancer Center, utilising CGA in 279 patients with gastric and OG junction adenocarcinoma undergoing gastrectomy showed that ECOG-PS was the main modifiable variable associated with gastrectomy outcome (Pujara et al. 2015). There are treatment guidelines supporting neoadjuvant chemotherapy and chemoradiotherapy prior to gastrectomy, which allow a window of opportunity for prehabilitation during this time and may reduce postoperative complications.

In a Japanese study assessing the impact of GA on postoperative survival in 544 older persons with gastrointestinal cancers, it was found that GA as well as age, type of cancer, clinical stage, performance status and body mass index (BMI) were independent predictors of postoperative overall survival (Yamasaki et al. 2019). By predicting postoperative prognosis, GA may help determine treatment strategies for older persons with gastrointestinal cancer.

Based on the current evidence, it is prudent to utilise GA tools in UGIC surgery to assist in case selection and identify those with limited organ reserves, functional and cognitive impairment, frail and malnourished older persons with UGIC for preoperative optimisation and rehabilitation.

14.2.3 Transdisciplinary or Multidisciplinary Team with Geriatric Care Emphasis

In about 2010, in the United Kingdom, perioperative care of elderly surgical patients was found to be fragmented and managed poorly, resulting in potentially avoidable morbidity and mortality. Hence, a 10-point summary of Perioperative Care of Elderly 2014 Guidelines was published by the Association of Anaesthesia of Great Britain and Ireland (AAGBI), with the members of working party consisted of the College of Emergency Medicine, British Geriatrics Society, Age Anaesthesia Association, Intensive Care Society and the Royal College of Surgeons (Griffiths et al. 2014). The guidelines remain practical and applicable to this day, particularly multidisciplinary care improves outcomes for elderly surgical patients. The AAGBI strongly supports an expanded role for senior geriatricians in coordinating perioperative care for older persons, with input from senior anaesthetists and surgeons.

An Italian study looking at the effect of geriatric co-management with targeted interventions during daily geriatrician-led ward rounds in 207 older persons undergoing surgery for gastrointestinal cancer showed a significant reduction in Clavien-Dindo grade I–V complications and in 1-year readmissions with no difference in 1-year mortality (Giannotti et al. 2022).

A group of multidisciplinary Spanish experts in oncogeriatric, digestive tumours and cancer treatment reviewed the existing scientific evidence of 96 published articles in older persons (age ≥65 years old) with gastric cancer and provided a series of recommendations that allow optimisation of management during all phases of the disease. The recommendations were summarised in Table 4 of the article which can beaccessibleonlineathttps://www.geriatriconcology.net/action/showPdf?pii=S1879-4068%2823%2900554-4 (Paredero-Pérez et al. 2024).

Based on the current global evidence, it is prudent to collaborate in a transdisciplinary or multidisciplinary team for holistic UGIC management in older persons with geriatric care emphasis during their continuum of cancer care from the hospital to the community.

14.3 Prehabilitation

Prehabilitation is the process of enhancing a patient's functional capacity before surgery, with the aim of improving postoperative outcomes. Ageing is associated with reduced lean body mass, increased body fat, decreased total body water, reduced bone density (Lugli et al. 2008) and decreased physiological and mental reserve (Carli and Baldini 2021). Prehabilitation can improve the physiological reserve by optimising cardiorespiratory capacity, muscle strength and mental resiliency in anticipation of surgery (Carli and Baldini 2021).

Preoperative interventions, including medical optimisation, physical exercise, nutritional support and psychological support, may enhance the overall fitness of those with poor health, likely contributing to better postoperative outcomes (Kow 2019). A multimodal rehabilitation programme in older persons before major surgery with the duration between 4 and 8 weeks is required to be effective (Banugo and Amoako 2017). Rehabilitation with shorter duration may be ineffective, while longer duration may have compliance issue.

14.3.1 Why Use Multimodal Prehabilitation in UGIC?

A systematic review and meta-analysis of nine randomised controlled trials (RCTs) totalling 823 patients by the National University Hospital, Singapore, showed that multimodal rehabilitation in older persons before major abdominal surgery increases perioperative functional capacity and potentially decreases postoperative complications (Pang et al. 2022).

A Japanese group citing 84 references in a review article found emerging evidence that prehabilitation in both exercise and nutritional support can improve preoperative functional capacity, postoperative recovery and surgical outcomes in these groups of frail older persons with gastrointestinal cancers by preventing or minimising functional decline after surgery (Mima et al. 2022).

An American meta-analysis of 11 RCTS totalling 929 patients, analysing prehabilitation programmes in gastrointestinal cancer surgery, found improvement in exercise capacity both before and after surgery, with no significant difference in hospital length of stay (LOS), rates of postoperative complications, 30-day readmission and mortality (Lau and Chamberlain 2020).

Interestingly, a British group that performed a meta-analysis of nine RCTs and six uncontrolled trials determining the impact of prehabilitation on patient outcomes in hepatobiliary, colorectal and UGIC surgery showed that prehabilitation was associated with reduced hospital LOS but had no effect on functional capacity, postoperative complications or mortality rate (Lambert et al. 2021).

A school of nursing in China performed a systematic review and meta-analysis of eight studies with 902 participants, investigating the impact of prehabilitation in frail older persons, and found a reduction in total complications and 6-min walking test (6MWT) after surgery, with no difference in mortality and readmission rates (She et al. 2024).

A Chinese RCT investigated the effectiveness of prehabilitation in improving the physical and nutritional status in 136 patients undergoing gastric cancer resection (Li et al. 2024). The intervention consisted of preoperative exercise and nutrition optimisation. The prehabilitation training included abdominal breathing exercises, deep inspiration training with a breathing coach, aerobic exercise and strengthening exercise. When compared to the control group, the prehabilitation group exhibited improved functional capacity both before and after surgery in 6MWT. In addition, the prehabilitation group demonstrated significantly higher levels of albumin and prealbumin before and after surgery than the control group.

14.3.2 Role of Telehealth Prehabilitation in UGIC

With the advancement in telehealth technology, there are two studies confirming the feasibility and effectiveness of telehealth prehabilitation programme in OG cancer patients before and during COVID-19 pandemic, respectively.

In the first study from Belgium involving 23 patients, Internet-based tele-prehabilitation including aerobic, resistance and inspiratory muscle training was conducted over 2–4 weeks with a rate high in recruitment, retention and satisfaction. There was a good attendance to exercise sessions with no exercise-related adverse events. After prehabilitation, the participants significantly improved their fatigue, quality of life, physical well-being, emotional well-being and anxiety (Piraux et al. 2020).

The second study from United Kingdom involving 31 patients showed that digital prehabilitation can be delivered effectively to patients with OG cancer, with high engagement and retention rates. There were observed improvements in some physical and psychological parameters with the digital service, with comparable clinical outcomes to the in-person prehabilitation (Moorthy et al. 2023).

14.3.3 Sarcopenia in UGIC

Sarcopenia is defined as the severe loss of muscle mass and function.

In a Japanese retrospective single-centre study, 199 patients who underwent oesophagectomy for oesophageal cancer had their skeletal muscle mass analysed using CT scans at the third lumbar vertebra level (L3) (Nishigori et al. 2016). The study showed sarcopenia as an independent predictor of pulmonary complications after oesophagectomy.

In a Canadian retrospective single-centre study, 141 patients with oesophageal cancer undergoing trimodality therapy were investigated using staging CT scan (Jogiat et al. 2023). Sarcopenia classified by the staging CT was present in 20 (17.0%) patients, which increased to 45 (38.1%) patients by the post-neoadjuvant scan and 44 (37.3%) by the surveillance scan. In a multivariable analysis, sarcopenia at the post-neoadjuvant scan was significantly associated with overall survival (OS) and disease-free survival (DFS). The net change in skeletal muscle index was associated with OS and DFS.

Similarly, in an Australian single-centre retrospective study, 62 patients who underwent gastrectomy for gastric cancer showed sarcopenia as an independent predictor for major postoperative complications and decreased recurrence-free survival (RFS) (Alnimri et al. 2021).

In a Chinese meta-analysis of 11 cohort studies totalling 2149 patients, the effect of sarcopenia in digestive carcinoma showed sarcopenia prevalence ranging from 11.6 to 33.0%. Sarcopenia was associated with an increased risk of total and major complications, readmissions, total infection and severe infections, 30-day mortality, longer hospital LOS and increased hospitalisation expenditures (Hua et al. 2019). However, the limitation of the study includes heterogeneity related to different gastrointestinal cancer and muscle mass measurements.

A systematic review and meta-analysis of 40 retrospective and prospective studies totalling 5669 patients with sarcopenia undergoing oesophagectomy or oesophago-gastrectomy for cancer by the Brazilian group concluded that sarcopenia was significantly associated with postoperative complications, severe complications and pneumonia. Patients with sarcopenia had a lower chance of long-term survival (Park et al. 2023).

Based on the current global evidence, sarcopenia in UGIC is an independent risk factor for postoperative complications, especially infection and reduced overall long-term survival. Hence, preoperative exercise and nutrition are important to reduce the risks from sarcopenia.

14.3.4 Why Use Perioperative Nutrition in UGIC?

In older persons with or at risk of malnutrition, European Society for Parenteral and Enteral Nutrition (ESPEN) guidelines recommend enteral nutrition, preferably oral route, than tube feeding to improve nutritional status and to reduce mortality (Volkert et al. 2006).

A Japanese retrospective study evaluating the impact of preoperative Geriatric Nutritional Risk Index (GNRI) on short- and long-term outcomes in 303 older persons with gastric cancer who underwent laparoscopy-assisted gastrectomy showed that GNRI is an important predictor of postoperative complications and overall survival (Hirahara et al. 2021). It is a reliable and cost-effective prognostic indicator that should be routinely evaluated. In another Japanese retrospective study of 206 older persons undergoing emergency gastrointestinal surgery, it was found that GNRI may be a predictor of postoperative infection (Takano et al. 2024).

A systematic review of 15 articles looking at preoperative nutrition and postoperative outcome in older persons undergoing general surgery by the Dutch group revealed that the two preoperative predictors of postoperative outcome are weight loss $\geq$10% in previous 6 months and serum albumin (van Stijn et al. 2013).

A systematic review and meta-analysis investigated the effect of nutrition-based rehabilitation on postoperative outcomes in 661 patients who underwent oesophagectomy and gastrectomy. The Chinese study group found that unimodal (nutrition only) and multimodal prehabilitation collectively decreased the risk of any postoperative complication by 23% (Shen et al. 2024).

In a review article with 68 references on oral nutritional supplements (ONS) and enteral nutrition (EN) in patients undergoing gastrointestinal surgery, the German authors provided a list of perioperative nutrition recommendations (Wobith and Weimann 2021):

(a) Preoperative assessment of the nutritional status is mandatory.
(b) Surgery should be postponed if there is a high metabolic risk/severe malnutrition.
(c) Nutritional therapy should be administered enterally for 10–14 days.
(d) Prehabilitation should be considered.
(e) Preoperative use of ONS for at least 7 days may diminish the rate of infectious complications and the length of hospital stay.
(f) Preoperative immunonutrition for 5–7 days may lead to a reduction in infectious complications in gastrointestinal cancer patients.
(g) Early oral intake is also feasible after oesophagectomy and gastrectomy.
(h) If the oral calorie intake is insufficient (<50% for more than 7 days), ONS and enteral supplementation may be indicated.
(i) Metabolic risk patients should receive dietary counselling at the time of discharge and follow-up nutritional care.
(j) Follow-up on the nutritional status and nutrition therapy after discharge may be necessary, especially after surgery in the UGIC due to prolonged weight loss with high metabolic risk.

Based on the current global evidence, it is prudent to implement a standardised pathway in multimodal prehabilitation programme in UGIC surgery for medical optimisation, physical exercise, nutritional support and psychological support prior to surgery.

14.4 Minimally Invasive Surgery (MIS)

MIS is a surgical approach involving smaller incisions to produce less tissue trauma and potentially reduce pain, complications and recovery time. MIS creates less inflammatory response when compared to open surgery.

14.4.1 Why Use MIS in UGIC?

Several studies have shown that MIS (Fig. 14.12a–j) that includes laparoscopy, thoracoscopy or robotic surgery can improve postoperative outcomes, compared to open surgery, with less postoperative pain, early postoperative recovery, lower rates of complications and mortality in oesophagectomy and robotic-assisted gastrectomy (Zhou et al. 2015; Gottlieb-Vedi et al. 2019; Müller-Stich et al. 2021; Kikuchi et al. 2021).

Similarly, RCTs in laparoscopic gastrectomy have reported reduced wound complications, blood loss, postoperative pain, time to first bowel movement and length

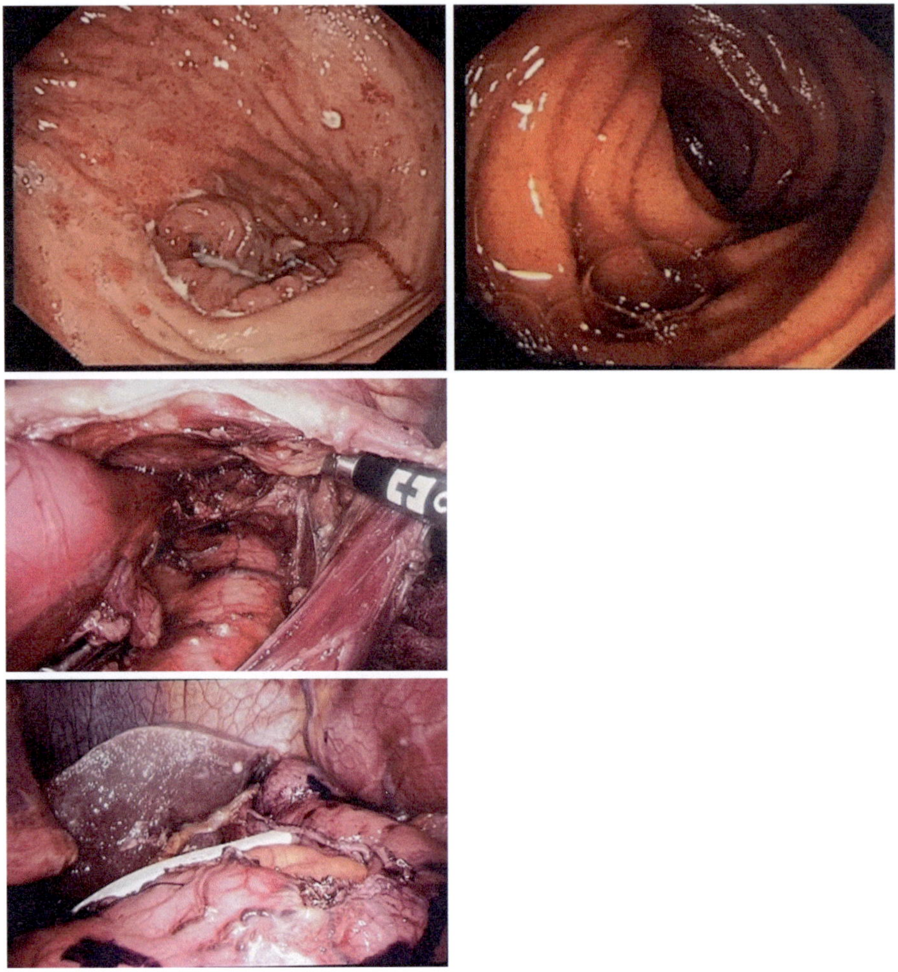

Fig. 14.12 (**a**) Endoscopic view of gastrojejunostomy following a laparoscopic subtotal gastrectomy. (**b**) Endoscopic view of alimentary jejunal limb with some bile reflux following laparoscopic subtotal gastrectomy and Roux-en-Y reconstruction. (**c**) Laparoscopic trans-hiatal view of posterior mediastinum following mobilisation of OG junction and thoracic oesophagus in a supine position. (**d**) Laparoscopic view of abdominal gastric tube conduit creation (Stage 1 of Ivor-Lewis oesophagectomy) in preparation for thoracic phase (Stage 2 of Ivor-Lewis oesophagectomy). (**e**) Thoracoscopic view of pleural space with the oesophagus between the thoracic vertebrae, aorta and the lung in a semi-prone position. (**f**) Thoracoscopic view of mobilised oesophagus and lymph nodes from posterior mediastinum and trachea–bronchial region. (**g**, **h**) Thoracoscopic view of a transected proximal oesophagus using a linear stapler. (**i**) Thoracoscopic view of gastric conduit pull-up in the thoracic cavity in preparation for transection of proximal stomach. (**j**) Thoracoscopic view of an oesophagogastric anastomosis creation

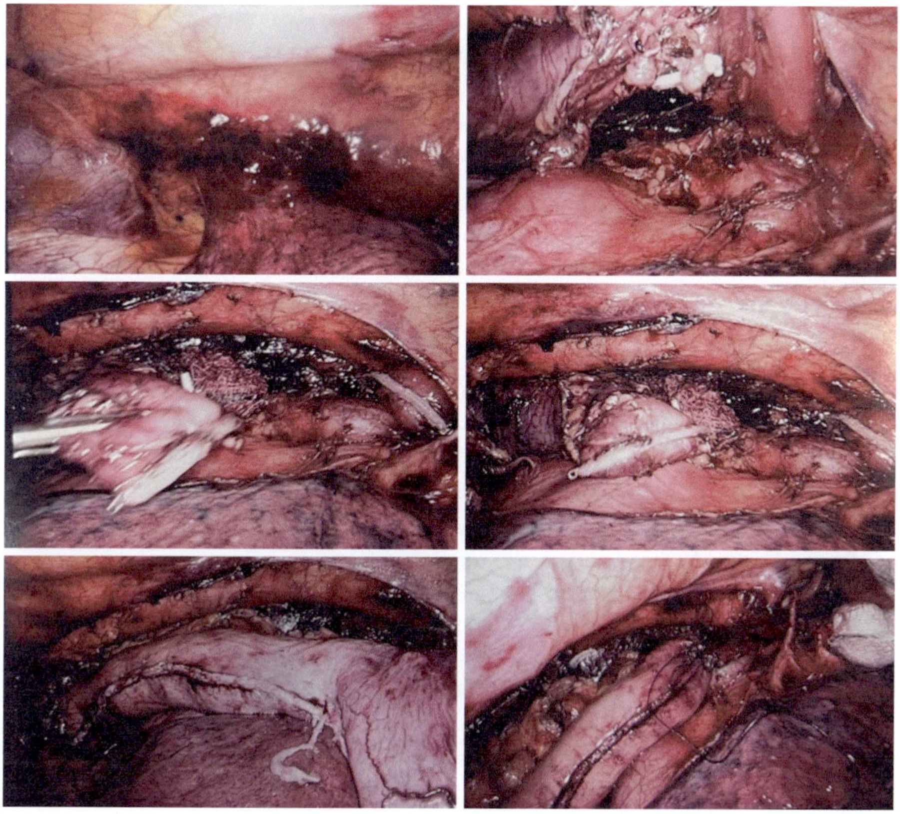

Fig. 14.12 (continued)

of hospital stays, in addition to better quality of life and equally good oncological outcomes (Deng et al. 2015; Kim W et al. 2016; Kim HH et al. 2019).

While there are many advantages of MIS, open surgery skills remain a safe necessity and should form part of surgical armamentarium. Open surgery may allow rapid access and better exposure to the surgical field and provides tactile sensation in such conditions like emergency, challenging cases and patients with compromised state under general anaesthesia with or without prior MIS (Zhao and Gu 2022).

There is an important concept of limited surgery for older persons with gastric cancer (Mikami et al. 2018). This Japanese retrospective study included 267 older persons with gastric cancer who were divided into either standard gastrectomy with nodal dissection (standard group) or gastrectomy with reduced nodal dissection (limited group). The limited group had significantly poorer nutrition status and a significantly higher proportion with comorbidities. However, the morbidity and mortality were similar in both groups. A multivariate analysis showed that the overall survival rates were significantly worse in patients with advanced age, male gender, low BMI, low Onodera prognostic nutritional index and a higher tumour stage.

This chapter highlights the importance of modifiable risk of sarcopenia and malnutrition which should be addressed prior to standard gastrectomy.

14.4.2 Timing of Surgery

The timing of operative surgery in acute versus elective is essential in determining whether it is appropriate for preoperative optimisation. It is possible to divert immediate crisis into temporary stabilisation while addressing nutrition, prehabilitation and optimisation of organ function. Initial non-operative management of UGIC bleed utilizing endoscopic haemostasis, interventional radiology angioembolization and radiation therapy may be considered in a suitable scenario. Similarly, non-operative management of UGIC partial obstruction utilizing endoscopically or radiologically inserted fine bore nasogastric or nasojejunal tube is useful for preoperative enteral nutrition. In completely obstructed UGIC, total parenteral nutrition should be considered. In perforated UGIC, the majority would require emergent or urgent operative intervention. The use of temporary stents and suction drains to control perforated leaks may be considered case by case in the expert hands.

Based on the current evidence, it is prudent to adopt MIS techniques and instruments in UGIC surgery such as endoscopy, laparoscopy, thoracoscopy or robotic-assisted surgery as appropriate. Consider initial non-operative management of UGIC crisis such as in partial obstruction and bleeding, by allowing opportunity for perioperative optimisation or prehabilitation.

14.5 Enhanced Recovery After Surgery (ERAS)

ERAS is a multimodal perioperative evidence-based care within the fast-track methodology that significantly enhances postoperative recovery and reduces morbidity (Kehlet and Wilmore 2008). Transdisciplinary or multidisciplinary engagement is therefore required to make it work successfully.

14.5.1 Why Use ERAS in UGIC?

Many centralised UGIC units have established standardised care pathways for the management of patients undergoing oesophagectomy. An example of institutional standardised clinical pathway for oesophagectomy is from the Virginia Mason Medical Centre, United States of America (Zylstra et al. 2018).

In oesophagectomy, the operative components to consider are the timing of surgery (6–8 weeks after neoadjuvant chemotherapy and up to 10 weeks after neoadjuvant chemoradiotherapy), surgical techniques (MIS, extent of lymphadenectomy, choice of conduit and its route and stapled versus hand-sewn anastomosis), surgical drains (early removal of drains when no longer needed or <100–150 mL/day), nasogastric tube (early removal of drain when no contraindication in Day 2) and anaesthetic management (shorter-acting neuromuscular blockers, lung-protective ventilation, reduced driving pressure and duration of single lung ventilation, early extubation and balanced intravenous fluid therapy).

Post-oesophagectomy components to consider are the care level (ICU or HDU), pain control (multimodal analgesic agents with local and regional anaesthetics such as paravertebral block and thoracic epidural), mobilization (early on Day 1), nutrition (early enteral tube feed or oral feed) and pharmacological prophylaxis (thromboprophylaxis, antiemetics, antibiotics <24 h, bowel stimulation, glycaemic and arrhythmia control).

ERAS programme in United Kingdom have resulted in improved short-term outcomes after surgery such as reduced length of stay and readmissions to hospital after surgery and have widely been integrated into surgical–oncology pathways as best practice (Preston et al. 2013).

A systematic review of nine studies with pooled analysis of 1240 patients on the effect of standardised ERAS protocol in oesophagectomy patients reported improved outcomes including anastomotic leaks, pulmonary complications and hospital LOS with no significant change in postoperative mortality and readmission rate (Markar et al. 2015). Similarly, in an Italian study of 207 older persons undergoing surgery for gastrointestinal cancer, incorporating ERAS programme onto CGA and geriatric co-management showed a significant reduction in Clavien-Dindo grade I–V complications and in 1-year readmissions with no difference in 1-year mortality rate (Giannotti et al. 2022).

A Chinese meta-analysis of 25 RTCs comprising 2809 patients, looking at the application of ERAS in minimally invasive gastrectomy for gastric cancer, showed shorter postoperative hospital LOS, hastened first postoperative flatus, reduced medical costs and overall postoperative complication rate without increasing readmission rates (Jin et al. 2022).

Based on the current global evidence, it is prudent to implement ERAS protocol for UGIC surgery focusing on the care level, pain control, early mobilisation, enteral nutrition, pharmacological prophylaxis and most importantly rehabilitation.

14.5.2 Why Rehabilitation in UGIC?

Rehabilitation is a set of interventions designed to optimise function, reduce disability in individuals with poor health conditions, allowing them to interact normally with their environment. Rehabilitation is patient-centred with the help of health workers such as physiotherapist, occupational therapists, speech and language therapists and physical rehabilitation doctors. Rehabilitation can help reduce the length of hospital stay, prevent readmission, increase the ability to return to work and remain independent in the community.

A Danish controlled clinical trial study looking at the effects of high-intensity exercise after 49 oesophagectomies for stage I–III OG junction cancer reported 12 weeks of postoperative aerobic and resistance training increased muscle strength and cardiorespiratory fitness to pretreatment levels. However, there was no difference in health-related quality of life when compared to the usual care control group (Simonsen et al. 2020).

Based on the evidence, it is prudent to integrate rehabilitation within the ERAS protocol in UGIC.

14.6 Conclusion

The management of curative UGIC remains challenging, in the form of a multimodal therapy including chemotherapy, radiotherapy and surgery. Older persons' ability to withstand the rigours of multimodal therapy can be similarly challenging due to their limited physiological reserves, cognitive and functional decline, frailty and malnutrition.

Based on the current evidence, it is prudent to adopt multimodal strategies (Fig. 14.13) to promote better outcomes that include the following: (1) apply GA tools to select the most appropriate and safe medical and surgical interventions in older persons with UGIC diagnosis; (2) collaborate with a transdisciplinary or multidisciplinary team for holistic UGIC management in older persons with geriatric care emphasis during their continuum of cancer care from the hospital to the community; (3) implement a standardised pathway in multimodal prehabilitation programme for medical optimisation, physical exercise, nutritional support and psychological support; (4) adopt MIS techniques and instruments such as endoscopy, laparoscopic, thoracoscopy or robotic-assisted surgery as appropriate. Consider initial non-operative management of UGIC crisis, allowing opportunity

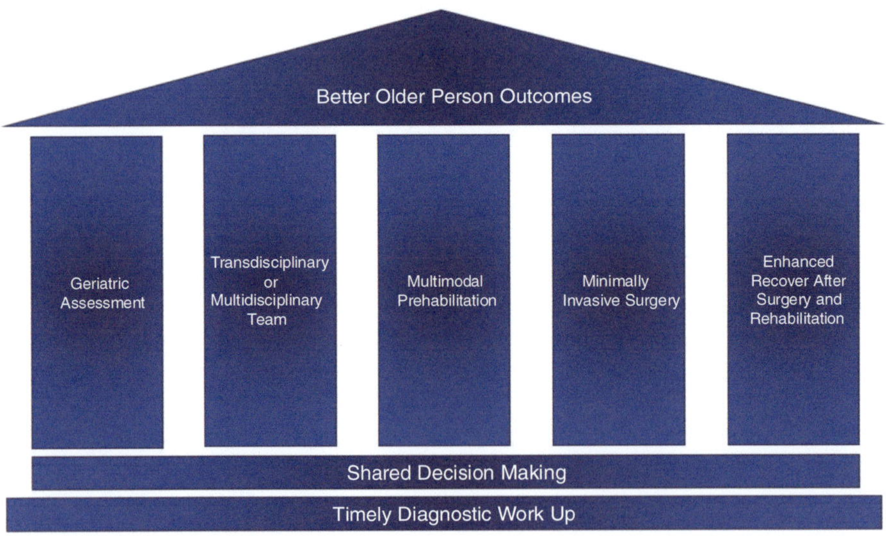

Fig. 14.13 Strategies for better older person outcomes in upper gastrointestinal cancer surgery is supported by the two stepping stones and five pillars of perioperative management

for perioperative optimisation or prehabilitation; and (5) implement ERAS protocol in UGIC surgery focusing on pain control, nutrition and rehabilitation.

The management of palliative-intent UGIC should focus on respecting older persons' preferences and wishes during the end-of-life journey in shared decision-making.

14.7 Case Scenario

An 89-year-old widow presented with a history of dyspepsia and acid reflux symptoms for 3 years. She has been taking omeprazole 20 mg daily for symptoms control. Her past history included hypertension, hyperlipidaemia and left mastectomy for breast cancer. An UGIE was performed which showed severe pangastritis with some mucosal irregularity at the incisura, which was biopsied (Fig. 14.14). The histology revealed a moderate to poorly differentiated adenocarcinoma and *Helicobacter pylori*-associated chronic active gastritis (Fig. 14.15a, b). A staging CT chest, abdomen and pelvis scan showed a large hepatic cyst in the left liver lobe measuring about 11 cm (Fig. 14.16). There was no significantly enlarged perigastric lymph nodes and no evidence of intra-thoracic or intra-abdominal metastasis. In view of poorly differentiated adenocarcinoma, it was not suitable for ESD. She was treated with triple therapy and referred to Geriatric Surgery Service (GSS), a transdisciplinary team for GA and preoperative optimisation and prehabilitation. She was counselled in the presence of two children for a laparoscopic D2 subtotal gastrectomy.

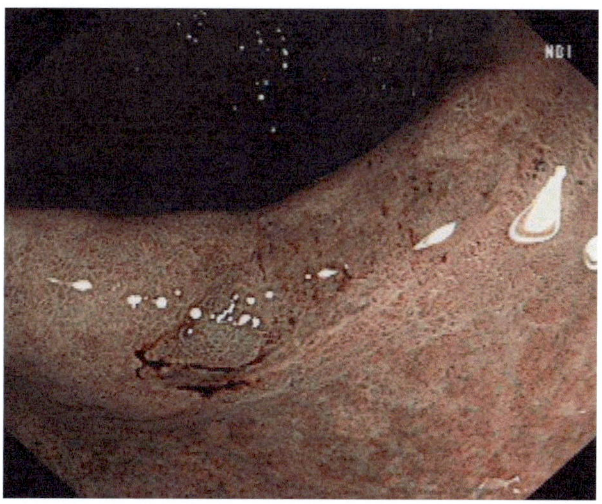

Fig. 14.14 UGIE view of gastric incisura mucosal abnormality

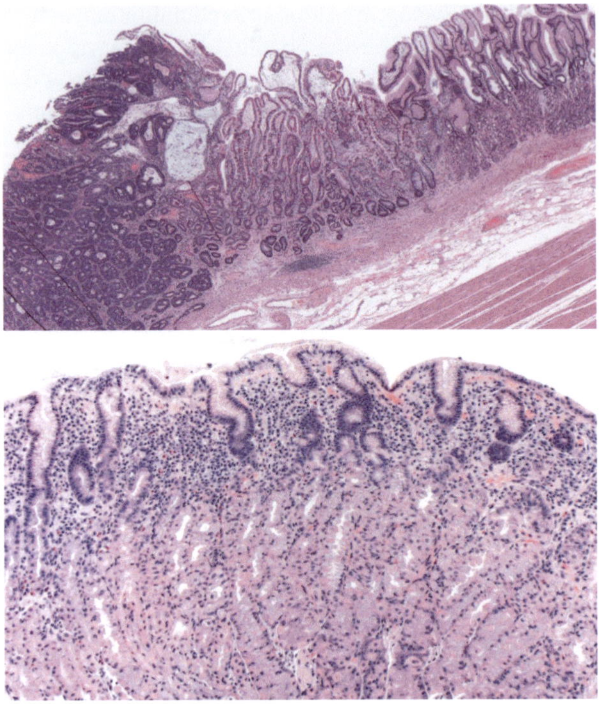

Fig. 14.15 (**a**) Microscopic histological view of adenocarcinoma of gastric incisura biopsy. (**b**) Microscopic histological view of *Helicobacter pylori*-associated chronic active gastritis from gastric antrum biopsy

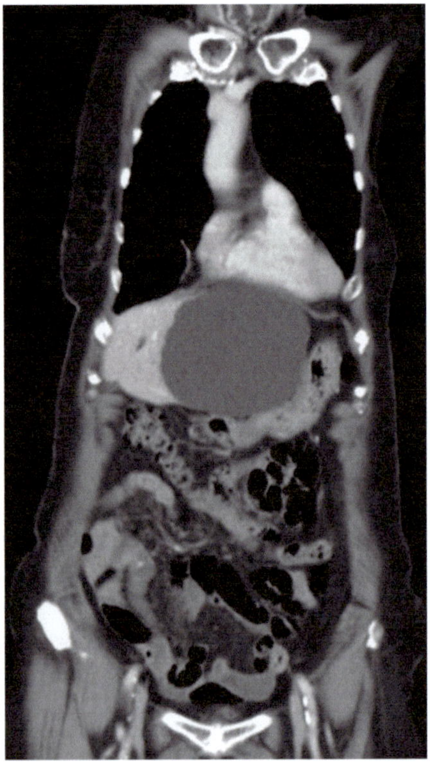

Fig. 14.16 Coronal view of CT scan of chest, abdomen and pelvis showing a large left lobe of liver cyst creating an external compression onto the gastric body

GSS Assessment	
Age, Gender	89, Female
Social	Widow, lives with two children and a domestic helper.
Activity of Daily Living (ADL)	Independent, community ambulant. Does brisk walking and Yoga for 40 min/day.
Barthel Index (BI)	100/100
Charlson Comorbidity Index (CCI)	2
Fried Frailty Index	Prefrail (grip strength and exhaustion)
Rockwood CFS	2
Abbreviated Mental Test (AMT)	10/10
Surgeon	Laparoscopic subtotal gastrectomy with date in 2–3 weeks.
Dietician	Subjective Global Assessment (SGA) A, well nourished. 1. Phone call follow-up weekly. 2. Aim to meet 100% requirement and weight maintenance.
Physiotherapist	Time Up and Go Test (score is best of 2 attempts) 10.04 s—normal for age group. Gait Speed (Normal) Average: 10.78 s, 20 steps, 0.93 m/s. Gait Speed (Fast) Average 8.69 s, 19.5 steps, 1.15 m/s. (score is best of 2 attempts) 8.65 s, 19 steps, 1.15 m/s.
Anaesthetist	Stand by GXM 2 units PCT for surgery. Avoid IV access to left arm if previous left axillary clearance. Admit 1 day pre-surgery. Book surgical HDU.
Cardiologist	Low cardiac risk.
GRM	Nifedipine LA on the morning of surgery and discontinue thereafter. Consider changing ACEI for microalbuminaemia if renal function is stable postoperative, otherwise change to amlodipine (may have issue with modified release medication post gastric surgery). Check Vitamin D level. Consider BMD and osteoporosis treatment if required.
MSW	NA.
Nursing	Left arm precaution in view of previous left mastectomy.
Pharmacist	NA.

She underwent laparoscopy and required decompression of large benign liver cyst and marsupialisation to provide exposure to the whole of stomach. Laparoscopic subtotal gastrectomy, D2 lymphadenectomy and Roux-en-Y reconstruction were performed with intraoperative UGIE check. P-POSSUM score was operative morbidity risk of 21.6% and mortality risk of 1%. The total operative time was 359 min. Inpatient surgical recovery and rehabilitation were uneventful and was discharged home. The hospital LOS was 10 days.

The final histology of the specimens reported: (1) Benign simple biliary cyst. (2) pT1aN0 (0/52LN positive) diffuse or poorly cohesive adenocarcinoma with signet ring of gastric incisura. G3, LVI and PNI negative. R0 (Fig. 14.17a, b).

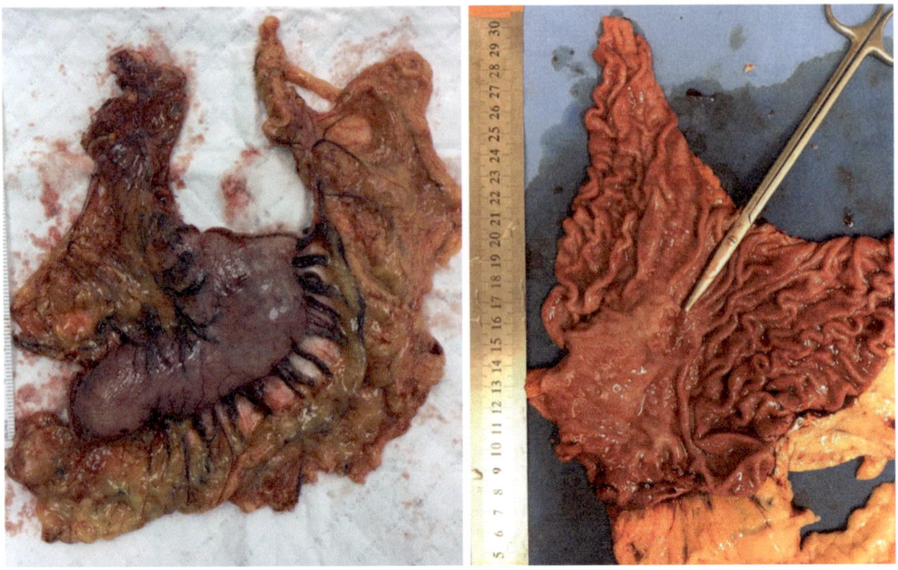

Fig. 14.17 (**a**) Macroscopic view of the resected subtotal gastrectomy and adjacent lymph nodes with lesser and greater omentum. (**b**) Macroscopic view of gastric lumen with pointed instrument showing the site of gastric incisura cancer

At 3-monthly clinic review, she remained well in physical and cognitive function, and has returned to her baseline ADL and has no cancer recurrence at 1 year follow-up.

References

Al-Batran SE, Homann N, Pauligk C, Goetze TO, Meiler J, Kasper S, Kopp HG, Mayer F, Haag GM, Luley K, Lindig U, Schmiegel W, Pohl M, Stoehlmacher J, Folprecht G, Probst S, Prasnikar N, Fischbach W, Mahlberg R, Trojan J, Koenigsmann M, Martens UM, Thuss-Patience P, Egger M, Block A, Heinemann V, Illerhaus G, Moehler M, Schenk M, Kullmann F, Behringer DM, Heike M, Pink D, Teschendorf C, Löhr C, Bernhard H, Schuch G, Rethwisch V, von Weikersthal LF, Hartmann JT, Kneba M, Daum S, Schulmann K, Weniger J, Belle S, Gaiser T, Oduncu FS, Güntner M, Hozaeel W, Reichart A, Jäger E, Kraus T, Mönig S, Bechstein WO, Schuler M, Schmalenberg H, Hofheinz RD, FLOT4-AIO Investigators (2019) Perioperative chemotherapy with fluorouracil plus leucovorin, oxaliplatin, and docetaxel versus fluorouracil or capecitabine plus cisplatin and epirubicin for locally advanced, resectable gastric or gastro-oesophageal junction adenocarcinoma (FLOT4): a randomised, phase 2/3 trial. Lancet 393(10184):1948–1957. https://doi.org/10.1016/S0140-6736(18)32557-1

Alnimri F, Sivakumar J, Sutherland T, Johnson MA, Ward S, Chong L, Hii MW (2021) Preoperative low muscle mass is associated with major complications and lower recurrence-free survival after gastric cancer surgery. ANZ J Surg 91(3):316–322. https://doi.org/10.1111/ans.16590

Bang YJ, Van Cutsem E, Feyereislova A, Chung HC, Shen L, Sawaki A, Lordick F, Ohtsu A, Omuro Y, Satoh T, Aprile G, Kulikov E, Hill J, Lehle M, Rüschoff J, Kang YK, ToGA Trial Investigators (2010) Trastuzumab in combination with chemotherapy versus chemotherapy alone for treatment of HER2-positive advanced gastric or gastro-oesophageal junction cancer (ToGA): a phase 3, open-label, randomised controlled trial. Lancet 376(9742):687–697. https://doi.org/10.1016/S0140-6736(10)61121-X. Erratum in: Lancet 2010 Oct 16;376(9749):1302

Banugo P, Amoako D (2017) Prehabilitation. BJA Educ 17(12):401–405. https://doi.org/10.1093/bjaed/mkx032

Bracken-Clarke D, Farooq AR, Horgan AM (2018) Management of locally advanced and metastatic esophageal cancer in the older population. Curr Oncol Rep 20(12):99. https://doi.org/10.1007/s11912-018-0745-3

Bray F, Laversanne M, Sung H, Ferlay J, Siegel RL, Soerjomataram I, Jemal A (2024) Global cancer statistics 2022: GLOBOCAN estimates of incidence and mortality worldwide for 36 cancers in 185 countries. CA Cancer J Clin 74(3):229–263. https://doi.org/10.3322/caac.21834

Cady B (1997) Basic principles in surgical oncology. Arch Surg 132(4):338–346. https://doi.org/10.1001/archsurg.1997.01430280012001

Carli F, Baldini G (2021) From preoperative assessment to preoperative optimization of frail older patiens. Eur J Surg Oncol 47:519–523

Deng Y, Zhang Y, Guo TK (2015) Laparoscopy-assisted versus open distal gastrectomy for early gastric cancer: a meta-analysis based on seven randomized controlled trials. Surg Oncol 24(2):71–77. https://doi.org/10.1016/j.suronc.2015.02.003

Ethun CG, Bilen MA, Jani AB, Maithel SK, Ogan K, Master VA (2017) Frailty and cancer: implications for oncology surgery, medical oncology, and radiation oncology. CA Cancer J Clin 67:362–377

Feeney C, Hussey J, Carey M, Reynolds JV (2010) Assessment of physical fitness for esophageal surgery, and targeting interventions to optimize outcomes. Dis Esophagus 23(7):529–539. https://doi.org/10.1111/j.1442-2050.2010.01058.x

Fried TR, Bradley EH, Towle VR, Allore H (2002) Understanding the treatment preferences of seriously ill patients. N Engl J Med 346(14):1061–1066. https://doi.org/10.1056/NEJMsa012528

Giannotti C, Massobrio A, Carmisciano L, Signori A, Napolitano A, Pertile D, Soriero D, Muzyka M, Tagliafico L, Casabella A, Cea M, Caffa I, Ballestrero A, Murialdo R, Laudisio A, Incalzi RA, Scabini S, Monacelli F, Nencioni A (2022) Effect of geriatric comanagement in older patients undergoing surgery for gastrointestinal cancer: a retrospective, before-and-after study. J Am Med Dir Assoc 23(11):1868.e9–1868.e16. https://doi.org/10.1016/j.jamda.2022.03.020

Glance LG, Osler TM, Neuman MD (2014) Redesigning surgical decision making for high-risk patients. N Engl J Med 370(15):1379–1381

Gottlieb-Vedi E, Kauppila JH, Malietzis G, Nilsson M, Markar SR, Lagergren J (2019) Long-term survival in esophageal cancer after minimally invasive compared to open esophagectomy: a systematic review and meta-analysis. Ann Surg 270:1005–1017

Griffiths R, Beech F, Brown A, Dhesi J, Foo I, Goodall J, Harrop-Griffiths W, Jameson J, Love N, Pappenheim K, White S (2014) Association of anesthetists of Great Britain and Ireland. Peri-operative care of the elderly 2014: Association of Anaesthetists of Great Britain and Ireland. Anaesthesia 69(Suppl 1):81–98. https://doi.org/10.1111/anae.12524

Guchelaar NAD, Nasserinejad K, Mostert B, Koolen SLW, van der Sluis PC, Lagarde SM, Wijnhoven BPL, Mathijssen RHJ, Noordman BJ (2024) Intraperitoneal chemotherapy for peritoneal metastases of gastric origin: a systematic review and meta-analysis. Br J Surg 111(5):znae116. https://doi.org/10.1093/bjs/znae116

van Hagen P, Hulshof MC, van Lanschot JJ, Steyerberg EW, van Berge Henegouwen MI, Wijnhoven BP, Richel DJ, Nieuwenhuijzen GA, Hospers GA, Bonenkamp JJ, Cuesta MA, Blaisse RJ, Busch OR, ten Kate FJ, Creemers GJ, Punt CJ, Plukker JT, Verheul HM, Spillenaar Bilgen EJ, van Dekken H, van der Sangen MJ, Rozema T, Biermann K, Beukema JC, Piet AH, van Rij CM, Reinders JG, Tilanus HW, van der Gaast A, CROSS Group (2012) Preoperative chemoradiotherapy for esophageal or junctional cancer. N Engl J Med 366(22):2074–2084. https://doi.org/10.1056/NEJMoa1112088

Hirahara N, Tajima Y, Fujii Y, Kaji S, Kawabata Y, Hyakudomi R, Yamamoto T, Taniura T (2021) Prediction of postoperative complications and survival after laparoscopic gastrectomy using preoperative Geriatric Nutritional Risk Index in elderly gastric cancer patients. Surg Endosc 35(3):1202–1209. https://doi.org/10.1007/s00464-020-07487-7

Hua H, Xu X, Tang Y, Ren Z, Xu Q, Chen L (2019) Effect of sarcopenia on clinical outcomes following digestive carcinoma surgery: a meta-analysis. Support Care Cancer 27(7):2385–2394. https://doi.org/10.1007/s00520-019-04767-4

Itami T, Yamamoto K, Kurokawa Y, Saito T, Takahashi T, Momose K, Yamashita K, Tanaka K, Makino T, Yasunobe Y, Akasaka H, Fujimoto T, Yamamoto K, Nakajima K, Eguchi H, Doki Y (2024) Assessing the risk of postoperative delirium through comprehensive geriatric assessment and eastern cooperative oncology group performance status of elderly patients with gastric cancer. Ann Surg Oncol 31(13):9039–9047. https://doi.org/10.1245/s10434-024-16034-w

Jin H, Song S, Lu T, Ma S, Wang Y, Fu L, Zhang G, Han X, Zhang L, Yang K, Cai H (2022) The application of enhanced recovery after surgery in minimally invasive gastrectomy for gastric cancer: a meta-analysis of randomized controlled trials. Expert Rev Gastroenterol Hepatol 16(11–12):1089–1100. https://doi.org/10.1080/17474124.2022.2145944

Jogiat UM, Baracos V, Turner SR, Eurich D, Filafilo H, Rouhi A, Bédard A, Bédard ELR (2023) Changes in sarcopenia status predict survival among patients with resectable esophageal cancer. Ann Surg Oncol 30(12):7412–7421. https://doi.org/10.1245/s10434-023-13840-6

Joharatnam-Hogan N, Shiu KK, Khan K (2020) Challenges in the treatment of gastric cancer in the older patient. Cancer Treat Rev 85:101980. https://doi.org/10.1016/j.ctrv.2020.101980

Kehlet H, Wilmore DW (2008) Evidence-based surgical care and the evolution of fast-track surgery. Ann Surg 248(2):189–198. https://doi.org/10.1097/SLA.0b013e31817f2c1a

Kenig J, Zychiewicz B, Olszewska U, Richter P (2015) Screening for frailty among older patients with cancer that qualify for abdominal surgery. J Geriatr Oncol 6:52–59

Kikuchi K, Suda K, Shibasaki S, Tanaka T, Uyama I (2021) Challenges in improving the minimal invasiveness of the surgical treatment for gastric cancer using robotic technology. Ann Gastroenterol Surg 5:604–613

Kim HH, Han SU, Kim MC, Kim W, Lee HJ, Ryu SW, Cho GS, Kim CY, Yang HK, Park DJ, Song KY, Lee SI, Ryu SY, Lee JH, Hyung WJ, Korean Laparoendoscopic Gastrointestinal Surgery Study (KLASS) Group (2019) Effect of laparoscopic distal gastrectomy vs open distal gastrectomy on long-term survival among patients with stage I gastric cancer: the KLASS-01 randomized clinical trial. JAMA Oncol 5(4):506–513. https://doi.org/10.1001/jamaoncol.2018.6727

Kim W, Kim HH, Han SU, Kim MC, Hyung WJ, Ryu SW, Cho GS, Kim CY, Yang HK, Park DJ, Song KY, Lee SI, Ryu SY, Lee JH, Lee HJ, Korean Laparo-endoscopic Gastrointestinal Surgery Study (KLASS) Group (2016) Decreased morbidity of laparoscopic distal gastrectomy compared with open distal gastrectomy for stage I gastric cancer: short-term outcomes from a multicenter randomized controlled trial (KLASS-01). Ann Surg 263(1):28–35. https://doi.org/10.1097/SLA.0000000000001346

Klevebro F, Garritano S, Scandavini CM, Shetye A, Coppola A, Kamiya S, Nilsson M, Lundell L, Rouvelas I (2019) Surgical outcomes of oesophagectomy or gastrectomy due to cancer for patients ≥75 years of age: a single-centre cohort study. ANZ J Surg 89(3):228–233. https://doi.org/10.1111/ans.14761

Koppert LB, Lemmens VE, Coebergh JW, Steyerberg EW, Wijnhoven BP, Tilanus HW, Janssen-Heijnen ML (2012) Impact of age and co-morbidity on surgical resection rate and survival in patients with oesophageal and gastric cancer. Br J Surg 99(12):1693–1700. https://doi.org/10.1002/bjs.8952

Kow AW (2019) Prehabilitation and its role in geriatric surgery. Ann Acad Med Singap 48(11):386–392

Lambert JE, Hayes LD, Keegan TJ, Subar DA, Gaffney CJ (2021) The impact of prehabilitation on patient outcomes in hepatobiliary, colorectal, and upper gastrointestinal cancer surgery: a PRISMA-accordant meta-analysis. Ann Surg 274(1):70–77. https://doi.org/10.1097/SLA.0000000000004527

Lau CSM, Chamberlain RS (2020) Prehabilitation programs improve exercise capacity before and after surgery in gastrointestinal cancer surgery patients: a meta-analysis. J Gastrointest Surg 24(12):2829–2837. https://doi.org/10.1007/s11605-019-04436-1

Li L, Liu J, Zhang Y, Wang J, Li S (2024) Clinical study of preoperative prehabilitation synchronized neoadjuvant chemotherapy for gastric cancer patients. Eur J Cancer Care 2024:9494994. https://doi.org/10.1155/2024/9494994

Lugli AK, Wykes L, Carli F (2008) Strategies for perioperative nutrition support in obese, diabetic and geriatric patients. Clin Nutr 27(1):16–24. https://doi.org/10.1016/j.clnu.2007.10.002

Markar SR, Karthikesalingam A, Low DE (2015) Enhanced recovery pathways lead to an improvement in postoperative outcomes following esophagectomy: systematic review and pooled analysis. Dis Esophagus 28(5):468–475. https://doi.org/10.1111/dote.12214

Mikami K, Hirano K, Futami K, Maekawa T (2018) Gastrectomy with limited surgery for elderly patients with gastric cancer. Asian J Surg 41(1):65–72. https://doi.org/10.1016/j.asjsur.2016.09.002

Mima K, Nakagawa S, Miyata T, Yamashita YI, Baba H (2022) Frailty and surgical outcomes in gastrointestinal cancer: integration of geriatric assessment and prehabilitation into surgical practice for vulnerable patients. Ann Gastroenterol Surg 7(1):27–41. https://doi.org/10.1002/ags3.12601

Moorthy K, Halliday LJ, Noor N, Peters CJ, Wynter-Blyth V, Urch CE (2023) Feasibility of implementation and the impact of a digital prehabilitation service in patients undergoing treatment for oesophago-gastric cancer. Curr Oncol 30(2):1673–1682. https://doi.org/10.3390/curroncol30020128

Morgan E, Soerjomataram I, Rumgay H, Coleman HG, Thrift AP, Vignat J, Laversanne M, Ferlay J, Arnold M (2022) The global landscape of esophageal squamous cell carcinoma and esophageal adenocarcinoma incidence and mortality in 2020 and projections to 2040: new estimates from GLOBOCAN 2020. Gastroenterology 163(3):649–658.e2. https://doi.org/10.1053/j.gastro.2022.05.054

Müller-Stich BP, Probst P, Nienhüser H, Fazeli S, Senft J, Kalkum E, Heger P, Warschkow R, Nickel F, Billeter AT, Grimminger PP, Gutschow C, Dabakuyo-Yonli TS, Piessen G, Paireder M, Schoppmann SF, van der Peet DL, Cuesta MA, van der Sluis P, van Hillegersberg R, Hölscher AH, Diener MK, Schmidt T (2021) Meta-analysis of randomized controlled trials and individual patient data comparing minimally invasive with open oesophagectomy for cancer. Br J Surg 108(9):1026–1033. https://doi.org/10.1093/bjs/znab278

Muro K, Chung HC, Shankaran V, Geva R, Catenacci D, Gupta S, Eder JP, Golan T, Le DT, Burtness B, McRee AJ, Lin CC, Pathiraja K, Lunceford J, Emancipator K, Juco J, Koshiji M, Bang YJ (2016) Pembrolizumab for patients with PD-L1-positive advanced gastric cancer (KEYNOTE-012): a multicentre, open-label, phase 1b trial. Lancet Oncol 17(6):717–726. https://doi.org/10.1016/S1470-2045(16)00175-3

NCCN (2024a) NCCN clinical practice guidelines in oncology (NCCN Guidelines®) esophageal and esophagogastric junction cancers version 5.2024 — December 20, 2024. NCCN.org. https://www.nccn.org/guidelines/guidelines-detail?category=1&id=1433

NCCN (2024b) NCCN clinical practice guidelines in oncology (NCCN Guidelines®) gastric cancer version 5.2024 — December 20, 2024. NCCN.org. https://www.nccn.org/guidelines/guidelines-detail?category=1&id=1434

Nishigori T, Okabe H, Tanaka E, Tsunoda S, Hisamori S, Sakai Y (2016). Sarcopenia as a predictor of pulmonary complications after esophagectomy for thoracic esophageal cancer. J Surg Oncol 113(6):678–84. https://doi.org/10.1002/jso.24214. Epub 2016 Mar 3. PMID: 26936808.

Pang NQ, Tan YX, Samuel M, Tan KK, Bonney GK, Yi H, Kow WCA (2022) Multimodal prehabilitation in older adults before major abdominal surgery: a systematic review and meta-analysis. Langenbeck's Arch Surg 407(6):2193–2204. https://doi.org/10.1007/s00423-022-02479-8

Paredero-Pérez I, Jimenez-Fonseca P, Cano JM, Arrazubi V, Carmona-Bayonas A, Covela-Rúa M, Fernández-Montes A, Martín-Richard M, Gironés-Sarrió R (2024) State of the scientific evidence and recommendations for the management of older patients with gastric cancer. J Geriatr Oncol 15(3):101657. https://doi.org/10.1016/j.jgo.2023.101657

Park A, Orlandini MF, Szor DJ, Junior UR, Tustumi F (2023) The impact of sarcopenia on esophagectomy for cancer: a systematic review and meta-analysis. BMC Surg 23(1):240. https://doi.org/10.1186/s12893-023-02149-6

Piraux E, Caty G, Reychler G, Forget P, Deswysen Y (2020) Feasibility and preliminary effectiveness of a tele-prehabilitation program in esophagogastric cancer patients. J Clin Med 9(7):2176. https://doi.org/10.3390/jcm9072176

Preston SR, Markar SR, Baker CR, Soon Y, Singh S, Low DE (2013) Impact of a multidisciplinary standardized clinical pathway on perioperative outcomes in patients with oesophageal cancer. Br J Surg 100(1):105–112. https://doi.org/10.1002/bjs.8974
Pujara D, Mansfield P, Ajani J, Blum M, Elimova E, Chiang YJ, Das P, Badgwell B (2015) Comprehensive geriatric assessment in patients with gastric and gastroesophageal adenocarcinoma undergoing gastrectomy. J Surg Oncol 112(8):883–887. https://doi.org/10.1002/jso.24077
Rostoft S, O'Donovan A, Soubeyran P, Alibhai SMH, Hamaker ME (2021) Geriatric assessment and management in cancer. J Clin Oncol 39(19):2058–2067. https://doi.org/10.1200/JCO.21.00089
She KY, Huang L, Zhang HT, Gao Y, Yao KR, Luo Q, Tang X, Li L, Zhao L, Wang ZH, Yang XJ, Yin XH (2024) Effect of prehabilitation on postoperative outcomes in the frail older people: a systematic review and meta-analysis. Geriatr Nurs 55:79–88. https://doi.org/10.1016/j.gerinurse.2023.10.027
Shen Y, Cong Z, Ge Q, Huang H, Wei W, Wang C, Jiang Z, Wu Y (2024) Effect of nutrition-based prehabilitation on the postoperative outcomes of patients with esophagogastric cancer undergoing surgery: a systematic review and meta-analysis. Cancer Med 13(14):e70023. https://doi.org/10.1002/cam4.70023
Simonsen C, Thorsen-Streit S, Sundberg A, Djurhuus SS, Mortensen CE, Qvortrup C, Pedersen BK, Svendsen LB, de Heer P, Christensen JF (2020) Effects of high-intensity exercise training on physical fitness, quality of life and treatment outcomes after oesophagectomy for cancer of the gastro-oesophageal junction: PRESET pilot study. BJS Open 4(5):855–864. https://doi.org/10.1002/bjs5.50337
Smyth EC, Verheij M, Allum W, Cunningham D, Cervantes A, Arnold D, ESMO Guidelines Committee (2016) Gastric cancer: ESMO Clinical Practice Guidelines for diagnosis, treatment and follow-up. Ann Oncol 27(suppl 5):v38–v49. https://doi.org/10.1093/annonc/mdw350
van Stijn MF, Korkic-Halilovic I, Bakker MS, van der Ploeg T, van Leeuwen PA, Houdijk AP (2013) Preoperative nutrition status and postoperative outcome in elderly general surgery patients: a systematic review. JPEN J Parenter Enteral Nutr 37(1):37–43. https://doi.org/10.1177/0148607112445900
Takano Y, Kobayashi Y, Kudo T, Takahashi S, Kanno H, Hanyu N (2024) The role of geriatric nutritional risk index as a predictor for postoperative outcomes in gastrointestinal emergencies. World J Surg 48(1):40–47. https://doi.org/10.1002/wjs.12001
United Nations (2023) Department of Economic and Social Affairs. Leaving no one behind in an ageing world. World Social Report 2023. https://www.un.org/development/desa/pd/sites/www.un.org.development.desa.pd/files/undesa_pd_2023_wsr-fullreport.pdf. Accessed 10 Nov 2024
Varkey B (2021) Principles of clinical ethics and their application to practice. Med Princ Pract 30(1):17–28. https://doi.org/10.1159/000509119
Volkert D, Berner YN, Berry E, Cederholm T, Coti Bertrand P, Milne A, Palmblad J, Schneider S, Sobotka L, Stanga Z, DGEM (German Society for Nutritional Medicine), Lenzen-Grossimlinghaus R, Krys U, Pirlich M, Herbst B, Schütz T, Schröer W, Weinrebe W, Ockenga J, Lochs H, ESPEN (European Society for Parenteral and Enteral Nutrition) (2006) ESPEN guidelines on enteral nutrition: geriatrics. Clin Nutr 25(2):330–360. https://doi.org/10.1016/j.clnu.2006.01.012
Wobith M, Weimann A (2021) Oral nutritional supplements and enteral nutrition in patients with gastrointestinal surgery. Nutrients 13(8):2655. https://doi.org/10.3390/nu13082655
World Health Organization (2024) Global cancer burden growing, amidst mounting need for services. https://www.who.int/news/item/01-02-2024-global-cancer-burden-growing%2D%2Damidst-mounting-need-for-services#:~:text=Projected%20cancer%20burden%20increase%20in,20%20million%20cases%20in%202022. Accessed 10 Nov 2024
Yamasaki M, Maekawa Y, Sugimoto K, Mizushima T, Eguchi H, Ogihara T, Shintani A, Rakugi H, Mori M, Doki Y (2019) Development of a geriatric prognostic scoring system for predicting survival after surgery for elderly patients with gastrointestinal cancer. Ann Surg Oncol 26(11):3644–3651. https://doi.org/10.1245/s10434-019-07687-z

Zhao Z, Gu J (2022) Open surgery in the era of minimally invasive surgery. Chin J Cancer Res 34(1):63–65. https://doi.org/10.21147/j.issn.1000-9604.2022.01.06

Zhou C, Zhang L, Wang H, Ma X, Shi B, Chen W, He J, Wang K, Liu P, Ren Y (2015) Superiority of minimally invasive oesophagectomy in reducing in-hospital mortality of patients with resectable oesophageal cancer: a meta-analysis. PLoS One 10(7):e0132889. https://doi.org/10.1371/journal.pone.0132889

Zylstra J, Boshier P, Whyte GP, Low DE, Davies AR (2018) Peri-operative patient optimization for oesophageal cancer surgery - from prehabilitation to enhanced recovery. Best Pract Res Clin Gastroenterol 36–37:61–73. https://doi.org/10.1016/j.bpg.2018.11.006

Strategies for Older Patients Undergoing Emergency Laparotomy

15

Min-Li Kang, Kurihara Hayato, and Jerry Tiong-Thye Goo

Take-Home Messages

- The worldwide phenomenon of a rapidly aging population poses significant challenges for patients requiring emergency laparotomy. Older patients face increased perioperative morbidity and mortality due to inherent factors such as frailty, sarcopenia, and multiple comorbidities.
- A multidisciplinary approach is essential. The ideal team would consist of specialists familiar with the complex needs of the geriatric population, including surgeons, anesthesiologists, and geriatricians.
- The use of a dedicated perioperative pathway can improve outcomes with the use of standardized protocols, risk assessment tools, continuous audit, and quality improvement.

Clinical Scenario

A 72-year-old woman with a past medical history of atrial fibrillation on warfarin and end-stage renal failure requiring hemodialysis presents with a worsening periumbilical bulge and severe abdominal pain and vomiting. Physical examination reveals a tender, discolored periumbilical swelling, concerning for a strangulated hernia.

M.-L. Kang · J. T.-T. Goo (✉)
Emergency Surgery and Trauma Unit, Department of General Surgery, Khoo Teck Puat Hospital, Singapore, Singapore
e-mail: kang.min.li@ktph.com.sg; goo.jerry.tt@ktph.com.sg

K. Hayato
Emergency Surgery and Trauma Unit, Department of Surgery, Humanitas Clinical and Research Center, Rozzano, Milan, Italy

K.-Y. Tan et al. (eds.), *Mastering Geriatric Surgery*,
https://doi.org/10.1007/978-981-95-0665-1_15

What are the perioperative considerations for this patient?

- What other subspecialties should be involved in her care?
- What tools can be used to perform the preoperative risk assessment?
- How should the patient be counselled regarding her perioperative course?
- What technical considerations are there? What is the preferred surgical approach?
- Where should the patient be monitored postoperatively? And for how long?
- How should the patient's nutrition be managed?

15.1 Emergency Laparotomy in Older Patients

There is an increasing proportion of elderly patients being admitted for acute surgical conditions as populations around the world age (Figs. 15.1 and 15.2). Data from the National Emergency Laparotomy Audit (NELA), including all patients

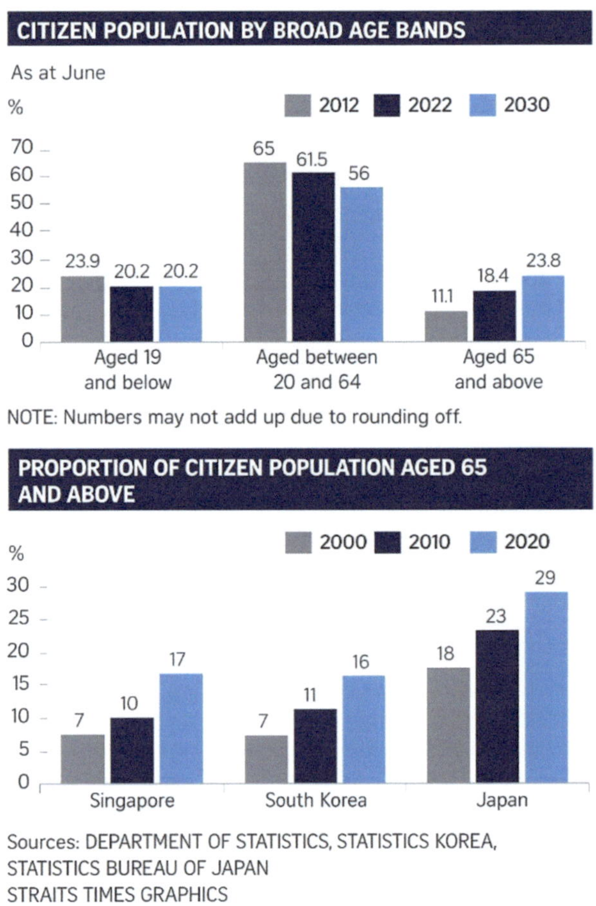

Fig. 15.1 Number of Singapore, South Korea, and Japan citizens aged 65 and above (Straits Times 2022)

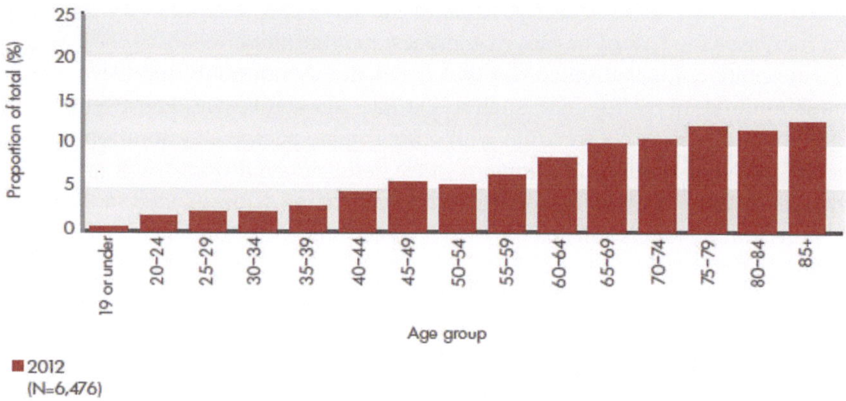

Fig. 15.2 Age distribution of patients with high-risk emergency general surgery diagnosis who underwent a major general surgical procedure, 2012. From Emergency General Surgery Report (April 2016), Royal College of Surgeons (Watson et al. 2016)

undergoing emergency laparotomy (EL) from 2013 to 2017, shows a predominance of older persons, with 57% aged 65 years and older (Aitken et al. 2020), while similar data from Australian and New Zealand Emergency Laparotomy Audit-Quality Improvement (ANZELA-QI) from 2018 to 2020 showed 63% of EL patients aged 65 years and older. It is anticipated that this proportion will rise in the coming decades as life expectancies rise. Emergency surgery in this group bears significant risks of mortality and morbidity, with EL patients experiencing an overall mortality of almost one in ten patients within 30 days after surgery, rising to one in four over the age of 80 years (Tian et al. 2023). Patients at the extremes of age such as centenarians and nonagenarians are also presenting with surgical emergencies, where there is limited evidence-based treatment.

Elderly patients who undergo EL are at a higher risk of suffering adverse outcomes and longer hospital stays due to factors that are especially prominent in older persons, such as frailty, poorer nutrition, and cognitive decline. This leads to poorer functional recovery and decreased quality of life, with a reduced number of patients returning to independence postoperatively (Fig. 15.4).

15.1.1 Increased Risk of Postoperative Complications and Mortality

Definitive management of the elderly patient with a surgical emergency may be hindered by delayed diagnosis. Acute surgical conditions may present in an atypical fashion due to factors such as dementia and delirium, with less clinical markers to guide the clinician on initial primary evaluation. For example, analysis of the NELA dataset shows that patients more than 65 years of age are less likely to present with a raised white cell count or tachycardia. In the acute care setting, delay in management increases the risk of negative outcomes and mortality.

Postoperative adverse outcomes that occur more commonly in elderly patients include multiorgan dysfunction such as cardiac and cerebrovascular events, occurring individually or in conjunction with other organ-specific deterioration. They are especially at risk for constellations of other geriatric syndromes such as delirium, functional decline, as well as complications associated with reduced mobility such as skin breakdown, urinary tract infections, pneumonia, and venous thromboembolism.

Advanced age is a predictor of both 30-day and 90-day mortality in patients undergoing EL, with patients more than 85 years of age being more than twice as likely to die as their younger counterparts in the group aged 65–74 years (Fig. 15.3).

The factors contributing to this are manifold, including atypical presentations in the geriatric age group leading to delays in diagnosis and intervention and an increased chance of presence of malignancy. Elderly patients are less tolerant of delays in care or prolonged trials of nonoperative management, due to reduced physiological reserve.

Protective factors included the presence of a consultant surgeon and anesthetist leading patient care and the involvement of a geriatrician for multidisciplinary comprehensive geriatric assessment (CGA).

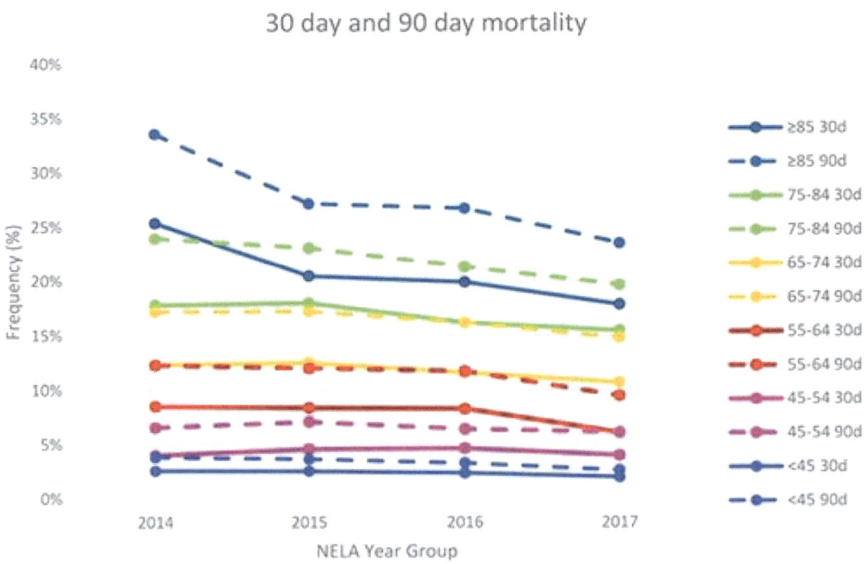

Fig. 15.3 The 30-day and 90-day mortality: age and NELA year (Aitken et al. 2020)

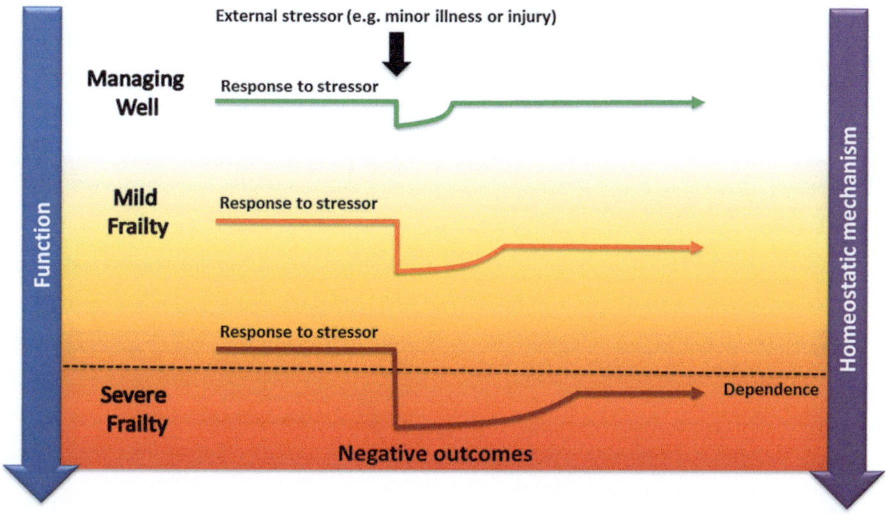

Fig. 15.4 Impact on the patient's functional outcome following surgery or stressor depending on the preoperative baseline frailty's status (Clegg et al. 2013)

15.1.2 Increased Prevalence of Frailty and Sarcopenia in Elderly Patients

Frailty is characterized by a physiological multisystem decline, resulting in greater vulnerability to stressors such as surgery, leading to higher rates of adverse postoperative outcomes. It is a powerful predictor of morbidity and mortality in elderly surgical patients (Fig. 15.4).

There are multiple tools for assessing frailty, such as the Rockwood Clinical Frailty Scale (Fig. 15.5), Emergency General Surgery-Specific Frailty Index (EGSFI), and the Comprehensive Geriatric Assessment (CGA), which are considered the benchmark but in practice may be less utilized preoperatively in the emergency setting as they are more time-consuming. These include a comprehensive history-taking and a multidisciplinary-guided assessment, culminating in goals for current and future (curative or palliative) management, based on five main age-friendly care principles:

1. What matters most to the patient
2. Multicomplexity management
3. Medication management
4. Mentation
5. Mobility

Geriatric patients are also more prone to sarcopenia. Lack of muscle mass and strength has been shown to correlate with negative outcomes such as postoperative falls, hospitalizations, infection, delirium, and death. Assessment of sarcopenia can

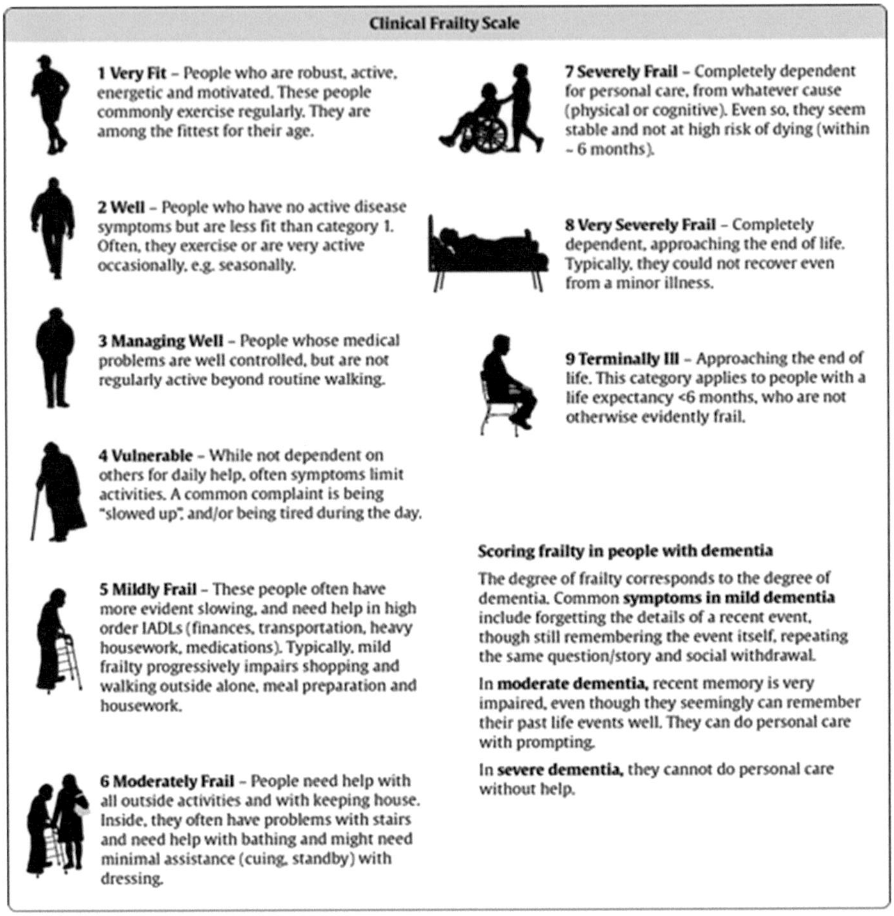

Fig. 15.5 Clinical frailty scale (CFS) (Moorhouse and Rockwood 2012)

be performed with the measurement of the psoas on computed tomography, handgrip strength testing, or the 6-m walk test (Guo et al. 2023).

15.1.3 Risk Assessment and Treatment Plan

P-POSSUM, NELA, and NSQIP may be used to prognosticate the postoperative morbidity and mortality for patients undergoing EL. The utility of risk assessment tools is manifold, such as in the preoperative period, where these can be used to determine the appropriate allocation of resources such as critical care monitoring, as well as adjuncts in a discussion of options with the patient, family, and other advocates. This should include anticipated outcomes in the domains of longevity, functional status, independence, and comfort to align with the patient's goals of care as best as possible.

15.2 Preoperative Care for Geriatric Patients Requiring EL

15.2.1 National Initiatives for Improving Perioperative Care for Emergency Laparotomy

The increased care needs and complexity of geriatric EL patients have led to further audit and the development of integrated pathways, taking into account the higher perioperative risks and the need for stratification of frailty and mortality to formulate a care plan. Examples of high-quality national clinical audit programs carried out on EL patients include the National Emergency Laparotomy Audit (NELA) and Australian and New Zealand Emergency Laparotomy Audit-Quality Improvement (ANZELA-QI). The principal standards of NELA and the key performance indicators (KPIs) of ANZELA-QI are reflected in Fig. 15.6.

The NELA preoperative standards also include the **timeliness of administration of antibiotics** as well as **frailty assessment for patients over 65 years of age**.

The overlap of general EL initiatives with geriatric surgery is an echo of the changing population demographic, with more than half of all EL patients in NELA and ANZELA-QI being aged 65 years and older. The emphasis on frailty care and the involvement of multidisciplinary care and postoperative geriatrician input as the standard of care in elderly patients is particularly apt, considering this trend.

These models of care have demonstrated improvements in the mortality rate and length of stay. Data from NELA shows a drop in 30-day mortality from 11.8% to

Before surgery

KPI 1: *Proportion of all emergency laparotomy patients who received a preoperative CT scan by a consultant radiologist*

KPI 2: *Proportion of patients for whom a risk assessment was documented preoperatively*

KPI 3: *Proportion of patients arriving in theatre within a time appropriate for the urgency of surgery*

During surgery

KPI 4: *Proportion of patients with a calculated preoperative risk of death ≥5% for whom a consultant surgeon and consultant anaesthetist were present in theatre*

KPI 5: *Proportion of patients with a calculated preoperative risk of death ≥5% for whom a consultant surgeon was present in theatre*

KPI 6: *Proportion of patients with a calculated preoperative risk of death ≥5% for whom a consultant anaesthetist was present in theatre*

After surgery

KPI 7: *Proportion of patients with a preoperative risk of death ≥10% who were directly admitted to critical care postoperatively*

KPI 8: *Proportion of patients age 65 years or over who were assessed by a specialist in gerontology*

Fig. 15.6 ANZELA-QI: eight key performance indicators (ANZELA-QI Working Party et al. 2020)

9.2% and a shortened average length of stay from 19.2 days to 16.6 days. This has yielded substantial economic benefits for the NHS by saving over 108,000 bed days and £344 million (approximately $470 million USD) in 2017 alone.

The presence of a national audit is also able to highlight the variability of care between institutions, such as in the ANZELA-QI, where in-hospital mortality was 7.1%, with significant interhospital variation (2.3% to 13.3%), and those with unknown preoperative risk assessments had higher complication rates. This underscores the need for changes in policy at the national level to improve adherence to evidence-based standards and improve outcomes across all institutions.

15.2.2 Developing a Dedicated Perioperative EL Pathway

The presence of a structured approach to perioperative care has been shown to decrease adverse outcomes across emergency surgery patients. Geriatric EL patients, often with pre-existing multimorbidity and frailty, are particularly vulnerable to delays in coordinating care and lack of holistic management (Fig. 15.7).

The creation of a defined pathway of care is the backbone of emergency geriatric surgery. It brings together multidisciplinary clinical leads in geriatric care and enables prioritization of resources within the hospital. The team should involve the general surgical team, geriatricians, nursing, physiotherapists, occupational therapists, dieticians, speech and language therapists, as well as a clinical coordinator who may also participate with research and audit.

NELA has shown a demonstrable improvement in consultant-led care with the involvement of specialists from surgery, anesthesia, and intensivists at each appropriate step of care. There is also mounting evidence that collaboration with geriatricians should be the standard of care postoperatively.

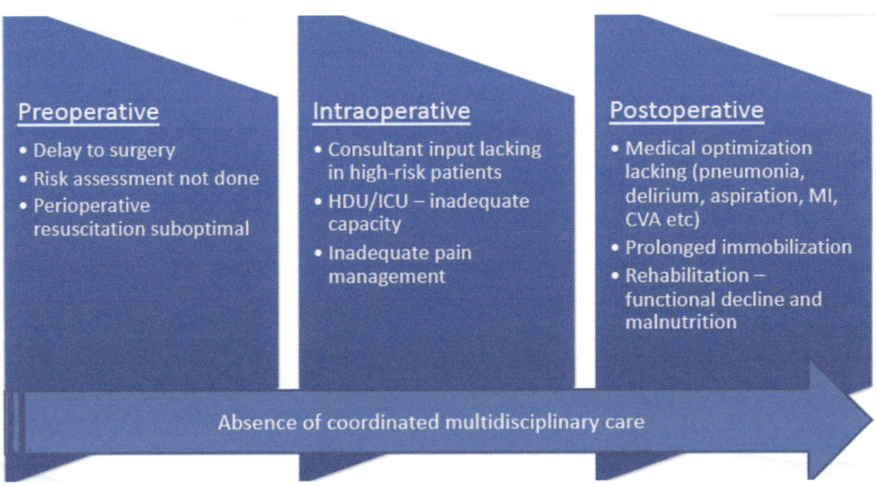

Fig. 15.7 Traditional care in emergency laparotomy

The geriatric EL unit may exist within or separately from a dedicated emergency surgical ward, adequately equipped with nursing and ancillary healthcare staff who are familiar with the management of common geriatric postoperative syndromes such as delirium, pressure injury, and reduced mobility.

Table 15.1 outlines a framework for establishing a dedicated perioperative pathway in EL that leverages on data-driven quality improvement within an institution.

The authors' department developed a standardized Emergency Laparotomy (ELAP) pathway based on the above principles, one of the first pathways targeting emergency surgery in elderly patients in Singapore. It was implemented in 2019 in Khoo Teck Puat Hospital, Singapore, and was designed to be a holistic framework of care with recommended assessment tools, protocolized intervention, and postoperative geriatrician-led care. Table 15.2 shows a tracked process timeline for patients proceeding through the ELAP pathway.

The key timestamps include early warning score assessment within 30 min of admission, sepsis management within 1 h, surgical review within 2 h, preoperative risk assessment via NELA, surgery within 2–4 h for high-risk patients, and postoperative geriatric assessment for all patients 65 years and older, or significant frailty. All acute abdominal cases requiring emergency laparotomy followed this pathway.

Initial data and outcomes from the use of the ELAP pathway across 2019–2020 showed overall improvement in the 30-day mortality rate, with a statistically significant drop in 30-day mortality for patients aged 65 years and older, from 8.8% to 4.6%. The postoperative complication rate for severe complications (Clavien-Dindo IV) decreased significantly from 11.2% to 3.1%, and unplanned radiological interventions dropped from 12.5% to 1.9% ($p < 0.01$). Other outcomes, including hospital stay length, costs, unplanned critical care needs, reoperation rates, and 30-day readmissions, improved but were not statistically significant.

Table 15.1 Key principles in establishing an emergency laparotomy pathway (Ong et al. 2021)

Key principles	Description
Dedicated pathway	Establish a clear pathway for each surgical procedure, outlining best practices from presurgical assessment to post-discharge follow-up.
Data-driven quality improvement	Implement a robust system for collecting and analyzing perioperative data to identify areas for improvement and measure the impact of interventions.
Regular audits	Conduct regular audits to ensure adherence to the pathway and identify optimization opportunities. Foster a shared responsibility for continuous improvement among the perioperative team.
Effective multidisciplinary teamwork	Promote open communication and shared decision-making among surgeons, anesthesiologists, nurses, and other healthcare professionals.
Local leadership	Appoint dedicated local leads in each department to champion the pathway implementation and serve as a point of contact and resource.
Culture of continuous improvement	Cultivate a culture that encourages innovation, celebrates successes, and fosters a learning environment.
Benchmarking	Benchmark results against other leading centers to identify best practices and continuously improve the quality of care.

Table 15.2 Key timestamps and objectives in ELAP (Ong et al. 2021)

Preoperative
1. Time of admission to Emergency department
2. Time of review by Emergency medicine physician
3. Time of antibiotic administration
4. Time of CT imaging
5. Preoperative risk assessment (NELA)
6. Time of review by the surgical team
7. Proportion of patients reviewed by the surgical consultant
8. Time of decision for laparotomy
Intraoperative
9. Consultant surgeon present during operation
10. Consultant anesthetist present during operation
Postoperative
11. Proportion of patients admitted to critical care unit if mortality risk >10%
12. Proportion of patients >65 years old reviewed by geriatrician

The improved outcomes in the authors' study of a single-institution dedicated EL pathway echo previous research that protocolized care shows the potential to reduce mortality rates, shorten hospital stays, and ultimately save lives through collaborative quality improvement efforts.

15.2.3 Intraoperative Considerations for EL

15.2.3.1 Optimizing Surgical Approach

The technical considerations in surgery for older patients vary considerably between institutions, practitioners, and patients. The core dictum is that wherever possible, a simpler operation that achieves a good outcome should be prioritized. This minimizes tissue trauma, reduces surgical stress, and decreases time under anesthesia. Surgical intervention should be led by the most experienced member of the surgical team, who should ideally be familiar with emergency surgical care in the geriatric population. While it is beyond the scope of this book to explore all possible approaches and techniques that may be performed in EL, there should be sufficient versatility in the surgical conduct to accommodate more complex procedures should it be deemed necessary.

The use of damage control surgery has been often touted as improving outcomes in emergency surgery, and no less in the elderly population due to reduced physiological reserves. The concepts in damage control surgery include prioritizing the source control of sepsis over definitive treatment in high-risk patients with deranged physiology. This may include a staged procedure with temporary abdominal closure or fecal diversion procedures such as stoma creation over primary anastomosis in the first setting.

15.2.3.2 Anesthetic Considerations

A close collaboration between surgeons and anesthesiologists is paramount in ensuring optimal outcomes for older surgical patients. Careful intraoperative management is essential to minimize complications and promote timely recovery.

Geriatric patients often have pre-existing comorbidities that make maintenance of organ-specific homeostasis more fragile, such as reduced cardiac function and lung reserve, limiting oxygen delivery.

Preoperative measures to preserve homeostasis include reducing rapid fluid shifts by judicious fluid resuscitation and the application of oxygen therapy. An anesthetic specialist familiar with emergency geriatric surgery should be involved closely at the earliest possible juncture to perform pre-anesthesia assessment and preparation. Early use of antibiotic therapy and prioritization of resources to achieve surgical source control should be prioritized as well (Fig. 15.8).

The intraoperative environment should be optimized with measures to reduce physiological stress to the patient, such as maintaining thermoregulation with warming blankets, intravenous fluid warmers, and maintaining a warm operating room environment. Hypothermia can significantly impair physiological function in elderly patients, increasing the risk of bleeding, infection, and delayed wound healing. Preoperative application of skin care bundle can also assist with the avoidance of pressure injury.

Maintaining normotension is also crucial for adequate tissue perfusion and oxygenation. This may be more difficult in patients with known cardiovascular comorbidities or new-onset dysfunction such as stress-related cerebrovascular events, arrhythmias such as atrial fibrillation, where a normal blood pressure may be considered relative hypotension, and under-delivery of oxygen.

The use of multimodal analgesia in the perioperative period is a keystone of geriatric anesthesia. Opioid use has long been known to lead to adverse effects, including respiratory depression, nausea, vomiting, and constipation. A

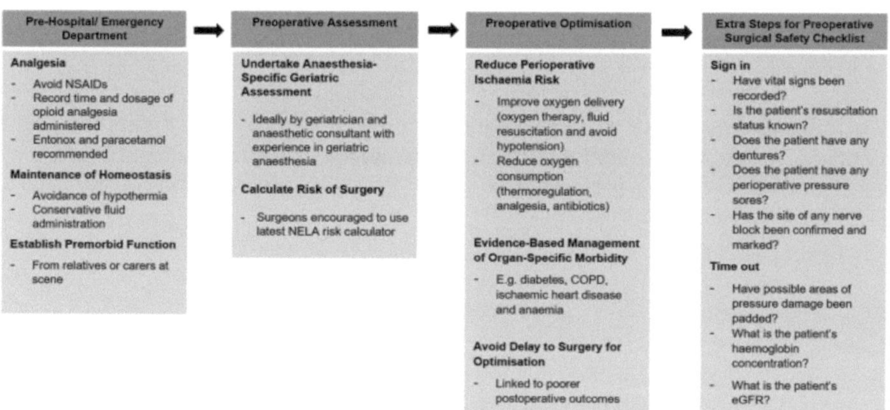

Fig. 15.8 Recommendations for the management of elderly patients before emergency surgery (Foss and Kehlet 2020)

combination of methods such as regional anesthesia such as epidurals, local anesthetics such as pre-peritoneal blocks, and non-opioid analgesics may effectively manage postoperative pain while minimizing opioid-related side effects.

15.2.4 Geriatric Medicine in Perioperative Care

The geriatric medicine specialist should be involved as early as possible in elderly patients with acute surgical conditions requiring EL. The presence of a geriatrician is central to tailoring the perioperative assessment of geriatric surgical patients, investigating the presence of chronic comorbidities, polypharmacy, and treating cognitive impairment and physical immobility (Fig. 15.9). This can improve postoperative outcomes, decrease mortality, and length of hospital stay, with the postoperative geriatrician review being associated with reduced mortality in the analysis of the NELA dataset from 2014 to 2017.

15.2.4.1 Preoperative Care

Early review by a geriatrician following identification of an elderly patient needing EL can utilize various instruments for assessment and optimization.

The Guideline for Preoperative Care for People Living with Frailty Undergoing Elective and Emergency surgery outlines some key principles:

1. Obtain a thorough history of the patient, including comorbidities, living arrangements, level of mobility and any aids used, functional status, mood, and mental status, as soon as possible.
2. Optimize the management of physiological derangements and pain according to age and polypharmacy.
3. Share decision-making and treatment escalation planning with the patient, relatives, and carers, using the appropriate legal framework.
4. Assess frailty with the Rockwood clinical frailty scale.
5. Screen for delirium using a validated tool, and manage and prevent it according to available guidelines.

The initial assessment of an elderly patient with an acute surgical condition is often hindered by the time-critical nature of EL, as well as the prevalence of cases presenting outside of office hours. Some of the other barriers identified include a lack

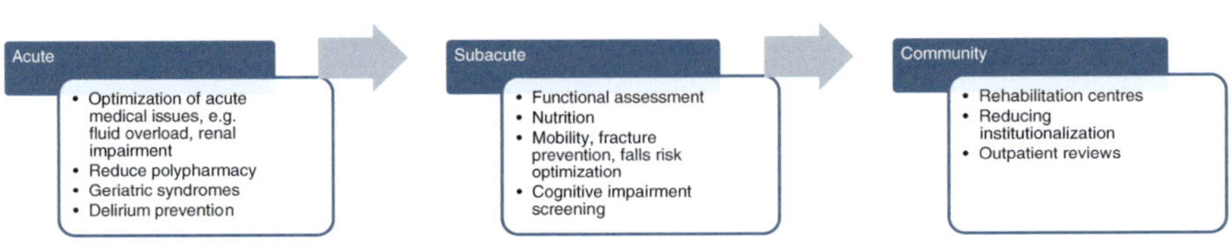

Fig. 15.9 Role of geriatric medicine in the perioperative setting

of trained staff, a severely ill patient with hemodynamic instability, as well as cognitive impairment. However, the following factors should be assessed and optimized as possible in the limited time frame, such as decreased physiological reserve, comorbidity, polypharmacy, and frailty.

15.2.4.2 Postoperative Care

The involvement of geriatricians can improve the postoperative care of patients with geriatric syndromes (e.g., dementia, delirium, propensity for falling, comorbidity, and polypharmacy) and frailty. This is done through patient-centered cognitive and physical rehabilitation, as well as addressing pre-existing issues such as polypharmacy, nutritional intervention, physical therapy strategies, and avoiding deleterious medications by optimizing opioid-sparing analgesia.

There is an association between frailty and postoperative delirium, and pre-emptive measures should be taken in patients who have been screened. Delirium risk reduction interventions should be implemented, such as orientation to staff and surroundings, sleep hygiene, early mobilization, and optimization of vision and hearing, avoiding medications with known deliriogenic side effects, such as opioids, benzodiazepines, antihistamines, atropine, and sedative hypnotics.

There has been increasing utilization of evidence-based elder-friendly practices as part of the postoperative pathway for acute cases, such as the Elder-Friendly Approach to the Surgical Environment (EASE) model, which reported a decrease in in-hospital major complications or death by 19%, the median LOS by 3 days, and patients requiring an alternative level of care at discharge. The Acute Care for the Elderly (ACE) model is an equivalent in acute medical wards, emphasizing a specialized environment, patient-centered care, medical review, and interdisciplinary care. It was associated with fewer falls, less delirium, less functional decline at discharge from the baseline 2-week prehospital admission status, shorter LOS, fewer discharges to a nursing home, lower costs, and more discharges to home.

Over 30% of older patients do not return to their own homes after EL. The role of a geriatrician in assessing care needs and then engaging community resources, such as senior centers and home care services, is essential to develop a long-term care plan that promotes independence and well-being. This may include physical and occupational therapy services, medication management support, and social engagement opportunities.

The collaboration between the geriatric and surgical team to address these considerations can significantly improve the outcomes of older persons after emergency surgery. The management of frailty, preventing complications, and optimizing long-term care is essential for ensuring a smooth recovery and a better quality of life for this vulnerable population.

15.3 Goals of Care

The goal of care is an ongoing discussion throughout the elderly patient's stay in hospital. In the emergency setting, it may be difficult to have a comprehensive discussion with patients, particularly if they are hemodynamically unstable or have cognitive impairment. Early engagement with the patient's family members is usually key to sharing management options, decisions on postoperative disposition, as well as having patients designate a surrogate decision-maker.

The concept of quantitative futility, as defined as the scientific assessment of the probability of the failure of treatment, should in clinical practice be based on best risk and frailty assessment in the preoperative phase. However, it is often difficult to deem the presenting surgical condition a terminal event, and there should be consideration of medical ethics, prior quality of life, and patient and family preferences of goals of care during the process of planning management. A standardized protocol of shared decision-making can be helpful to communicate goals as well as avoid nonbeneficial surgery.

The patient's goals of care may also change during the perioperative period, and realistic discussions of code status and treatment limitations should be introduced with the options of advanced care planning to ensure patients' wishes regarding future medical care are documented and respected.

15.3.1 Future Directions: Optimizing Emergency Surgery Care for Elderly Patients

The past goal-based audits such as NELA have sparked improvements in surgical outcomes for geriatric patients undergoing EL. However, there should be further expansion of domains to ensure a more patient-centered approach. The traditional focus on mortality and length of stay should be expanded to encompass patient-centric outcomes that reflect their overall well-being. This includes measuring a patient's ability to perform activities of daily living (ADLs) after surgery, understanding their experience throughout the surgical journey, considering their perceived benefits and risks of different surgical approaches, and evaluating the cost-effectiveness of interventions.

There is also a stronger role for empowering older persons through improved preoperative education. Informing patients and carers of postoperative progress and expectation of recovery can alleviate anxiety and promote active participation in their care plan.

The use of minimally invasive surgical techniques should be pursued where feasible to take advantage of the benefits such as reduced tissue trauma, faster recovery times, and less postoperative pain. This enables early mobilization after surgery to reduce complications and promote functional recovery.

The judicious use of glucocorticoids, a class of anti-inflammatory medications, shows promise in reducing postoperative complications in some older surgical patients. Further research is needed to determine the optimal timing and dosage of glucocorticoids for this population.

Creating dedicated geriatric surgical wards staffed with personnel specifically trained in the care of older persons can significantly enhance outcomes. These units would provide an environment tailored to the unique needs of this population, fostering faster recovery and improved patient experiences.

15.4 Conclusion

Effective management of older persons undergoing emergency laparotomy demands a multidisciplinary approach tailored to their unique vulnerabilities. Emphasis on standardized perioperative pathways, risk assessment, and continuous quality improvement can significantly enhance patient outcomes, reducing morbidity and mortality. Future efforts should prioritize patient-centered and functional outcome assessment, more use of minimal invasive surgery and postoperative medical optimization, and rehabilitation to address the complex challenges associated with aging populations in emergency surgical care.

References

Aitken RM, Patridge JSL, Oliver CM, Murray D, Hare S, Lockwood S, Beckley-Hoelscher N, Dhesi JK (2020) Older patients undergoing emergency laparotomy: observations from the National Emergency Laparotomy Audit (NELA) years 1–4. Age Ageing 49(4):656–663

ANZELA-QI Working Party, Aitken RJ, Griffiths B, Acker JV, O'Loughlin EO, Fletcher D, Treacy JP, Watters D, Babridge WJ (2020) Australian and New Zealand Emergency Laparotomy Audit – quality improvement (ANZELA-QI). First ANZELA-QI program summary report 1 June 2018 to 30 June 2020

Clegg A, Young J, Iliffe S, Rikkert MO, Rockwood K (2013) Frailty in elderly people. Lancet 381(9868):752–762

Foss NB, Kehlet H (2020) Challenges in optimizing recovery after emergency laparotomy. Anaesthesia 75(Suppl 1):e83–e89

Guo K, Wang X, Lu X, Yang Y, Lu W, Wang S, Tang X, Wu Y, Xu Y, Chen Q, Liu SJ (2023) Effects of sarcopenia and frailty on postoperative recovery in elderly patients. J Cachexia Sarcopenia Muscle 14(6):2642–2652. https://doi.org/10.1002/jcsm.13337

Moorhouse P, Rockwood K (2012) Frailty and its quantitative clinical evaluation. J R Coll Physicians Edinb 42:333–340

Ong MW, Goh SNS, Tung JWM, Lim WW, Hu HH, Lim CY, Ng P, Tan KY, Goo JTT (2021) Initial emergency laparotomy outcomes following a transdisciplinary perioperative care pathway in Singapore. Acute Med Surg 8(1):e702

Straits Times (2022, May 10) Singapore's population ageing rapidly: nearly 1 in 5 citizens is 65 years and older. https://www.straitstimes.com/singapore/singapores-population-ageing-rapidly-184-of-citizens-are-65-years-and-older

Tian BWCA, Stahel PF, Picetti E, Campanelli G, Di Saverio S, Moore E, Bensard D, Sakakushev B, Galante J, Fraga GP, Koike K, Di Carlo I, Tebala GD, Leppaniemi A, Tan E, Damaskos D, De'Angelis N, Hecker A, Pisano M, Cui Y, Maier RV, De Simone B, Amico F, Ceresoli M, Pikoulis M, Weber DG, Biffl W, Beka SG, Abu-Zidan FM, Valentino M, Coccolini F, Kluger Y, Sartelli M, Agnoletti V, Chirica M, Bravi F, Sall I, Catena F (2023) Assessing and managing frailty in emergency laparotomy: a WSES position paper. World J Emerg Surg 18(1):38. https://doi.org/10.1186/s13017-023-00506-7

Watson R, Crump H, Imison C, Currie C, Gaskins M (2016) Emergency general surgery: challenges and opportunities. Research report. Nuffield Trust

Driving Quality, Consistency, and Value in Surgery for Older Persons

16

Hui-Yu Tham and Kok-Yang Tan

Take-Home Messages
- Functional assessments serve as important indicators in the postoperative period.
- CUSUM methodology facilitates monitoring of the consistency of good postoperative outcomes.
- The utility of a patient value compass guides managing patients in a holistic manner.

16.1 Introduction

With surgeries being increasingly performed for a multitude of conditions, it is essential to maintain constant audits on surgical outcomes to ensure standard of practices are conformed to. As we perform surgeries of greater complexities, monitoring and improving surgical outcomes become increasingly important as we continue to pursue further clinical excellence. These outcomes are not limited to only postoperative mortality and morbidity, with postoperative functional outcomes and patient-reported outcomes being equally or, if not, more important. Hence, quality and value in surgery have a delicate balance between perioperative outcomes, cost effectiveness, and patient-centered goals.

H.-Y. Tham (✉)
National Healthcare Group General Surgery Residency, Singapore, Singapore
e-mail: huiyu.tham@mohh.com.sg

K.-Y. Tan
General and Colorectal Surgery, Khoo Teck Puat Hospital, Singapore, Singapore
e-mail: tan.kok.yang@geriatricsurgery.org.sg

K.-Y. Tan et al. (eds.), *Mastering Geriatric Surgery*,
https://doi.org/10.1007/978-981-95-0665-1_16

As defined by the World Health Organization (WHO), "Health is a state of complete physical, mental, and social well-being and not merely the absence of disease or infirmity" (World Health Organization 1946). While traditional postoperative metrics such as early discharge, reductions in major postoperative complications, and unplanned return to operating theater matter, the older patients place greater emphasis and value toward functional independence, quality of life, and preservation of cognition. Second, cost effectiveness is an important consideration for older patients, balancing patients' value toward a meaningful quality of life with financial and nonfinancial costs of surgery. Last but not the least, the gradual shift toward improving patient-centered care through shared decision-making, often with the involvement of family members allows patients to share their preferences for individualized care.

Functional decline in the older people is commonly observed after undergoing major surgery, often requiring a period of rehabilitation before they return close to their premorbid function. While the recovery of functional status tends to be overlooked and neglected in the initial perioperative counselling, these in fact serve as essential outcome measures in the older people (Yim and Tan 2024). It was previously highlighted that many patients were more fearful of postoperative disability and loss of independence than death (Tan 2017). Indeed, one needed to consider, "what good would surgery do for an elderly individual who survived, yet becomes debilitated and loses independence?" (Chia et al. 2023). It is therefore imperative to include functional outcome measurements as part of the pre- and postoperative assessment in elderly adults because it will be a true reflection of postoperative heath status in this group.

16.2 What Constitutes Meaningful Outcomes to Elderly Patients Undergoing Major Surgery

As we progress into an aging society with longer life expectancies coupled with low fertility rates in Singapore, family sizes have rapidly declined over the years. Globally, a combination of marriages and childbirth occurring at a later age along with increased longevity of the older population has led to a "sandwich" generation which concurrently provides and cares for both children and the older generation—contributing to increased care burden and overall caregiver stress (Lei et al. 2023).

A Singapore-based Population Health Survey of residents in the north of Singapore was carried out in 2022; 2499 residents were studied. It was found that 6.9% of residents were providing regular care or assistance to a friend or family member who had a health problem, long-term illness, or disability. Of the caregivers, 40.6% had at least one chronic medical condition themselves, and 34.8% expressed distress, anger, or depression. Another study from Singapore on caregiving experience typologies carried out in 2022 (Sung et al. 2022) suggests that a substantial proportion of family caregivers toward older adults beyond 75 years of age with at least one limitation in their activities of daily living report a negative caregiving experience, with a lower quality of life and higher level of depressive symptoms (Sung et al. 2022).

In addition, as the aging population increases globally, the number of frail individuals continues to trend upward, leading to increased healthcare and societal costs. While there is no clear definition or consensus on frailty, frail individuals have been shown to be at increased number of falls, hospitalization, disabilities, and mortalities (Yang et al. 2023). Previous research has suggested a plausible bi-directional correlation between social isolation and loneliness with frailty, although its exact mechanism is unclear (Ge et al. 2022). Older people are at increased risk for social isolation and loneliness as they are more likely to be living alone, suffer from underlying chronic illness, increased tendency for vision or hearing impairment, and reduced mobility (National Academies of Sciences, Engineering, and Medicine, et al. 2020).

Hence, as we integrate and embrace the challenges associated with an aging population, it is prudent to discuss and look beyond traditional surgical outcomes of postoperative complications, morbidities, and mortalities. In our midst of counselling older patients for surgery, it is instrumental to understand what they value in their life and what their goals are—not just for the upcoming surgery but their goals in life (Fig. 16.1). This is to ensure that the treatments offered are aligned with their goals. In fact, older patients value different outcomes as compared to younger patients, with previous studies suggesting that 70% of older patients would opt against treatments that may result in functional decline with a loss of independence or cognitive impairment, even if longevity may be achieved (Fried et al. 2002).

Geriatric-specific quality indicators have been designed and used to evaluate the quality of healthcare provided to older patients, with an emphasis on their unique healthcare challenges and requirements. These indices and indicators prioritize patients' functional status, cognitive health, and other age-related concerns (Aceto et al. 2020).

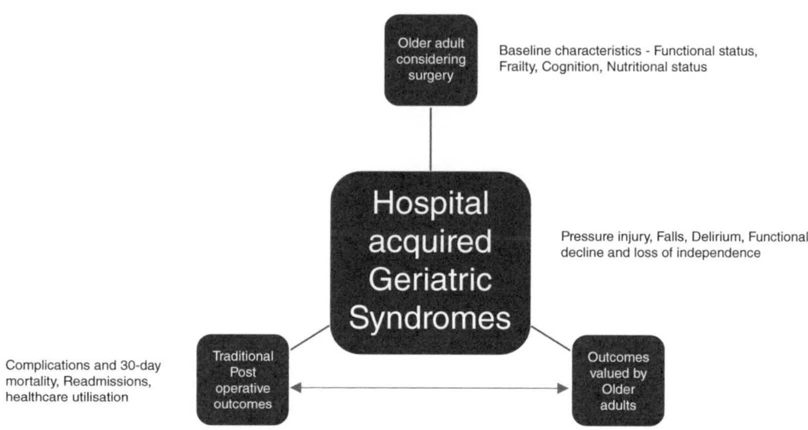

Fig. 16.1 Systemic diagram on the relationship between traditional postoperative outcomes and perioperative outcomes valued by the older adults

While we continue to track and audit traditional perioperative mortality and morbidity outcomes, the use of patient-centric measures such as patient-reported outcome measures (PROM) and patient-reported experience measures (PREM) provide a more holistic measurement and insight of a successful surgery. With greater emphasis toward functional independence over longevity in the older people, preoperative and postoperative functional assessments and evaluations should be considered to allow for adequate counselling and enable timely interventions to be carried out.

16.3 Types of Surgical Audit

Presently, there are different forms of surgical audits being practiced in our current healthcare system.

(a) Mortality and Morbidity (M&M)

First described by Dr. Ernest Codman in 1907 (Gregor and Taylor 2016), M&M processes and meetings involve retrospective peer-review processes of mortality or unfavorable outcomes in patient care and have become a mandated educational tool at institutions sponsoring residency training programs. However, these conferences may not always be sufficient for improvement in surgical quality control on its own due to time constraints and lack of comprehensive, in-depth discussion. In addition, in surgical departments which do not practice open communication, reporting bias may be present, stemming from clinician's concerns regarding professional or clinical repercussions. The common pitfalls of M&M meetings include emphasis over individual errors instead of systemic issues contributing to adverse events, creating a culture of fear and hesitancy to openly discuss any faults, and impeding growth and learning within the department (de Vos et al. 2023; Higginson et al. 2012). In addition, the lack of systemic analysis may result in inadequate root cause analysis, losing sight of areas for improvement. Second, M&M meetings tend to be held within departments and divisions and hence often do not include relevant specialties or allied health professionals involved in the care of patients, resulting in a fragmented discussion on patient care (Pagano and Lookinland 2006). Finally, many of these M&M meetings do not reach a clear conclusion for action plans to be established and followed upon (de Vos et al. 2023).

(b) Cohort Reviews and Retrospective Studies

Retrospective studies and surgical audits aim to improve clinical processes and outcomes by analyzing previous surgical records, reviewing data such as surgical techniques, perioperative outcomes, and complications to identify areas for improvement. However, these are sensitive to sample size and do not actively monitor the outcomes of current surgeries at real time.

Surgical audits such as Enhanced Recovery After Surgery (ERAS) protocol or American College of Surgeons' National Surgical Quality Improvement Program (ACS-NSQIP) are examples of systematic processes that collect and analyze data on patients' perioperative outcomes, with the aims to review and evaluate perioperative practices to identify gaps for improvement, ensuring quality of care. Since the implementation of ERAS protocols, few retrospective studies evaluating PROM demonstrate improved functional outcomes and patient satisfaction in recent years (Choi et al. 2022; Turaga 2023).

16.4 CUSUM Methodology

The cumulative sum (CUSUM) curve methodology looks at the cumulative summation of consecutive cases in a chronological order using a graphical representation (Novoa and Varela 2020). The CUSUM methodology allows for monitoring of important outcomes at real time. The CUSUM chart is then plotted based upon sequential, consecutive monitoring of cumulative performance or outcomes over time (Novoa and Varela 2020).

The CUSUM curve plots the learning curve of a process, describing the performance of each successive case in chronological order after adjusting for various physiological and operative factors. With every plotted point on the curve, sequential monitoring of cumulative performance is demonstrated over time; hence, any slow but constant change in quality of processes deviating from initially defined benchmark control can be identified. Through these methods, comparisons could be made between heterogeneous groups of patients when changes are applied. Any successful outcome would result in a positive curve being plotted (Novoa and Varela 2020).

The mathematical equation used is as follows (Tan et al. 2011):

$$C_n = X_n - K + C_{n-1},$$

where X is success or failure, K is the adjustment for risk.

$X = 1$ if failure occurs, while $X = 0$ if success is achieved, while K represents risk. As such, success in a high-risk patient will result in a large negative swing, while failure in a low-risk patient results in a large positive swing. A downward sloping graph suggests consistency in achieving successful outcomes. In this aspect, the use of CUSUM methodology may be utilized to track and evaluate outcomes in the older people. Within Singapore, CUSUM was first used to evaluate and track post-surgical outcomes in older patients who received dedicated collaborative transdisciplinary geriatric service, demonstrating excellent outcomes in these patients (Tan et al. 2011).

The use of CUSUM was first introduced within the General Surgery service in Khoo Teck Puat Hospital to track surgical outcomes in elderly patients undergoing major surgery via a transdisciplinary approach—a collaborative effort between surgeons, geriatricians, and allied health professionals (Tan et al. 2011; Chan et al. 2024).

The service tracked consecutive patients who underwent colorectal resection and were managed by the multidisciplinary team (Fig. 16.2).

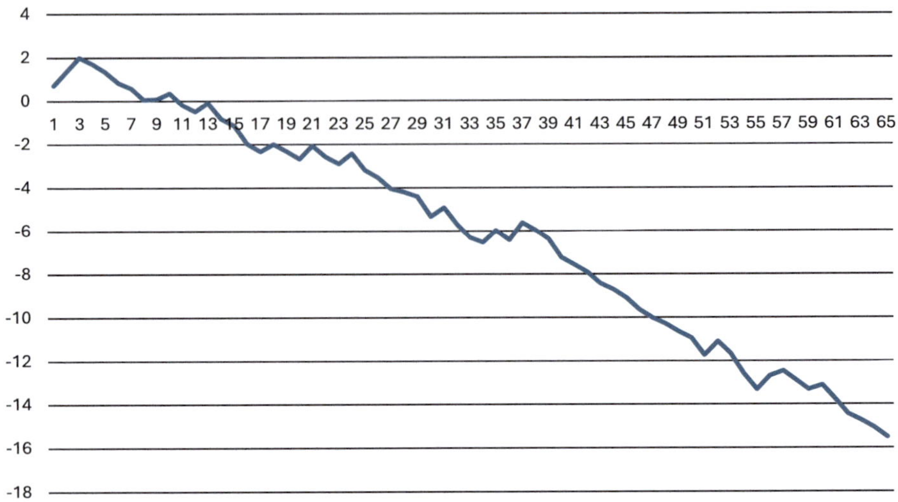

Fig. 16.2 Shows the plot for 65 consecutive patients

Failure was defined by:

- Perioperative mortality
- Unplanned prolonged hospital stay for any reason including morbidity
- Failure to achieve a functional score (Barthel's score) of premorbid status at 6 weeks

Risk adjustment was using the predicted morbidity using the P-POSSUM model.

This generally downward-sloping graph suggests that the service was consistent in achieving successful outcomes managed by the team in collaboration with geriatricians and allied health professionals.

This same service went on to track consecutive cases over the years, with the graph demonstrating a trend toward continued improvement and successful outcomes (Fig. 16.3).

In this graph (Fig. 16.3), the consistency of achieving successful outcomes reached a plateau phase during Jan 2016 to Feb 2019 due to expansion of the transdisciplinary geriatric service to include elderly patients with higher perioperative risks (Chan et al. 2024). Interventions and root cause analysis were then performed with subsequent improvements, achieving consistency in the following years.

Since its introduction, CUSUM has been used to track surgical performances via a three-way approach: (1) standardization of surgery and outcome variables, aligning them to a standardized set of four variables; (2) systematizing risk-adjusted CUSUM by adjusting for patients' morbidities when evaluating surgical outcomes, to allow for an accurate reflection of the surgeon's performance; and (3) automation of risk-adjusted CUSUM.

Overall, CUSUM methodology is quick to perform and may be applied to various processes with binary outcomes within a surgical system.

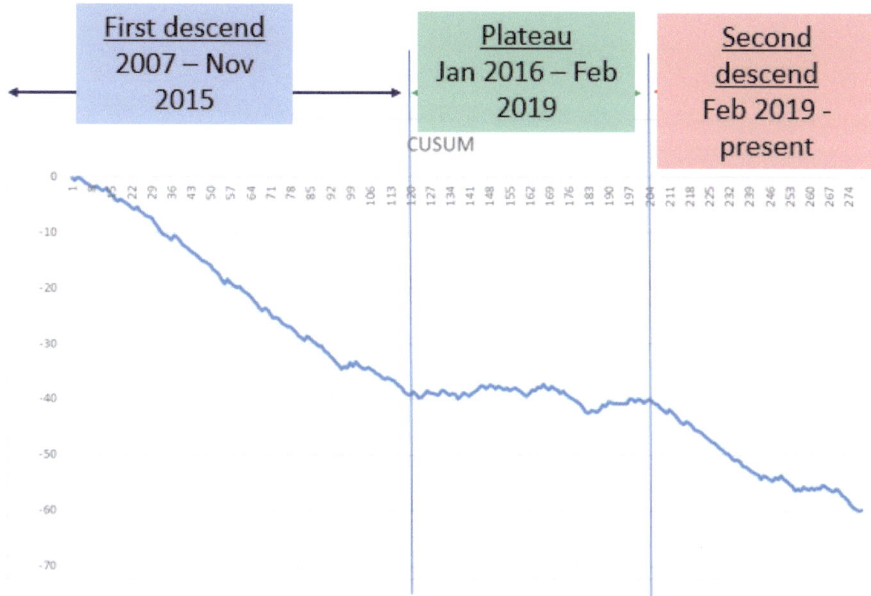

Fig. 16.3 Shows the CUSUM curve for the same service over years and more patients

16.5 Maintaining Patient-Centeredness

As physicians, it is important to approach and treat the patient as a whole individual, providing a holistic care, instead of treating the disease process only. This often involves understanding patients' wishes and goals, patients' perspective on their conditions, and knowing what patients value most. Over the past decade, healthcare has gradually shifted away from a paternalistic approach toward a more patient-centered approach for shared decision-making (Kilbride and Joffe 2018).

However, are we doing enough to promote a patient-centered approach toward healthcare? In Asia, the family unit plays a pivotal role toward various healthcare decisions, gradually leaning toward a family-centric healthcare instead (Mori and Morita 2020; Eddleston et al. 2020; Takimoto and Nabeshima 2022). These decisions are often made collectively, with various family members contributing and sharing their rationale and thought processes. Occasionally, family members would impose their decisions upon patients, while some patients would give up in exercising their decisions, leaving it solely to their family members.

The use of patient-value compass can be a guide that centers care on patients (Fig. 16.4). Factors to consider when managing older persons include—functional status, risk status, well-being, costs, satisfaction with health care, and its perceived benefits as well as the overall clinical outcomes (Chia et al. n.d.). Hence, a patient-centric model of care considers and integrates patients' psychosocial and functional

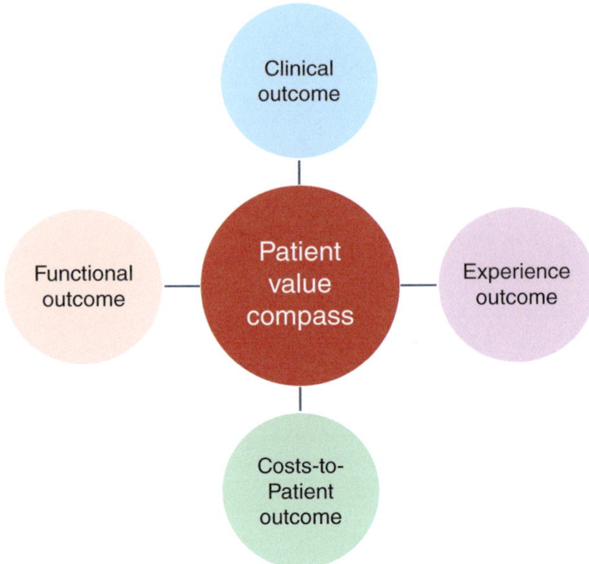

Fig. 16.4 Patient value compass

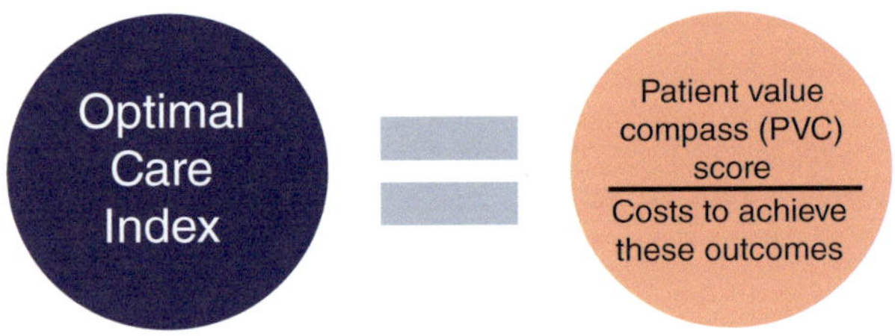

Fig. 16.5 Optimal care index

well-being apart from health conditions alone. These often require patients' involvement and understanding of their health, expressing their wishes and goals of care, and working together with physicians to provide a holistic care.

With these values and considerations being taken into account when developing outcome tracking strategies, one can then assign different weights to the factors and derive an optimal care index.

The optimal care index (OCI) (Fig. 16.5) (Chia et al. n.d.) is a novel holistic index incorporating patient's function, cost, and experience into the traditional clinical model, to quantify value delivered to patients through holistic outcome measurement. It aims to integrate clinical and administrative arms of the hospital in creating a holistic healthcare model.

Last but not the least, it is imperative to understand that every patient, every older patient, holds different values and compass toward life, where a "one-size-fits-all" mentality is often not feasible and not sustainable. With lower physiological reserves and increased frailty in the older people, we need to consider the value of every intervention proposed, likelihood to achieve the intended outcome, risks of functional decline, as well as the role of palliation.

References

Aceto P, Antonelli Incalzi R, Bettelli G, Carron M, Chiumiento F, Corcione A, Crucitti A, Maggi S, Montorsi M, Pace MC, Petrini F, Tommasino C, Trabucchi M, Volpato S, Società Italiana di Anestesia Analgesia Rianimazione e Terapia Intensiva (SIAARTI), Società Italiana di Gerontologia e Geriatria (SIGG), Società Italiana di Chirurgia (SIC), Società Italiana di Chirurgia Geriatrica (SICG) and Associazione Italiana di Psicogeriatria (AIP) (2020) Perioperative management of elderly patients (PriME): recommendations from an Italian intersociety consensus. Aging Clin Exp Res 32(9):1647–1673. https://doi.org/10.1007/s40520-020-01624-x. Erratum in: Aging Clin Exp Res 2020 Sep;32(9):1907

Chan KS, Lee DJK, Kok Y et al (2024) A 10-year review on older patients undergoing colorectal cancer surgery: surgeon-led geriatric service and good quality surgery are drivers of good outcomes. J Gastrointest Surg 28(1):40–46

Chia CLK, Lim WW, Liu NY, Ng YF, Tang T, Tan KY, Goo TT (n.d.) Optimal care index (OCI): a novel healthcare index showing holistic outcomes improvement for acute cholecystitis by an Acute Surgical Care Model. Virtual. https://corp.nhg.com.sg/QnS/Documents/2021%20QIA%20Winner%20Poster/Cat%20A%20-%20Improving%20and%20Sustaining%20Quality%20and%20Safety/(Merit)%20Acute%20Surgical%20Care%20Model%20Improves%20Outcomes%20Holistically%20for%20Acute%20Cholecystitis.pdf. Accessed 1 Mar 2025

Chia CLK, Yong NTWM, Ong MWJ, Lam XY, Soon BLL, Tan KY (2023) Frailty, meeting challenges, and beyond in geriatric surgery – 10 years' experience from Singapore's first geriatric surgery service. Topics Geriatr Rehabil 39(2):79–97

Choi YS, Kim TW, Chang MJ, Kang SB, Chang CB (2022) Enhanced recovery after surgery for major orthopedic surgery: a narrative review. Knee Surg Relat Res 34(1):8

Eddleston KA, Jaskiewicz P, Wright M (2020) Family firms and internationalization in the Asia-Pacific: the need for multi-level perspectives. Asia Pac J Manag 37:345–361

Fried TR, Bradley EH, Towle VR, Allore H (2002) Understanding the treatment preferences of seriously ill patients. N Engl J Med 346(14):1061–1066

Ge L, Yap CW, Heng BH (2022) Associations of social isolation, social participation, and loneliness with frailty in older adults in Singapore: a panel data analysis. BMC Geriatr 22:26

Gregor A, Taylor D (2016) Morbidity and mortality conference: its purpose reclaimed and grounded in theory. Teach Learn Med 28:439–447

Higginson J, Walters R, Fulop N (2012) Mortality and morbidity meetings: an untapped resource for improving the governance of patient safety? BMJ Qual Saf 21(7):576–585

Kilbride MK, Joffe S (2018) The new age of patient autonomy: implications for the patient-physician relationship. JAMA 320(19):1973–1974

Lei L, Leggett AN, Maust DT (2023) A national profile of sandwich generation caregivers providing care to both older adults and children. J Am Geriatr Soc 71(3):799–809

Mori M, Morita T (2020) End-of-life decision-making in Asia: a need for in-depth cultural consideration. Palliat Med 34(2):NP4–NP5

National Academies of Sciences, Engineering, and Medicine, Division of Behavioral and Social Sciences and Education, Health and Medicine Division, Board on Behavioral, Cognitive, and Sensory Sciences, Board on Health Sciences Policy, Committee on the Health and Medical Dimensions of Social Isolation and Loneliness in Older Adults (2020) Social isolation and loneliness in older adults: opportunities for the health care system. National Academies Press (US), Washington (DC). https://www.ncbi.nlm.nih.gov/books/NBK557972/

Novoa NM, Varela G (2020) Monitoring surgical quality: the cumulative sum (CUSUM) approach. Media 4:4

Pagano LA, Lookinland S (2006) Nursing morbidity and mortality conferences: promoting clinical excellence. Am J Crit Care 15:78–85

Sung P, Goh VS, Azman ND, Visaria A, Malhotra R (2022) Types of caregiving experience and their association with caregiver depressive symptoms and quality of life. J Aging Health 34(4–5):591–601

Takimoto Y, Nabeshima T (2022) Ethical healthcare attitudes of Japanese citizens and physicians: patient-centered or family-centered? AJOB Empir Bioeth 14(3):125–134

Tan KY (2017) Geriatric surgery service – our journey piloting in colorectal surgery and future challenges. Ann Acad Med Sing 46:317–320

Tan K-Y, Tan P, Tan L (2011) A collaborative transdisciplinary "geriatric surgery service" ensures consistent successful outcomes in elderly colorectal surgery patients. World J Surg 35:1608–1614

Turaga AH (2023) Enhanced recovery after surgery (ERAS) protocols for improving outcomes for patients undergoing major colorectal surgery. Cureus 15(7):e41755

de Vos MS, Verhagen MJ, Hamming JF (2023) The morbidity and mortality conference: a century-old practice with ongoing potential for future improvement. Eur J Pediatr Surg 33(2):114–119

World Health Organization (1946) Constitution of the World Health Organization. https://apps.who.int/gb/bd/PDF/bd47/EN/constitution-en.pdf. Accessed 1 Feb 2025

Yang Z-C, Lin H, Jiang G-H, Chu Y-H, Gao J-H, Tong Z-J, Wang Z-h (2023) Frailty is a risk factor for falls in the older adults: a systematic review and meta-analysis. J Nutr Health Aging 27(6):487–495

Yim THJYZ, Tan KY (2024) Functional outcomes after abdominal surgery in older adults - how concerned are we about this? Eur J Surg Oncol 50(6):108347

Value-Based Care Outcomes Measurement and Improvement for Surgical Teams

17

Yeuk-Fan Ng

Redefining Value in Surgical Care: Traditional healthcare metrics often focus on process indicators rather than what truly matters to patients. The Patient Value Compass (PVC) provides a more holistic, patient-centered measurement across four domains: functional outcomes, clinical outcomes, patient experience outcomes, and cost-to-patient outcomes. This helps reframes surgical care effectiveness.
Patient Value Compass Score (PVC Score): The PVC Score is a weighted composite index aggregating selected indicators from the four domains, using customized baselines and targets to reflect actual clinical and practice context. It is standardized yet flexible, allowing teams to evaluate and track value delivered to patients over time.
Optimal Care Index (OCI): The OCI complements the PVC Score by quantifying provider value as patient outcomes per dollar spent. This enables healthcare teams to evaluate how efficiently they deliver patient value, spotlighting opportunities to enhance care either through improved outcomes or cost reduction.

Y.-F. Ng (✉)
Khoo Teck Puat Hospital & Yishun Community Hospital, National Healthcare Group, Singapore, Singapore

Saw Swee Hock School of Public Health, National University of Singapore, Singapore, Singapore

Duke-NUS Medical School, National University of Singapore, Singapore, Singapore
e-mail: yeukfan@nus.edu.sg

K.-Y. Tan et al. (eds.), *Mastering Geriatric Surgery*,
https://doi.org/10.1007/978-981-95-0665-1_17

Steps of Systematic Improvement (SOSI): SOSI enables clinical teams to drive continuous value improvement using a simple four step process based on systematic theory of change methodologies such as the Clinical Logic Model (CLM) that is anchored on the PVC to enable and drive accountability for data driven continuous value improvement.

Implications for Health System Improvement: The **PVC** and **OCI** methodologies are more adaptable than conventional all-or-none indexes, and encourage tailored benchmarking and integration of subjective patient goals into value based care. Used together with **SOSI** methodology, they support continuous value improvement by clinical care teams with different experience levels and resource access by providing actionable insights to optimize value creation at scale.

The concept of value in healthcare was first described by Porter, defining "value" in healthcare as healthcare outcomes achieved per dollar spent (Porter and Teisberg 2006; Porter 2008) (Fig. 17.1).

For value to be measured meaningfully in relation to healthcare services delivery such as surgical care and services, surgical or healthcare outcomes must first be defined. Healthcare systems have conventionally focused on clinical performance indicators, such as door-to-balloon time and length of hospitalization. Such indices are not actually outcomes from the patient's perspective, although they may be important measures about the patient's care, that is, a process or output indicator.

Britten et al. in their elaboration of the Gothenburg model of person-centered care said that individuals' goals are often absent from clinical practice and are not usually measured in clinical trials and hence are also absent from the evidence base (Britten et al. 2017; Wicks 2015). For these reasons, and against the backdrop of an aging population (Chia et al. 2016), care teams have increasingly adopted patient function and experience indicators as part of outcomes measurement, including the use of patient-reported outcomes measurement (PROM) and patient-reported experience measurement (PREM) to expand the repertoire of healthcare outcome indices for different disease conditions.

However, depending on the measurement tools used, important functional and experience outcomes continue to be underemphasized, such as well-being, perceived quality, and perception of health benefit. Conventional services delivery outcomes measurement also tends to be divorced from the measurement of costs. Without practical ways to measure the value impact by clinical teams, and use value

$$\text{VALUE} = \frac{\text{OUTCOMES}}{\text{COST}}$$

Fig. 17.1 Michael Porter's value equation (Porter and Teisberg 2006) estimation and trending to continuously drive healthcare improvement, the concept of value-continuously driven care cannot be fully realized.

This has important consequences on the overall cost-to-patients, as well as on the overall healthcare system cost and sustainability, particularly for healthcare systems with very limited resources.

17.1 Patient Value Compass (PVC)

A novel patient value-based care measurement methodology that is more meaningful and value-driven for patients might be the Patient Value Compass (PVC) that has been modified and adopted by Yishun Health, a large regional hospital system in the north of Singapore, anchored by the Khoo Teck Puat Hospital.

The Patient Value Compass has many versions in the literature, all of which are adaptations of the original Clinical Value Compass by Nelson et al (Nelson et al. 1996). The version described is shown in Fig. 17.2, comprising four domains with the specified subdomains, for which outcome indicators may be selected to enable the measurement of patient value.

The first domain comprises patient functional outcomes which include physical mobility, cognitive function, and perceived well-being measured using patient-reported surveys. Patient function is deemed to be the "north star" amongst the variety of outcomes in the PVC.

The second domain comprises clinical outcomes such as mortality and complication rates. For example, relevant surgical-related clinical outcomes can include measures such as 30-day mortality rate, 1-year mortality rate, and/or important *surrogate* indicators of clinical outcomes such as 30-day readmission rate, surgical operation conversion rates, time to start of surgery, and operative duration.

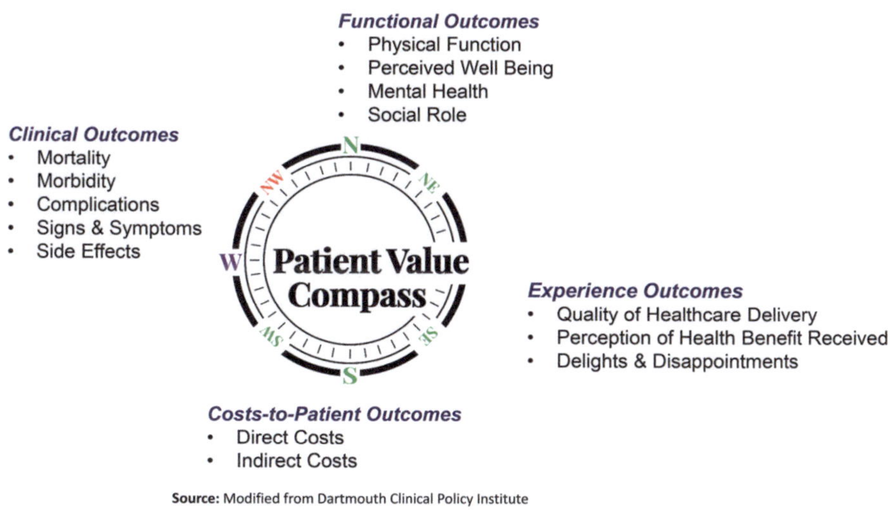

Fig. 17.2 Patient Value Compass adopted by Yishun Health

The third domain comprises patient experience outcomes such as the perceived quality of healthcare delivery and perception of health benefits received, both commonly measured using patient-reported surveys.

The last domain comprises cost-to-patient outcomes, which includes both direct and indirect costs. For direct costs, it might be common to use the patient's out-of pocket costs or the gross bill size after governmental subsidies as a surrogate. For indirect costs, the patient's length of hospital stay could be a useful surrogate of time away from work-life.

17.2 Patient Value Compass Score (PVC Score)

In order to derive a holistic amalgamation of important outcome indicators in all four domains of the PVC which include functional, clinical, experience, and cost-to-patient outcomes, the concept of a "PVC Score" could be employed. The PVC Score is a weighted composite of the PVC Outcome Points for different PVC outcome indicators calculated using our adaptation of the Combined Performance Index methodology from Business Performance Management Singapore (Business Management Singapore n.d.). Derivation of the PVC Score has two steps.

First, the PVC Outcome Points for each indicator were derived using the formula:

$$\text{Outcome Points} = \text{MIN}\left(\text{MAX}\left(80^* \frac{(\text{ACTUAL - BASE})}{(\text{TARGET - BASE})}, -20\right), 100\right)$$

Where *Base* refers to the setting of a baseline using the mean performance of that indicator in a specified year or the lowest acceptable performance for that indicator; *Target* refers to the internal target set for that indicator, for example, by the head of the department or by senior management; *Actual* refers to the actual performance for that indicator; the *Lower Limit* is defined as −20, which is the lowest PVC Score to be assigned if the actual performance falls below the baseline; and the *Upper Limit* is defined to be 100, which is the highest PVC Score to be assigned if the actual performance outperforms the target. In other words, the interpretation of a PVC Score of "−20 to 0" is that the performance is below both the "base" and "target"; a PVC Score of "1 to 80" represents the performance between the "base" and "target"; and finally, a PVC Score of "81 to 100" represents the performance above the "target".

Second, the weightage of the four PVC domains was set at a maximum of 30% for functional outcomes, 30% for clinical outcomes, 20% for experience outcomes, and 20% for costs-to-patient outcomes. In addition, each indicator in any of the four PVC domains was in turn given equal weightage that must add up to 100% in that domain.

$$\text{Weighted Outcome Points} = \text{Weightage} * \text{Outcome Points}$$

The sum total of all weighted outcome points for selected indicators in all four domains is also the PVC Score. For a given set of outcome indicators and its specified baseline and targets, the PVC Score is the aggregated measure of care outcomes delivered by a given care team in a given reporting period. This is conventionally referred to as the value that the patient receives from the care team, but notably, the cost it takes to deliver this value has not yet been taken into consideration.

17.3 Optimal Care Index (OCI): A Measurement of Value-Driven Care Impact

Next, in order to quantify the "provider value", which is the value provided by a given care team or service model, taking into consideration the cost, we used Porter's equation for value measurement, which requires outcomes to be divided by the cost it takes to deliver the outcome.

$$\text{Optimal Care Index} = \frac{\text{Sum of Weighted Outcome Points (i.e. PVC Score)}}{\text{Cost}}$$

For the numerator, we used the aforementioned PVC Score, and for the cost-to-deliver outcomes, we used the patient's bill size before government subsidy as a surrogate of our actual costs to deliver the patients' outcomes. The result of dividing the PVC Score by the cost it takes for the care team or services model to deliver the same outcomes is the "provider value". This is termed as the Optimal Care Index (OCI) (Fig. 17.3).

For a given set of outcome indicators and its specified baseline and targets, the OCI represents the measured outcomes per dollar of resource injected provided by the care team or healthcare system to a specified population of patients in a given reporting period.

Together, the patient value (PVC Score) and provider value (OCI) provides a fuller appreciation of the value-driven care impact that care teams bring to patients with different medical or surgical conditions.

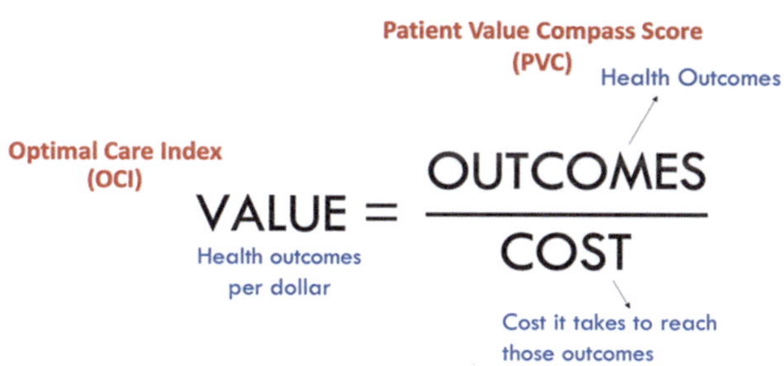

Fig. 17.3 Optimal care index, patient value compass score and cost

17.4 Discussion About Patient Value Compass and Optimal Care Index

Current value-based care methodologies insufficiently distinguish or account for the importance of both patient-perspective value measurement (Lee et al. 2016) versus provider or delivery system-perspective value creation and measurement. The former must take into account the fact that patients' subjective goals and preferences influence the value they perceive they receive and that the measurement of these patient perceptions, although subjective, can still be standardized by employing validated surveys or measurement instruments. For the latter, a provider or delivery system-perspective of value needs to take into account the team or system's ability to create value for a standardized population at a given cost; along with important standardizations to enable useful measurement, trending, and comparisons of the value created—such as population complexity, baseline and targets set, the team or system's experience, and its access to resources. Implicit in the latter is the (in)ability of current value-based care methodologies to aggregate value creation by different care teams to derive a whole systems perspective of healthcare system value creation.

For example, although there is increasingly a gradual usage of more patient-reported outcomes and experience outcomes, the Clinical Quality Index (CQI) commonly used by many Singapore hospitals to measure value for a range of disease conditions (En-Howe et al. 2024) (NUHS n.d.) managed by acute hospitals remains more focused on disease-related and institution-bounded clinical quality indicators as outcomes important to patients, rather than measuring the functional, experience, or cost outcomes of the patient's entire care journey or "whole-of-care-episode".

The PVC Score and OCI value-based care measurement methodologies present clinicians with more holistic value measurement and impact analysis tools that successfully combine both patient and provider/delivery system value measurement perspectives. Clinical teams can use these tools to standardize and incorporate appropriate indicators that measure the subjective or intangible but important patient perceptions in PVC domains such as Functional, Experience, and Cost-to-Patient outcome domains.

Incorporating patient experience and cost indicators into the PVC Score and the OCI is an ideal union of both clinical and administrative arms of the hospital coming together. For example, in high-performing teams where clinical outcomes have been fully optimized, provider value can still be enhanced by activities to bring down costs. Measuring and trending the total impact of care from the patient or providers' value perspective, taking into account a care team's baseline, targets set, their experience, and access to resources, becomes a holistic, approachable, and powerful opportunity for a care team/healthcare system to driving quality and value improvement.

First, most clinical quality indexes for outcome comparisons and institutional benchmarking include only a very small number of "must-have" or regulatory clinical or medical care process indicators and utilize an "all-or-none" binary methodology in deriving quality or value index scores. The PVC methodology allows for a larger variety of outcome indicators to be incorporated into the PVC Score, as well as providing the flexibility to adopt higher weightage for outcome domains/indicators that patients may value more, for example, functional domains/indicators. Internationally standardized indicators can still be included into the PVC Score, and indicator-level benchmarking activities can still proceed in parallel.

The use of a balanced basket of outcomes such as the PVC may reflect better the varied strategies/processes for patient value creation, while ensuring that all aspects of patient value are continuously optimized through the setting of an overall domain weightage, especially outcomes not otherwise emphasized in all-or-none indexes but which are meaningful to patients. Over time, as the care team's experience intensifies, more appropriate baseline, better outcome indicators (or surrogates), targets, and relative indicator weights can be adopted. Indicators and weightage can also be set by the management and care team, together in accordance with the care strategy of the organization.

Second, the limitations of all-or-none value index comparisons lie in the fact that the clinical experience and the level of resources available to each care team naturally vary from team to team and from institution to institution. The PVC Score and OCI methodology are better equipped to "meet the care team where they are currently at" in terms of patient value creation. It takes into account the care team's context, average experience, and available resources to set reasonable baselines and targets for calculating and tracking the care team's PVC Scores, which represent the patient value.

In a system that already produces a high patient value, this method reinforces the notion that patient value enhancement is an ongoing process of continuous improvement. It provides a more acceptable method of value measurement for clinicians and care teams, offering an alternative (and complementary) approach to all-or-none quality and value indexes that remain useful for governance and national benchmarking. At the organizational level, service leaders, department heads, or senior management can learn and decide on the appropriate indicators and standards to set and implement across care teams. They can also develop reasonable methods to account for variations in baselines, targets, and resources available to different care teams.

Third, the PVC Score itself can be a powerful motivator for continuous improvement. While it is possible to benchmark and compare **patient value** creation by different care teams using nationally standardized indicators, baselines, targets, and weightages, significant gains in patient value can be achieved simply by allocating additional resources. In the spirit of value-driven care, the challenge is to produce "excess" outcome improvement per dollar of resource, which can be measured and tracked by measuring and trending OCI. This can be accomplished by either increasing patient value or implementing initiatives to reduce costs. However, "excess" outcome is also influenced by patient complexity and team experience. Adopting average care team baselines, setting one-size-fits-all performance targets, and calculating **provider value** using national norm costs provide a provider value benchmark of sorts. However, such comparisons and the associated "opportunity indexes" may not be meaningful because they do not consider local realities. Of the two, comparing patient value is more objective if the appropriate indicator, baseline, weights, and targets are standardized. For provider value comparisons, it may be more meaningful to holistically assess a care team's efforts to improve patient value over time, taking into account the team's own baseline, setting realistic targets, and computing the provider value (OCI) using the actual costs the care team incurs to deliver the patient value.

Finally, the PVC and OCI value estimation methods combine different outcome indicators into a single PVC Score and OCI, and it is theoretically possible to aggregate these indices for ever-larger microsystems (populations) and ultimately the entire provider system, for example, the whole hospital or a regional population management system.

17.5 Ongoing Efforts and Approach to Systematic Value Improvement

Efforts are underway to implement and test the suitability of PVC Score and OCI measurements for a wide range of patient populations spanning acute heart failure, acute hip fracture, as well as elective patient populations undergoing total knee replacement.

Further development of the PVC and OCI concepts can also involve expanding their application to a more comprehensive value measurement and management system that incorporates a systematic value improvement methodology. This could involve designing and integrating Clinical Logic Models (CLMs) at the core of all value-based care systems. CLMs are uniquely suited to support care teams in measuring and improving processes that enhance PVC scores. By integrating CLMs into a holistic and systematic value improvement approach, such as the Steps of Systematic Improvement (SOSI) methodology (Fig. 17.4), we can enhance the effectiveness of value improvement initiatives.

The SOSI methodology is adapted from "Microsystems Thinking: 7 Questions Showing the Way" by the Qulturum Institute (Jonkoping, Sweden). The four-step methodology emphasizes the following:

1. Clear articulation of clinical team purpose: Use a Clinical Logic Model (CLM) with outcomes anchored in the PVC.
2. Development of relevant metrics: Based on the CLM, develop input, process, output, and outcome metrics. Create value-based care team dashboards to track performance.
3. Assign ownership and accountability: Assign and facilitate clinical team individual and group ownership and accountability for key metrics and targets.
4. Adoption of systematic improvement of science methods and quality improvement tools: Drive focused improvements that ultimately improve outcomes or reduce costs, ultimately improving value (OCI) for patients.

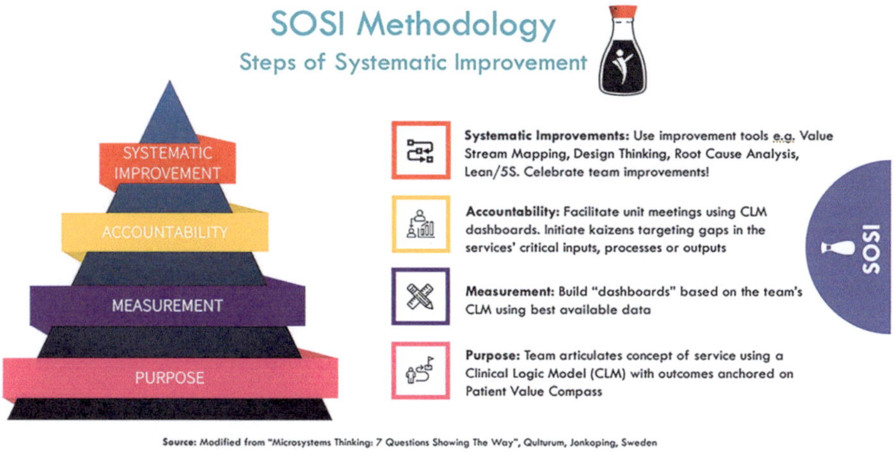
SOSI Methodology
Steps of Systematic Improvement
SYSTEMATIC IMPROVEMENT
ACCOUNTABILITY
MEASUREMENT
PURPOSE
Systematic Improvements: Use improvement tools e.g. Value Stream Mapping, Design Thinking, Root Cause Analysis, Lean/5S. Celebrate team improvements!
Accountability: Facilitate unit meetings using CLM dashboards. Initiate kaizens targeting gaps in the services' critical inputs, processes or outputs
Measurement: Build "dashboards" based on the team's CLM using best available data
Purpose: Team articulates concept of service using a Clinical Logic Model (CLM) with outcomes anchored on Patient Value Compass
SOSI
Source: Modified from "Microsystems Thinking: 7 Questions Showing The Way", Qulturum, Jonkoping, Sweden

Fig. 17.4 Steps of systematic improvement (SOSI) methodology

17.6 Conclusion

In essence, redefining value in surgical care can greatly benefit from aligning it with what truly matters to patients. The Patient Value Compass (PVC) presents a more comprehensive and patient-centered approach to evaluating the effectiveness of surgical care across four key domains: functional outcomes, clinical outcomes, patient experience, and cost-to-patient. The PVC Score, a weighted composite index, aggregates selected indicators from these domains. The Optimal Care Index (OCI) further complements the PVC Score by quantifying the provider value as patient outcomes per dollar spent. The Steps of Systematic Improvement (SOSI) is a systematic value improvement methodology that empowers clinical teams to drive continuous value enhancement through a straightforward four-step process. By combining these systematic approaches, surgical care teams of diverse experiences and resources can continuously improve value for their patients and populations.

References

Britten N et al (2017) Elaboration of the Gothenburg model of person-centred care. Health Expect 20(3):407–418. https://doi.org/10.1111/hex.12468

Business Management Singapore (n.d.) Combined performance index. https://bpmsg.com/combined-performance-index/. Accessed 21 Feb 2020

Chia CLK, Mantoo SK, Tan KY (2016) "Start to finish trans-institutional transdisciplinary care": a novel approach improves colorectal surgical results in frail elderly patients. Color Dis 18(1):O43–O50

Ivan Tan En-Howe et al (2024) Cost avoidance achieved through value-driven care practices. https://www.singhealthacademy.edu.sg/Documents/SHM2024/SHM2024%20Posters/Finance/SHM_FN005%20-%20Ivan%20Tan%20En-Howe_SHHQ%20-%20Cost%20Avoidance%20Achieved%20Through%20Value-Driven%20Care%20Practices.pdf

Lee VS et al (2016) Implementation of a value driven outcomes program to identify high variability in clinical costs and outcomes and association with reduced cost and improved quality. JAMA 316(10):1061–1072

Nelson EC, Mohr JJ, Batalden PB, Plume SK (1996) Improving health care, part 1: the clinical value compass. Jt Comm J Qual Improv 22(4):243–258

NUHS (n.d.) Value based care. https://www.nuhs.edu.sg/about-nuhs/value-based-healthcare

Porter ME (2008) Value-based health care delivery. Ann Surg 248:503–509

Porter ME, Teisberg EO (2006) Redefining healthcare: creating value-based competition on results. Harvard Business School Press, Boston

Wicks P (2015) Measuring what matters: the case for patient generated PROMS. BMJ 350:h54

Obtaining Informed Consent from Older Patients

18

James Alvin Low

Take-Home Messages

- The practice of obtaining consent from patients in order to provide care to them straddles the whole continuum of healthcare and forms the bedrock of ethical clinical practice, which in turn is founded upon patient autonomy and the right to self-determination.
- For a patient to possess autonomy, the following are the prerequisites: mental capacity, voluntariness and agency, material and relevant information.
- Informed consent should be obtained prior to any surgery, invasive procedure or complex treatment that carries risks of adverse effects or complications; from all patients who possess mental capacity, are able to act independently free of coercion and duress, are furnished with accurate, truthful and unbiased information and are able to make a decision that is in their best interest, in accordance to their beliefs and values.
- Shared decision-making (SDM) between patient, family and clinician is the key approach recommended when negotiating difficult conversations surrounding the acquisition of informed consent perioperatively.

J. A. Low (✉)
Department of Geriatric Medicine, Khoo Teck Puat Hospital, Singapore, Singapore
e-mail: low.james.yh@ktph.com.sg

K.-Y. Tan et al. (eds.), *Mastering Geriatric Surgery*,
https://doi.org/10.1007/978-981-95-0665-1_18

18.1 Introduction

Informed consent refers to the consent obtained from an individual with mental capacity, who on being provided with the necessary (material) information, voluntarily and independently, decides about whether to proceed with an intervention or treatment (Singapore Medical Council 2016). Consequently formal consent taking in the context of surgical preparation and planning is a process that involves a discussion or series of conversations between the patient and healthcare team that allows for the patient to be furnished with relevant information, assists the patient in understanding the information given, affords the opportunity for reflection and weighing of the information provided and, finally, documents the decision or choice made, in connection to a test, procedure, intervention or treatment that may be complex, carries certain risks or is invasive in nature.

The central tenet of this important activity is the principle of autonomy, which is one of the foundations or pillars of clinical ethics, espoused by Beauchamp and Childress (1979). In order to understand the significance and rationale for obtaining consent that is informed and independent, we will first need to understand the concept of autonomy and how it applies to the treatment and care of the patient within the clinical and healthcare setting. This is especially important in older patients who present with numerous comorbidities which may impact their cognitive state and decision-making capacity.

18.2 Autonomy

Autonomy refers to an individual's right to self-determination, which implies that a patient has the right to make decisions pertaining to what intervention, treatment or procedure could be applied to them or their body (Beauchamp and Childress 2019). In the healthcare setting, it would also mean that they have the right to decide on whether to consent or refuse tests, interventions or treatments that are offered to them. There are, however, certain prerequisites that are essential before a decision can be regarded as autonomous, and these include, the following (see Fig. 18.1):

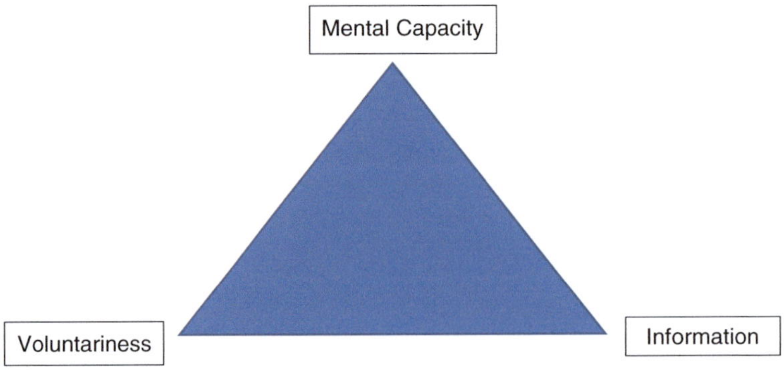

Fig. 18.1 Pre-requisites for autonomy

Table 18.1 Assessing mental capacity

The patient must fulfil the following criteria:	Remarks
1. Be informed and understand the information relevant to the decision to be made	Relevant or material information that can be understood and that the patient will use in the decision-making process
2. Register, retain, recollect and recall the information that is given	The whole mechanism or process of remembering the information should be intact
3. Utilise, weigh and consider the information that is given as part of the decision-making process	A seemingly unwise or irrational decision does not automatically indicate the loss of mental capacity
4. Communicate or convey the decision in a coherent and understandable manner (whether by talking, writing, using sign language or any other means)	The assessment of mental capacity is time-dependent and task-specific, i.e., context-specific (in terms of timing and treatment/intervention being considered)

- Mental capacity
- Voluntariness and agency
- Material information

Mental capacity is arguably the most important element or precondition of this construct as it incorporates the individual's ability to register, comprehend, retain and recall as well as to process by way of weighing the information provided by the healthcare team and to communicate the decision made in a coherent way (see Table 18.1) (Tan and Wong 2019; Singapore Statutes Online n.d.).

The principles and pitfalls encountered in the assessment of mental capacity are well promulgated in the statutes and laws of many jurisdictions (Ganzini et al. 2003). These may include any of the following:

- In the course of assessing a person's mental capacity, it is worth taking note that the latter is specific to the time it is conducted (time-specific) and the treatment or procedure that is being proposed (task-specific). To illustrate, a patient may have mental capacity just prior to developing delirium but loses it during the acute event, or to decide on a lower limb amputation but not for a Whipple's surgery, respectively. In the latter case, the threshold for passing a mental capacity test would be lower for a simple procedure (i.e. easily understood) as opposed to a complex operation.
- A person is assumed to possess mental capacity unless it can be proven otherwise, when all practicable measures have been undertaken to optimise their decision-making capability, as well.
- An irrational or unwise decision by the patient, as perceived by the healthcare team or any party for that matter, should not be taken at face value and be used to conclude that a patient lacks mental capacity. Likewise, a decision that does not conform to what is considered or being recommended by the healthcare team does not automatically constitute a lack of mental capacity.

- A diagnosis of dementia, cognitive impairment or any mental illness does not automatically preclude an individual from possessing or retaining mental capacity.

Voluntariness and freedom of choice are also important components of autonomy. Every human with agency has the right to make choices and decisions that are free of force, coercion, undue influence or duress. The skilled surgeon or physician should always be cognizant of the asymmetrical relationship between patient and clinician where the former is weak and vulnerable while the latter is 'strong', stands in a position of authority and is able to tip the decision-making scales in their favour. The surgeon or physician, in other words, has the power to influence the choices of the vulnerable patient who trusts them for better or for worse.

The information provided by the doctor or any healthcare worker in terms of what, how and why it is conveyed may also have a profound influence on the decisions of the patient. Hence, information provided to the patient should be accurate, truthful, timely and objectively relevant (or material) to the decision-making process. Certain skillsets are required to ascertain or discern what information would be 'material' to a patient when taking informed consent. Among these are empathy and a deeper understanding of the patient's values and beliefs, good communication skills and the ability to weigh and prioritise the importance of the information to be provided that would impact the patient's decision-making. It is indeed a fine balancing act between giving insufficient material information and (as opposed to) an overload of information ('information dump'), where the patient is 'inundated' by large amounts of minute and less relevant details, some of which may adversely influence or impair the patient's decision-making, to their detriment.

18.3 Substitute Judgement and Best Interest

As a general rule of thumb, when weighing and accepting decisions that are made relating to treatment and interventions, the following hierarchical framework is often assumed, in this order of preference: (1) patient's own autonomous and independent decision, (2) substitute judgement by the substitute decision-maker and (3) best interest judgement by the healthcare team. Decisions made by the patient would usually override those of the substitute decision-maker and healthcare team, while best interest judgements, while often emanating from the clinician, are very much predicated upon what the patient had indicated originally when decision-making capacity was intact, which in turn are based on the latter's values and beliefs.

Shared decision-making (SDM) is a hybrid model that incorporates all three decision-making principles, albeit applied at varying levels of weightage and that are subjected to the prevailing context or scenario.

18.4 Shared Decision-Making

SDM takes the principle of autonomy further and to a higher level, in the decision-making process. It is a collaborative effort in communication between the information giver (clinician) and the primary decision-maker (the patient) (Montori et al. 2022). Oftentimes, the patient's next-of-kin or family members are involved in these discussions as well. The patient's right to self-determination can be relational (relational autonomy) and cannot therefore be separated from the social dimension of the person, which thrives on connectedness, relationships and interdependencies (Mackenzie 2008). Autonomy can never be absolute as decisions made are influenced and, in turn, have a profound impact on the surrounding close circle of family members, friends and even the healthcare team. The fundamental concept of SDM is to confer agency to the patient by allowing them to make decisions and choices freely and independently, by way of providing information and facilitating or supporting the decision-making process. Utilising SDM in obtaining informed consent entails ascribing certain functions and tasks to the clinician as well as the patient and family members. The clinician or surgeon acts to lay out the options for treatment, the risk–benefit profile of the intervention and the alternatives which should include 'not doing anything' (foregoing the treatment). This should be conducted in an objective way so as to allow the patient to decide independently. However, the skilled surgeon should be able to guide or support decision-making based on the patient's values, beliefs and expressed preferences. These decisions are made on a background of what must be considered to be the patient's best interest.

Elwyn et al. propose a three-step approach to SDM which comprises choice talk, option talk and decision talk, where the clinician supports deliberation throughout the process (Elwyn et al. 2012). This is a communication tool that helps the clinician conduct SDM with the patient and/or their family members. In current healthcare practice, the patient's right to self-determination is gaining impetus, and many clinical ethical guidelines from the West attempt to promote this. However, the pendulum occasionally swings too much towards making rather than allowing the patient to make decisions based on their limited understanding of the options and choices at hand, where the clinician appears to be 'passing the buck' and in a way abrogating their responsibility towards advising the patient. Consequently, the uninformed patient could sense being abandoned and alone in the decision-making process.

The process of SDM requires much interpersonal and communication skills as well as empathy and compassion, that is, the ability to look at the issues from the patient and, at times, the family members' perspective.

18.5 Practice of Obtaining Informed Consent from the Older Patient

The act of obtaining informed consent should be based on sound ethical principles—autonomy, beneficence, non-maleficence, fiduciary duty (best interest) and veracity (truthfulness). And one of the key tenets of autonomy is the ability to make decisions or the right to self-determination (Beauchamp and Fadden 2014).

Unfortunately, the older patient often has multiple comorbidities which may affect their decision-making ability. Hence, the ascertainment of mental capacity may assume greater importance when discussing treatment plans with such patients. Although in most patients, mental capacity can be accurately assessed by the primary team, there are occasions when the decision-making capacity may not be clearly evident or unequivocal. Indeed, in borderline situations, such as in those with early-stage dementia, delirium or other psychological conditions, a formal assessment, usually by a trained specialist, would be indicated. Some pitfalls to avoid and good practice points to ponder are as follows:

- Consent should be obtained in almost all aspects of medical treatment and care (Shah et al. 2025). However, the rigour of consent-taking is commensurate with the complexity, risks for adverse outcomes and invasiveness of the intervention or treatment. Many minor and low-risk procedures, for example, venepunctures or urinary catheter insertion, require only oral or implied consent (by compliance), while a more invasive or complex procedure like an esophagogastroduodenoscopy will require complete, formal and documented informed consent. The need for obtaining informed consent may be waived if the patient is 'in extremis' or an emergency situation, when the clinician is compelled to act quickly, and the patient is indisposed to give consent. In such circumstances, the clinician will act in the patient's best clinical interest.
- The onus is on the clinician to ensure that informed consent-taking, which to a large extent is a communication process, is made optimal and conducive, especially for the patient; for example, language barriers can be resolved with the use of an interpreter while hearing impairment by a hearing aid.
- The clinician conducting the procedure or surgery should be the primary person directly obtaining informed consent from the patient. However, this may be delegated to a third party (e.g. a team member) who must be apprised, trained and supervised on how to obtain the informed consent in the specific context (for the specific procedure, intervention or surgery).
- Information regarding (1) the intervention or surgical procedure should be explained to some detail (omitting the use of medical jargon and without sounding too technical), in a way that can be understood by the lay person; (2) the purpose, potential risks of adverse outcomes, complications and side effects as well as benefits of undergoing the procedure; and (3) the risks and potential benefits of other treatment options or alternatives, one of which would be to forego the procedure or intervention altogether, should be provided to the patient so as to facilitate and assist them in the decision-making process. Qualitative and

quantitative measures could be provided to help the patient understand the probabilities of risks and benefits that may arise from the proposed intervention or procedure. For illustration, the surgeon could give the complication rates (quantitative) of the procedure while informing the patient of how their quality of life will be impacted by the surgery. The ultimate goal is to allow the patient to make an educated decision on whether to proceed with the intervention or procedure.

- Should there be possibility of a procedure (e.g. rescue or salvage surgery) being indicated or anticipated, based on the findings or events occurring at the main surgery and, within the same sitting, the patient should be informed in advance and prior consent obtained as far as practicable, because the patient would not be able to give consent under sedation or anaesthesia. This would also save the patient from an unnecessary second surgery and its attendant risks of complications (anaesthetic and surgical).
- Informed consent and discussions between the patient and clinician should be documented and signed by the relevant parties in the presence of a neutral witness. The patient should be reminded that they are allowed to review or change their minds regarding the procedure or surgery any time after signing the document but before the actual surgery itself.
- Collusion is defined as a secret agreement between two parties to hide information from a third party, frequently occurring in the Asian context when family members 'conspire' with the clinician to hide certain information (usually the diagnosis and prognosis of a life-threatening illness) from the patient. This may pose a problem whilst planning for surgery and obtaining informed consent, when providing material information is imperative in order for the patient to exercise their autonomy. The skilled clinician should use all means possible to address and resolve collusion, prior to obtaining informed consent unless, based on the principle of therapeutic exception or privilege, the disclosure of that information would be detrimental or harmful to the well-being of the patient (not in the patient's best interest) (Low et al. 2009; Shalak et al. 2022).

18.6 Informed Consent and the Refusal for Surgery

One of the commonest reasons for patient referral to the Clinical Ethics Committee is when the former refuses treatment that is deemed to be life-saving by the primary care team. An example of such a scenario would be in a patient with septicaemia from diabetic gangrene of the foot who refuses a below-knee amputation (which could potentially save their life). To many clinicians, this choice appears irrational and unreasonable and, therefore, puts the mental capacity of the patient into question. This counters one of the most important principles of assessing mental capacity, where it is stated that an unwise or irrational decision does not automatically make an individual mentally incompetent or lacking in mental capacity (Thirumoorthy and Loke 2013). While a decision may not make sense to the clinician, there will almost always be a plausible or 'personal' reason from the patient's perspective. This reason could be related to the latter's values, beliefs, character or personality. The clinician may attempt to change the patient's mind so that the decision aligns with that of the treating team. However, this endeavour may not always be successful, and the clinician has no recourse but to respect the patient's autonomy and accede to their wish. In this context, a surgeon who does otherwise and proceeds to perform the surgery on a patient with mental capacity, against their will (no informed consent obtained), could be considered to have committed assault and battery on the patient (maleficent).

18.7 Suspending a DNR Order or Advance Care Plans for Comfort Care Prior to Surgery

With increasing awareness of the importance of preplanning for one's future healthcare, especially towards the latter part of life, more patients are now making advance medical directives (AMD) and advance care plans (ACP) ahead of life-threatening or life-limiting illnesses.

The values of history, extent-of-care and goals-of-care conversations are iterations of the same pre-planning actions which allow the patient to state their wishes for future care plans, much of which are about foregoing burdensome and non-beneficial interventions which may be qualitatively or quantitatively futile or not in the patient's best interest. For a more in-depth discussion on the latter, the reader is advised to refer to the article by Schneiderman (2011). These tools allow the patient to express their wishes based on their values and beliefs and to exercise their (negative) right to refuse certain treatment such as cardiopulmonary resuscitation, endotracheal intubation, ICU care haemodialysis and so forth.

However, there are instances where a patient with a DNR order or ACP (choosing to forego CPR in the event of a cardiac arrest) suffers an acute but potentially reversible condition which requires treatment with surgery. Some surgeons and anaesthetists would loathe to offer surgery in such patients, especially if there is a risk of cardiorespiratory arrest intraoperatively, unless the DNR order is revoked or suspended. The reasons for the surgeon's or anaesthetist's inclination towards CPR are as follows (Shapiro and Singer 2019):

- The success rate of CPR in the operating room (OR) is deemed to be higher than in any other setting within or without the hospital. This is attributable to the fact that the patient is closely monitored in the OR at all times, and any decompensation in the haemodynamic status of the patient is rapidly detected and action taken immediately.
- Cardiac arrest in the OR could be a direct complication of the surgery or anaesthesia, in which case the condition may be easily reversed with CPR (in contradistinction to cardiac arrest from the underlying terminal illness which carries a much poorer prognosis).
- Much of the procedures related to the administration of general anaesthesia such as endotracheal intubation, sedation and infusions (via lines) are already in place and therefore would pre-empt their use for CPR. The only additional interventions to provide during CPR would be external cardiac compressions and/or defibrillation.

Based on our previous discussions which emphasise the primacy of patient autonomy in obtaining informed consent, it may not be ethically appropriate to adopt a blanket rule that DNR orders and ACPs be suspended in order to proceed with a surgical procedure. A more nuanced approach should be adopted that considers the patient's views and wishes on CPR in the OR when preparing for surgery. In addition, it cannot be assumed that consent for surgery automatically includes consent for CPR. Neither can it be assumed that the patient who chooses DNR would never reverse this decision in certain circumstances. Concomitantly, the surgeon should not deny beneficial surgery (including palliative surgery) to a patient just because the latter chooses the DNR option in the event of a cardiac arrest in the OR. It would be ethically unacceptable as this amounts to coercion or compulsion.

As mentioned, a shared decision-making (SDM) approach should be undertaken between the patient, the next-of-kin and the healthcare team when deciding on whether to provide CPR in the OR. The patient should be informed of the risk, benefits and probability of 'success' of CPR in the context of a cardiac arrest resulting from the various possible causes that may be reversible or irreversible. Hence, the patient may decide to suspend, maintain or adapt the DNR order. Adapting the DNR order could mean making CPR contingent upon whether the cardiac arrest can or cannot be reversed in a meaningful way [i.e. to return the patient back to their pre-arrest functional state, as opposed to merely bringing about a physiological response (of the heartbeat and breathing) and a vegetative state (Fig. 18.2).

Scenario

Mr M was a 76-year-old gentleman who was partially blind from aged-related macular degeneration of the left eye, diabetes mellitus (DM) complicated by proliferative diabetic retinopathy and bilateral cataracts, chronic kidney disease from DM nephropathy, ischaemic heart disease, hyperlipidaemia, hypertension, mild cognitive impairment, osteoarthritis of the knee and depression. He was offered surgery for cataract of his right eye which he consented to after some persuasion by the clinician. Unfortunately for Mr M, the feared complication of endophthalmitis, occurred around the 7th post-op day. Despite the prompt treatment of this infection with systemic and intravitreal antibiotics and further surgery, Mr M lost most of the vision of his right eye. Several months after the surgery, when Mr M realised that the lost of vision on his right eye was permanent and irreversible, he became furious and claimed that he would not have agreed for surgery if he had been told that he could become blind from this rare complication of cataract removal surgery.

The reader is now invited to reflect on the following:

1. How could the surgeon have ascertained the information that would be considered 'material' to the patient, to help the latter decide about whether to go for surgery?
2. Should the surgeon have informed the patient of most, if not, all of the potential complications that may have resulted from this surgery regardless of severity or probability?
3. Was there any 'negligence' on the surgeon's part in not informing the patient about this rare but possibly serious complication?

Previously, a doctor could be found negligent in making a wrong diagnosis or providing wrong or inappropriate treatment to a patient. However, with the Montgomery Rule, a doctor could also be found negligent if they did not provide information that was considered material or important by the patient for the latter to make an 'informed' decision. Herein lies the problem for the doctor- how would the doctor ever know what is important or material for the patient, without having the ability to read the patient's mind? (Austin LV 2019)

The latest guidelines by the courts in Singapore to address the above scenario where defensive medicine would be overly emphasised and where 'information dumping' would be the result, an extension or refinement of the above prinicple now includes that, in order to ascertain what would be material information, apart from what is articulated by the patient, as that which is decided by 'a responsible body of medical men skilled in that particular art.' (the Bolam Bolitho Standard), ie. accepted by a respectable body of medical opinion (peer professional opinion) as reasonable professional practice in the circumstances and that the peer professional opinion is logical. (Thamotharampillai et al. 2021).

Fig. 18.2 A hypothetical case study

References

Austin LV (2019) Hii Chii Kok v (1) Ooi Peng Jin London Lucien; (2) National Cancer Centre: modifying montgomery. Med Law Rev 27(2):339–351. https://doi.org/10.1093/medlaw/fwy044

Beauchamp TL, Childress JF (1979) Principles of biomedical ethics. Oxford University Press, New York

Beauchamp TL, Childress JF (2019) Principles of biomedical ethics: marking its fortieth anniversary. Am J Bioeth 19(11):9–12. https://doi.org/10.1080/15265161.2019.1665402

Beauchamp TL, Fadden RR (2014) Informed consent. In: Jennings B (ed) Bioethics, 4th edn. Cengage Learning, pp 1682–1686

Elwyn G, Frosch D, Thomson R, Joseph-Williams N, Lloyd A, Paul Kinnersley P et al (2012) Shared decision making: a model for clinical practice. J Gen Intern Med 27(10):1361–1367. https://doi.org/10.1007/s11606-012-2077-6

Ganzini L, Volicer L, Nelson W, Derse A (2003) Pitfalls in assessment of decision-making capacity. Psychosomatics 44(3):237–243

Low JA, Sim LK, Main N, Koh KL, Pang WS, Lim M (2009) Reducing collusion between family members and clinicians of patients referred to the palliative care team. Perm J 13(4):11–15. https://doi.org/10.7812/TPP/09-058

Mackenzie C (2008) Relational autonomy, normative authority, and perfectionism. J Soc Philos 39(4):512–533. https://doi.org/10.1111/j.1467-9833.2008.00440.x

Montori VM, Ruissen MM, Hargreaves IG, Brito JP, Kunneman M (2022) Shared decision-making as a method of care. BMJ Evid Based Med 28(4):213–217. https://doi.org/10.1136/bmjebm-2022-112068

Schneiderman LJ (2011) Defining medical futility and improving medical care. J Bioeth Inq 8(2):123–131. https://doi.org/10.1007/s11673-011-9293-3

Shah P, Thornton I, Kopitnik NL, Hipskind NE (2025) Informed consent. Statpearls Publishing. https://www.ncbi.nlm.nih.gov/books/NBK430827/

Shalak M, Shariff MA, Doddapaneni V, Suleman N (2022) The truth, the whole truth, and nothing but the truth: therapeutic privilege. Postgrad Med 68(3):152–155. https://doi.org/10.4103/jpgm.jpgm_1146_21

Shapiro ME, Singer EA (2019) Perioperative advance directives: do not resuscitate in the operating room. Surg Clin North Am 99(5):859–865. https://doi.org/10.1016/j.suc.2019.06.006

Singapore Medical Council (2016) Ethical code and ethical guidelines, 2016 edn. Brought. https://www.healthprofessionals.gov.sg/smc/guidelines/smc-ethical-code-and-ethical-guidelines-(2002-and-2016-editions)-and-handbook-on-medical-ethics-(2016-edition); https://www.healthprofessionals.gov.sg/docs/librariesprovider2/guidelines/2016-smc-ethical-code-and-ethical-guidelines%2D%2D-(13sep16).pdf?sfvrsn=80e05587_4; https://link.springer.com/article/10.1007/s11019-006-9000-z

Singapore Statutes Online (n.d.) Mental Capacity Act (Chapter 177A). https://sso.agc.gov.sg/Act/MCA2008

Tan G, Wong J (2019, Sep) Assessment of mental capacity - key points. Singapore Medical Association News - Insight. https://www.sma.org.sg/UploadedImg/1630651979_2019SepInsight%203.pdf

Thamotharampillai T, Shen J, Seah JY (2021) Lessons from the Lim Lian Arn case: duty to advise and consent taking. Singapore Med J 64(12):739–741. https://doi.org/10.11622/smedj.2021175

Thirumoorthy T, Loke P (2013, Aug) Consent in medical practice 3–dealing with persons lacking capacity. SMA Centre for Medical Ethics & Professionalism. SMA News, pp 16–19

19 Rational Approach to Surgery in Older Persons

Junde Lu and Kok-Yang Tan

Take-Home Messages

- Older individuals present with multiple comorbidities and reduced physiological reserves. A rational approach to surgery should align with their health status, functional capacity, and goals of care. Physicians must balance advocacy for patients' best interests while respecting their values and expectations of care.
- Open communication and shared decision-making improve patient satisfaction, outcomes, and trust. Recognizing cultural, emotional, and psychological aspects ensures personalized and compassionate care.
- A thorough, contextualized assessment of health status, comorbidities, and functional capacity is critical for older surgical patients. In addition, physicians must embrace uncertainty, involve multidisciplinary teams, and adapt care plans based on evolving patient needs and conditions. Transparency about risks, benefits, and uncertainties allows informed decisions aligned with patient values and goals.
- True person-centered care integrates medical evidence with individualized, contextualized decision-making. Understanding and respecting older patients' diverse experiences and values ensure compassionate and effective care.

J. Lu · K.-Y. Tan (✉)
General and Colorectal Surgery, Khoo Teck Puat Hospital, Singapore, Singapore
e-mail: tan.kok.yang@geriatricsurgery.org.sg

K.-Y. Tan et al. (eds.), *Mastering Geriatric Surgery*,
https://doi.org/10.1007/978-981-95-0665-1_19

19.1 Introduction

The aging population presents a unique set of challenges in the surgical realm. With advancements in modern medicine, individuals are living longer, albeit with multiple comorbidities and diminished physiological reserves. Singaporeans have one of the highest life expectancies in the world with an average life expectancy of 84.8 years. However, the Healthy Life Expectancy—the number of years a person can expect to live in good health—is significantly lower, at 74.2 years. On average, Singaporeans spend approximately 10.6 years living with some form of disability or illness before death (Singapore Ministry of Health 2017) owing to the increased prevalence of chronic conditions such as cardiovascular diseases, diabetes, and musculoskeletal disorders in the older population (Dicker et al. 2017). Adopting a rational approach to surgery in older persons must involve careful consideration of their overall health, function, and personal preferences. This chapter aims to provide a rational approach to surgical decision-making in older patients, taking into consideration the complex interplay of their physiology, comorbidities, and goals of care. It will delve into the pivotal concept of person-centered care and emphasize on the importance of a holistic approach. It hopes to remind the practicing surgeon to align their patient's values, beliefs, and sociocultural background to the goals of their treatment.

19.2 Pathology Versus Person: Advocating for a Paradigm Shift

There exists a fundamental distinction between treating a disease and treating the patient. Both approaches aim to treat the pathology and ultimately improve health outcomes. However, they diverge in their understanding of the individual's experience and factors influencing health.

The biomedical model of illness emerged in the early twentieth century to understand health and disease. It viewed illness as the result of the disruption of specific biological mechanisms (Wade and Halligan 2004). It emphasized the importance of identifying and treating these underlying biological factors to restore health. This approach led to significant advancements in medical science and technology which revolutionized and shaped the practice of modern medicine. Today, it still forms the bedrock and foundation of medicine, and it is an indispensable tool in a doctor's arsenal. However, the patient can often be seen as a passive recipient of treatment, with little emphasis on the broader psychological, social, or environmental factors that may influence their health.

Increasingly, there has been a paradigm shift with a call for the adoption of a more holistic model. The biopsychosocial model of illness was first conceptualized by George Engel in 1977. It acknowledged the intricate interplay of biological, psychological, and social factors in health and illness (Engel 1977). This holistic approach emphasized on the importance of understanding the patient's unique circumstances, integrating treatment with psychological support, social interventions, and lifestyle modifications to promote overall well-being.

The biomedical model, though still relevant in today's practice, may relegate and reduce the patient to only their pathology. The nuances of individual experiences can become eclipsed by the dogma of clinical algorithms, investigations, and treatments, potentially neglecting other important dimensions of an illness which may not be easily quantified. The biopsychosocial approach of "treating the patient" encompasses a broader and more holistic notion that deals with "softer" metrics. It acknowledges the patient as a complex and multifaceted individual, recognizing that the manifestation and presentation of disease are not solely determined by biological factors alone but rather influenced by many other circumstances. Therefore, contextualizing care becomes important. In recent years, there has been a notable surge in interest to quantify such "softer" metrics, leading to a growing development of instruments of measure such as quality of life assessments through SF-36 and EQ-5D scores (Ware Jr and Sherbourne 1992; EuroQol Research Foundation 2023).

While modern medicine has made remarkable strides in understanding and treating various pathologies, there is a growing recognition that focusing solely on the disease process may overlook the broader needs and preferences of patients. This becomes especially evident in the setting of tumor board meetings where the discourse often revolves predominantly around pathology, with limited consideration given to the broader context of the patient's values and preferences. While tumor board meetings serve as crucial forums for multidisciplinary collaboration to discuss and formulate treatment plans, these discussions frequently center on the intricacies of tumor histology, molecular markers, and treatment algorithms. Oftentimes, there is minimal attention paid to the unique circumstances and preferences of the individual. Adopting a holistic approach within tumor board meetings will mean broadening the scope of discussions to encompass not only the pathology of the tumor but also the broader context of the patient's life. This might include considerations such as the patient's functional status, comorbidities, psychosocial support, financial means, and cultural or religious beliefs—all of which can profoundly impact treatment decisions and outcomes.

19.3 Holistic Healthcare: From Patient-Centered to Person-Centered Care

While great lengths have been taken to ensure patient-centric care, it would be myopic to ignore the next most important stakeholder in the care of an older patient—the caregiver. Adopting person-centered care offers an expanded perspective which offers the integration of social, emotional, and caregiver dimensions of health. Older patients do not exist in isolation and are part of a complex ecosystem that includes

Table 19.1 Patient- vs. person-centered care

	Patient-centered care	Person-centered care
Focus of care	Patient as the central unit of care	The individual within their social context as central unit of care
Extent of care	Disease management and treatment	Holistic care, i.e., medical, emotional, social, and functional needs
Stakeholders	Shared decision-making between clinician and patient	Collaborative decision-making involving patient, caregivers, family, and healthcare providers
Role of caregivers	Limited consideration of caregiver needs	Active inclusion of caregiver well-being and roles
Measurement of success	Focused on clinical outcomes	Emphasis on patient, caregivers, and overall quality of life
Example	Optimizing oncological surgery in an older patient	Considering the impact of an oncological surgery on the individual's functional status, caregiver burden, and subsequent quality of life

caregivers, family members, and their social environment. Caregivers shoulder significant responsibilities such as daily care, medication management as well as logistical needs such as ensuring older patients attend their medical appointments. As such, it becomes essential to shift our perspective beyond the patient alone and adopt a person-centered approach that acknowledges the important role of caregivers. Caregiving itself carries significant burdens such as physical, emotional, and financial strain (Janssen et al. 2020) which can directly impact the quality of care that older patients receive and, ultimately, their outcomes (Lwi et al. 2017). By considering the needs of both the patient and their caregivers, we can foster a more balanced and sustainable system of care that supports the entire ecosystem surrounding older surgical patients. Hence, the integration of caregiver well-being into surgical decision-making is vital. Recognizing caregivers as active collaborators in the care process ensures that their needs and perspectives are incorporated. In an older patient undergoing major surgery, the recovery plan should include caregiver education, support services, and respite care to mitigate caregiver burnout. Surgical decisions must consider the social environment, such as housing arrangements, caregiver availability, and financial limitations. This reflects the broader principle of the Institute for Healthcare Improvement (IHI) Triple Aim Framework, first described by Berwick and colleagues (Berwick et al. 2008), emphasizing on improving the older patient's health outcomes, enhancing caregiver and social wellbeing, as well as optimizing the healthcare system's efficiency. Table 19.1 succinctly shows the difference between patient-centered versus person-centered care.

19.4 Contextualization of Care in Older Persons: Getting the Perspective Right

The contextualization of care involves the delicate task of balancing advocacy for the patient's best interests with the expectations of care. When the physician's treatment intentions align with the patient's and/or their family members' expectations, it allows trust to be fostered, enhancing and promoting a collaborative approach to a patient's health. However, in the situations where it does not, finding a middle ground becomes imperative. This means that physicians need to consider the overall clinical picture and take a nuanced approach to treatment. For example, in an older patient with severe dementia who is uncommunicative and bedridden amidst multiple comorbidities, pursuing a curative oncological surgery for a newly diagnosed colorectal cancer may not always be the most appropriate or beneficial. Instead, surgical interventions, if any, should be made under the intention to temporize any emergencies, palliate, and improve symptoms. In contrast, a 90-year-old individual who otherwise only has diabetes with preserved functional status and is still independent with their activities of daily living, pursuing curative oncological surgery merits serious consideration.

In a similar vein, contextualizing diagnostic investigations and workup in older persons involves discerning when to adopt an aggressive or conservative approach. While diagnostic investigations play a pivotal role in surgical decision-making, their utility must be contextualized within the broader management strategy. Rather than indiscriminately pursuing diagnostic tests or following through as "part of the workup," clinicians should prioritize investigations that align with the likely management plan and contribute meaningfully to informed decision-making processes. There exists an ethical and professional dilemma of "under-investigating" which may make a doctor apprehensive of a perceived failure of duty of care and fearful of the associated medicolegal repercussions. Nevertheless, it is important to understand that the judicious and appropriate use of medical investigations is the hallmark of a discerning clinician. It can help reduce costs and fatigue from over-investigation which oftentimes leads to uncertainty and frustration. Furthermore, it can increase the complexity of care where patients with chronic or complex medical conditions may undergo numerous investigations and consultations with different healthcare providers. This can lead to a cumulative burden of appointments and tests which further fatigues the patient, their caregivers, and the healthcare system.

Some of the difficulties in decision-making can be illustrated in Fig. 19.1, highlighting the case of Mr. TSG who was 95 years of age at the time of the diagnosis of his sigmoid cancer.

In 2023, Singapore's Health Minister had pointed out during his speech at the Ministry of Health Committee Supply Debate the growing aging population in Singapore and how healthcare costs have been burgeoning. The Singapore government had tripled its healthcare expenditure over the last 10 years, and this is projected to triple in the next decade (Ministry of Health 2022). A similar picture is likely in many developed countries. To that end, there is an imperative need to re-examine the way medicine is being practiced and to identify systemic inefficiencies to help alleviate the financial strain on the healthcare system.

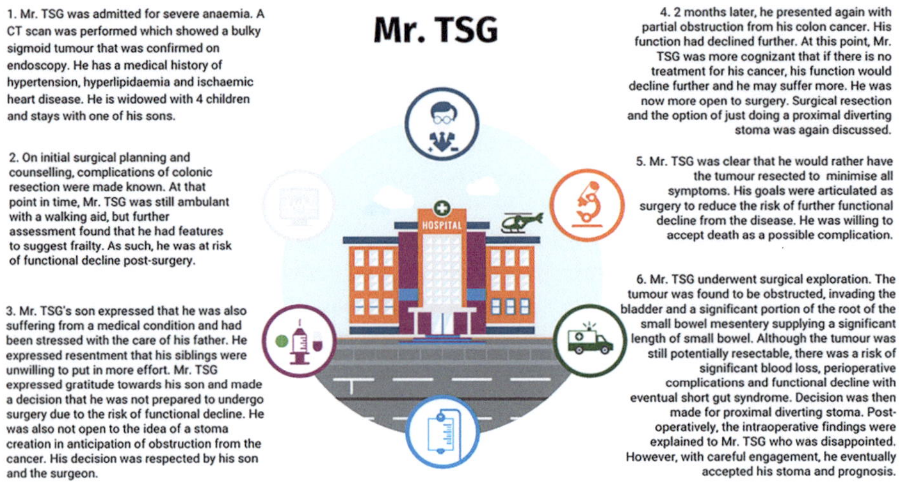

Fig. 19.1 Case of Mr. TSG

19.5 Making it Right: Empowering Self-Advocacy

Cultivating open communication channels and adhering to evidence-based practices can serve as a guide to ensure that medical care remains tailored, appropriate, and steadfastly person-centric. This may involve communicating to patients information about their diagnosis and treatment options, actively involving them in decision-making processes, and respecting their autonomy in choosing the course of their care. Studies have highlighted notable discrepancies between patient wishes, familial expectations, and healthcare provider perspectives, underscoring the necessity of robust communication and shared decision-making processes. Suen et al. found significant differences in treatment preferences between older adults and their caregivers, emphasizing the importance of understanding and respecting individual preferences in decision-making processes regarding life-sustaining treatments, illuminating the cultural nuances in shaping healthcare preferences (Suen et al. 2013). In addition, taking on a person-centric approach can translate to lower rates of unnecessary imaging tests and invasive procedures, leading to cost savings and better patient experiences (Bertakis and Azari 2011). It has been shown that comprehensive assessment and tailored management plans can result in better patient outcomes and satisfaction (Kuipers et al. 2019). This is best illustrated by the findings from the COMPASS (Cost and Medical Care of Patients with Advanced Serious Illness in Singapore) study. The COMPASS study is a longitudinal study in Singapore that studied healthcare utilization, cost, quality of care, and quality of life indicators among patients with advanced cancer (Teo et al. 2018). It highlighted significant knowledge gaps in patient and caregiver preferences for end-of-life care (Ozdemir et al. 2021), the quality of communication with physicians (Malhotra

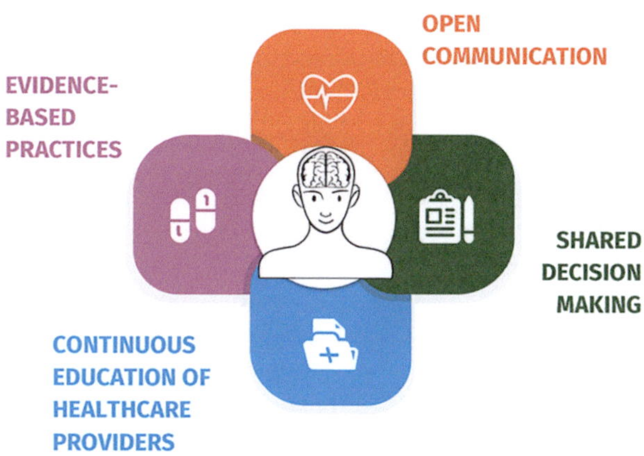

Fig. 19.2 Tenets of person-centric care

et al. 2021), and the management of pain and other symptoms (Shafiq et al. 2022). Pertinently, it showed that lower involvement of patients in their own care than preferred can lead to a poorer perceived quality of physician communication and care coordination. This may be extrapolated to be associated with poorer care outcomes (Malhotra et al. 2021). Further data also suggested that many advanced cancer patients had undergone costly medical treatments during the final months of their lives and that there were more institutional deaths (rather than dying at home) compared to other developed countries (Malhotra et al. 2022).

The approach of a person-centric care involves recognizing and addressing the emotional and psychological aspects of the patient's experiences. This means creating a supportive environment where patients can feel heard and understood, elevating them from a passive recipient to an active collaborator of their own medical care. This can significantly impact patients' overall well-being and trust in the healthcare system. Fostering a culture of continuous improvement is also essential for maintaining high standards of clinical care. Focus should be drawn to regularly reviewing and updating clinical practices based on the latest research and patient feedback, as well as investing in the training and development of healthcare professionals to enhance their communication and interpersonal skills. Figure 19.2 provides a simple illustration to showcase the above.

19.6 Rational Approach to Surgery

As the discussion of care will invariably lead to the subsequent discussion of a definitive management, offering surgery to an older person will require a thorough assessment of their overall health status and a collaborative decision-making process involving the patient, their family or caregivers, and the healthcare team. In other words, a rational approach to surgery demands a contextualized evaluation. The extent and strategy of a planned surgery in an older person must be carefully studied, accounting factors such as the patient's overall health status, comorbidities, and functional capacity. This ensures that surgical interventions are tailored to the individual's specific needs and circumstances. This can optimize the likelihood of successful outcomes and minimize any unnecessary risks.

Additionally, the use of diagnostic investigations must be contextualized to align with the likely management strategy and plan. Rather than blindly pursuing extensive diagnostic tests for better delineation of pathology, investigations should be judiciously selected based on their potential to inform treatment decisions and contribute meaningfully to the overall care plan. By adopting this rational approach, clinicians can navigate the complexities of surgical decision-making in older patients with more wisdom and insight.

Embracing uncertainty is another important skill that involves acknowledging the inherent unpredictability and complexities in treating older patients. Physicians must recognize that despite thorough evaluations and well-planned strategies, outcomes can vary due to numerous factors beyond their control. This acceptance of uncertainty does not equate to a lack of preparedness but rather a realistic approach to patient care that prioritizes adaptability and continuous reassessment. One crucial aspect of embracing uncertainty is the emphasis on shared decision-making. Engaging patients and their families in transparent conversations about potential risks, benefits, and uncertainties will allow patients and their families to make an informed decision. This fosters a collaborative environment where all parties can contribute to the decision-making process. This approach ensures that patients' values and preferences are central to the care plan, ultimately leading to more personalized and satisfactory outcomes. Furthermore, ongoing education is essential in adapting to and embracing uncertainty. Clinicians should stay abreast of the latest research and advancements in geriatric surgery so that they can integrate new knowledge into their practice to further refine and improve their patient care. Flexibility in adapting treatment plans based on evolving patient conditions and emerging evidence is also of paramount importance in managing the dynamic nature of surgical outcomes in older patients. A transdisciplinary approach also enhances the management of uncertainty. Collaborating with specialists from various fields will provide a comprehensive perspective on the patient's health and facilitates well-rounded decision-making. This collective expertise can help to address the multifaceted challenges that will arise in an older patient's surgical care.

19.7 Closing Thoughts: Achieving Balance in Evidence-Based Medicine and Patient Preference

Mastering geriatric surgery necessitates a paradigm shift toward person-centered care, where the individual's values, beliefs, and social context are prioritized alongside pathological considerations. By embracing a holistic approach that transcends disease processes, the surgeon can foster meaningful engagement with their patients to optimize patient outcomes while respecting their dignity and autonomy. Achieving a true appreciation of an older patient's health extends beyond managing symptoms and medical conditions; it requires understanding the complex interplay of medical, psychosocial, and emotional factors. To foster meaningful clinical decision-making, we must recognize and address inherent biases in medical care and embrace the diverse experiences and values each patient has. Medicine should evolve from a strict evidence-based approach to one that is personalized and contextualized. By doing so, we can make healthcare decisions that are not only medically sound but also deeply compassionate to the individual.

References

Bertakis KD, Azari R (2011) Patient-centered care is associated with decreased health care utilization. J Am Board Fam Med 24:229–239. https://doi.org/10.3122/jabfm.2011.03.100170

Berwick DM, Nolan TW, Whittington J (2008) The triple aim: care, health, and cost. Health Aff (Millwood) 27(3):759–769. https://doi.org/10.1377/hlthaff.27.3.759

Dicker D et al (2017) Global, regional, and national age-sex-specific mortality and life expectancy, 1950–2017: a systematic analysis for the Global Burden of Disease Study 2017. Lancet 392(10159):1684–1735

Engel GL (1977) The need for a new medical model: a challenge for biomedicine. Science 196(4286):129–136. https://doi.org/10.1126/science.847460

EuroQol Research Foundation (2023) EQ-5D-5L user guide [Internet]. EuroQol, Rotterdam. https://euroqol.org/wp-content/uploads/2023/11/EQ-5D-5LUserguide-23-07.pdf. Accessed 19 Dec 2024

Janssen TL, Lodder P, de Vries J et al (2020) Caregiver strain on informal caregivers when providing care for older patients undergoing major abdominal surgery: a longitudinal prospective cohort study. BMC Geriatr 20:178. https://doi.org/10.1186/s12877-020-01579-8

Kuipers SJ, Cramm JM, Nieboer AP (2019) The importance of patient-centered care and co-creation of care for satisfaction with care and physical and social well-being of patients with multi-morbidity in the primary care setting. BMC Health Serv Res 19:13

Lwi SJ, Ford BQ, Casey JJ, Miller BL, Levenson RW (2017) Poor caregiver mental health predicts mortality of patients with neurodegenerative disease. Proc Natl Acad Sci USA 114(28):7319–7324

Malhotra C, Chaudhry I, Ozdemir S, Teo I, Kanesvaran R (2021) Experiences with health care practitioners among advanced cancer patients and their family caregivers: a longitudinal dyadic study. Cancer 127:3002–3009. https://doi.org/10.1002/cncr.33592

Malhotra C, Koh LE, Teo I, Ozdemir S, Chaudhry I, Finkelstein E, on behalf of the COMPASS Study Team (2022) A prospective cohort study of stability in preferred place of death among patients with stage IV cancer in Singapore. J Natl Compr Cancer Netw 20(1):20–28. https://doi.org/10.6004/jnccn.2020.7795

Ministry of Health (2022) Speech by Minister for Health at the Ministry of Health Committee of supply debate 2022 [Internet]. Ministry of Health, Singapore. https://www.moh.gov.sg/news-highlights/details/speech-by-mr-ong-ye-kung-minister-for-health-at-the-ministry-of-health-committee-of-supply-debate-2022. Accessed 19 Dec 2024

Ozdemir S, Ng S, Malhotra C, Teo I, Finkelstein EA (2021) COMPASS Study Group, patient–caregiver treatment preference discordance and its association with caregiving burden and esteem. Innov Aging 5(3):igab020. https://doi.org/10.1093/geroni/igab020

Shafiq M, Malhotra R, Teo I, Ozdemir S, Kanesvaran R, Malhotra C (2022) Trajectories of physical symptom burden and psychological distress during the last year of life in patients with a solid metastatic cancer. Psychooncology 31(1):139–147. https://doi.org/10.1002/pon.5792

Singapore Ministry of Health (2017) The burden of disease in Singapore, 1990–2017 [Internet]. Ministry of Health, Singapore. https://www.moh.gov.sg/docs/librariesprovider5/default-document-library/gbd_2017_singapore_reportce6bb0b3ad1a49c19ee6ebadc1273b18.pdf?sfvrsn=edc74d4a_0. Accessed 19 Dec 2024

Suen LJ, Lee HH, Morris DL (2013) Life-sustaining treatment: a comparison of the preferences of Taiwanese older adults and their family caregiver. J Nurs Res 21(4):261–269. https://doi.org/10.1097/JNR.0000000000000006

Teo I, Singh R, Malhotra C et al (2018) Cost of medical care of patients with advanced serious illness in Singapore (COMPASS): prospective cohort study protocol. BMC Cancer 18:459. https://doi.org/10.1186/s12885-018-4356-z

Wade DT, Halligan PW (2004) Do biomedical models of illness make for good healthcare systems? BMJ 329(7479):1398–1401. https://doi.org/10.1136/bmj.329.7479.1398

Ware JE Jr, Sherbourne CD (1992) The MOS 36-item short-form health survey (SF-36). I. Conceptual framework and item selection. Med Care 30(6):473–483

20 Addressing the Person Who Needs Surgical Management

João Pärtel Araújo

Take-Home Messages

1. Introduction

    - Surgical care for older adults extends beyond medical conditions to encompass the whole person.
    - Human connection is impactful in the perioperative care experience.
    - Nonpharmacological, relationship-centered approaches are key in geriatric surgical care.

2. Humanitude Care Methodology

    - Humanitude is a care methodology that promotes the relationship between the person receiving care and the person providing care, based on four pillars: gaze, speech, touch, and verticality.
    - The Sensory Capture procedure establishes a systematic foundation to ensure positive interactions.
    - The Structured Sequence of Humanitude Care Procedures (SSHCP) provides validated measurements to assess and improve relationship-centered care.

J. P. Araújo (✉)
University of Coimbra, Coimbra, Portugal

Health Sciences Research Unit: Nursing (UICISA:E), Nursing School of Coimbra, Coimbra, Portugal

Humanitude International, Paris, France
e-mail: joaoaraujo@humanitude.pt

K.-Y. Tan et al. (eds.), *Mastering Geriatric Surgery*,
https://doi.org/10.1007/978-981-95-0665-1_20

- Personalized Care Prescription aligns the interdisciplinary team around common goals and nonpharmacological interventions.
- Humanitude research on its implementation in geriatric care suggests a reduction in delirium rates and improved outcomes.

3. Relationship-Centered Care in Perioperative Setting

- Relationship-centered care improves surgical outcomes by focusing on meaningful human connections.
- Understanding and addressing the person's broader concerns and core challenges can significantly impact recovery.
- Empathy is a crucial professional skill that can and should be systematically developed in healthcare settings.
- Relational competency can and needs to be developed by all healthcare professionals, through various means, including narrative medicine, simulation training, and hands-on practice.
- Humanitude techniques can enhance relational competency in perioperative care.

4. Particular Complexities of Geriatric Surgery

- Care refusal emerges from multiple determinants: personal, relational, environmental, and organizational factors.
- Postoperative delirium requires a relationship-centered approach focusing on identifying triggers, maintaining familiar connections, and ensuring safety and comfort throughout the surgical journey.
- Immobility syndrome prevention requires understanding psychological barriers, in both the person and the healthcare professionals, and building confidence through supportive relationships and relational handling practices.
- Failure to thrive often results from unmet emotional and social needs and compromised autonomy.
- Successful surgical outcomes depend on preserving the person's identity, dignity, autonomy, and social connections throughout the perioperative period.

5. Conclusion

- Relationship-centered care is fundamental to managing complex geriatric surgical syndromes.
- Humanitude methodology provides a structured framework for implementing relationship-centered perioperative care.
- Developing relational competency requires systematic training and organizational support.

- Nonpharmacological interventions based on human connection improve surgical outcomes.
- Approaches that preserve dignity and autonomy are essential for successful geriatric surgery.

20.1 Introduction

As our global population ages, surgical and perioperative care teams are increasingly confronted with surgical clients of older age, presenting unique challenges that extend far beyond the immediate surgical pathology. The landscape of modern postoperative care is evolving rapidly, particularly in geriatric care. Each surgical case brings not only a set of complex medical conditions but also a person with a life history, complex biopsychosocial needs, and unique expectations that profoundly impact on the surgical experience. Behind a surgical case, there is a person who ultimately depends on the healthcare team to improve their well-being, not only through surgery but also through perioperative care (Kehlet and Wilmore 2008; Petrescu et al. 2022).

As healthcare professionals, we must ask ourselves: are we curing pathologies, or are we caring for people? The renowned physician Abraham Verghese (2011) posits that the most important innovation in medicine to come in the next 10 years might be the power of the human hand and the power of human touch. Those 10 years have passed, and touch is far from being a professional tool in healthcare. This insight underscores a crucial point: while we have made remarkable strides in surgical techniques and technology, the missing link in truly impactful perioperative care may well be the human connection, which has been gradually considered elective (McGlone et al. 2024).

This chapter explores the complexities of addressing the person who needs surgical management in geriatric care, with a focus on nonpharmacological, relationship-centered approaches. We will examine the impact of care refusal, postoperative delirium, immobility syndrome, and failure to thrive on surgical outcomes in older adults, emphasizing the importance of comprehensive preoperative assessment, prehabilitation, and innovative strategies for managing common, yet neglected, challenges in the perioperative period (Araújo et al. 2025; Boechat et al. 2012; Dewar and Nolan 2013; Inouye et al. 2015; Roubenoff and Harris 1997; Soklaridis et al. 2016; Tsui et al. 2020).

Central to our discussion is the concept of relationship-centered care, including methodologies like Humanitude, which emphasizes the promotion of well-being through relational techniques. We will explore how this methodology may help to improve the surgical experience for older adults and consequently for healthcare professionals (Beach et al. 2006; Dewar and Nolan 2013; Gineste and Marescotti 2010; Soklaridis et al. 2016).

We will analyze the role of relational competency in perioperative care, examining how healthcare professionals can develop and refine these essential skills to build trust and potentially improve surgical outcomes for older adults (Kelm et al. 2014; Santana et al. 2018).

We begin with a fundamental principle: by preserving the person's Humanitude at every step of the perioperative path, we can elevate our practice and outcomes (Gineste et al. 2008). This chapter explores how relationship-centered care might improve the surgical experience for older adults. By integrating technical expertise with relational competencies, we may better address complex geriatric syndromes. In doing so, we can shift perioperative care from a task-centered enterprise to a specialized human practice, a service exchange between healthcare professionals and older adults who entrust their well-being to perioperative care.

20.2 The Humanitude Care Methodology

In 1979, when Yves Gineste and Rosette Marescotti were asked by a district hospital to join the healthcare team and help with the transfer and positioning of people receiving care, they could not be more foreign to the setting. While their background in physical education and occupational safety provided foundational knowledge of body mechanics and injury prevention, it did not prepare them for interactions with people receiving care. Although hospital management had envisioned them supporting healthcare professionals, the gap in interpersonal care skills became their main focus. Soon enough, they realized that the effectiveness of transferring and positioning of people was highly affected by the person's will to cooperate and understand instructions. Since then, Humanitude has been focused on how to connect and communicate with the person receiving care more efficiently, so that the care becomes more effective (Gineste and Pellissier 2007; Gineste and Marescotti 2010).

Imagine you are an 85-year-old surgical client, alone and frightened, a light gown covering your modesty, going through a cold air-conditioned environment, surround by masked strangers, under a glaring white bright light. The glaring lights, cold air, and sea of masked faces in green or blue make you feel vulnerable. Your survival instinct tells you that you are in danger, your amygdala gets startled, you get a discharge of cortisol and noradrenaline (Dhabhar 2014), your heart races, your blood pressure rises, and you consider refusing care to seek for safety. Suddenly, one of the staff comes to you and a pair of kind eyes comes to meet your gaze, with a slight smile visible behind the mask. In a soft, melodious tone, you hear: "Hello. I'm Sarah, I'll be your anaesthetist nurse today. We're here to take really good care of you. I can assure you that you're in good hands."

This simple act of human connection, grounded in the pillars of Humanitude (gaze, speech, and touch), can transform a person's surgical experience from fear and alienation to comfort and trust (Gineste and Pellissier 2007; Honda et al. 2016).

Humanitude is a care methodology that recognizes the inherent need of every person, regardless of age or health status, to feel safe, respected, validated, and

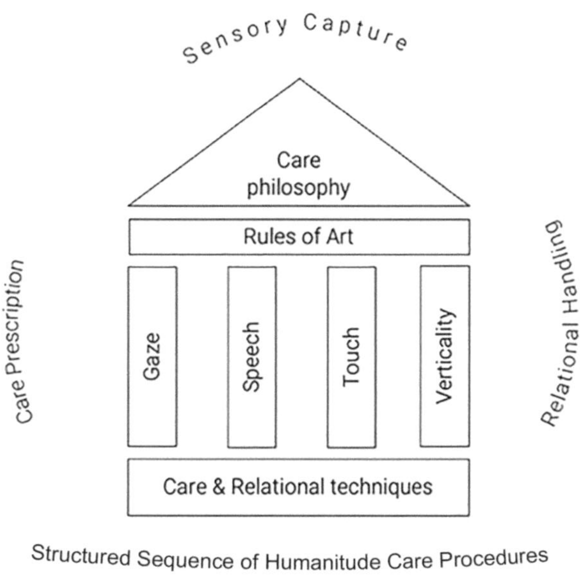

Fig. 20.1 Proposed Humanitude care methodology framework (Source: Original work by author)

cared for by other human beings. It is composed by a set of techniques, guided by a philosophy of care that views caregiving as a profound human emotional encounter that goes further than the immediate clinical interventions (Gineste et al. 2008; Melo et al. 2017a, b, 2020). A proposed framework for the Humanitude care methodology is illustrated in Fig. 20.1, which presents the interconnected components of the methodology, including care philosophy, relational techniques, and its tools.

20.2.1 The Four Pillars of Humanitude

Humanitude is an anthropological concept adapted to caregiving by Yves Gineste and Rosette Marescotti and defined as the set of characteristics that allow a human being to be recognized as a person and allow other people to recognize another person as a fellow member of the human species. This means that a person needs other people to feel validated, respected, and secure. As a social species, humans learn to interact with other humans, through a set of rituals, and can easily decode emotional meanings behind every eye contact, word spoken, touch used, and other nonverbal cues. There are specific neurological structures to give meaning to all these rituals and interactions, some quite primitive, that are matured in our human brain by thousands of interactions throughout our lives, from birth to death (Bales et al. 2018; Gineste and Pellissier 2007; Gineste et al. 2008; Gineste and Marescotti 2010; Honda et al. 2016).

Therefore, Yves Gineste and Rosette Marescotti established four fundamental pillars to promote and maintain a person's Humanitude: gaze, speech, touch, and verticality. These elements, when used intentionally and skillfully, have a significantly positive impact on the emotional meaning of an interaction and can help break through barriers of fear, confusion, and care resistance (Araújo et al. 2025; Giang et al. 2023; Gineste and Pellissier 2007; Gineste et al. 2008; Melo et al. 2017a, b).

1. Gaze: In the operating room scenario, Sarah's deliberate eye contact is a meaningful, eye-to-eye gaze that says, "I recognize you as a person." This gaze anchors Sarah to the person, fostering human bond. While brief glances and rapid eye contact between surgical team members are essential for efficient procedural coordination, the surgical client may interpret these quick exchanges as signs of concern or dismissal, potentially increasing their anxiety and affecting their trust in the medical team if not accompanied by clear explanation of this professional communication style. On the other hand, a long eye-to-eye contact gaze is associated to person's feeling validated, and a sense of confidence, and promotes the release of oxytocin, increasing bonds and trust in the person. Therefore, a simple, yet important, intentional Humanitude gaze may lead to better care acceptance and care compliance. On the other hand, a poorly executed gaze can trigger negative emotions enhancing fear and mistrust (Araújo et al. 2025; Giang et al. 2023; Honda et al. 2016; Melo et al. 2020; Petrescu et al. 2022; Sato et al. 2023; Uvnäs-Moberg et al. 2015).
2. Speech: Sarah's words, delivered in a low, melodic tone, do more than convey information. They create a soothing auditory stimulus that can activate the parasympathetic system and reduce heart rate and blood pressure. Introducing the name personalizes the interaction, reinforces the caregiver identity, and promotes the sense of trust. In a setting where it is easy to be a stranger and feel vulnerable, silence, strange loud noises, or inappropriate tones of voice can make the person feel more insecure. This sense of insecurity increases the release of cortisol, which in turn is linked to a higher inflammatory response and compromises the immune system (Altamirano et al. 2022; Gineste et al. 2008; Dhabhar 2014; Nilsson 2009).
3. Touch: A gentle touch in a socially accepted area, like hand or shoulder, is a powerful nonverbal communicator, conveying empathy, trust, and reassurance, sometimes more effectively than words alone. Research has shown that therapeutic touch can reduce stress hormones and alleviate pain perception. This is largely mediated through specialized nerve fibers called C-tactile (CT) afferents, which respond optimally to gentle stroking at speeds of 1–10 cm/s, with an adequate pressure. A tender touch contributes to social bonding and emotional well-being of the person; however, it requires consent. Understanding the complexity of these neurobiological mechanisms and the importance of a professionalized tender touch can help healthcare professionals deliver more effective therapeutic touch in clinical settings (Bales et al. 2018; Hertenstein et al. 2006; Liljencrantz and Olausson 2014; Mancini et al. 2015; McGlone et al. 2024).
4. Verticality: Upright posture and movement are fundamental to human physiology and neuropsychology. Our evolutionary adaptation to bipedalism has shaped not only our musculoskeletal system but also our cardiovascular, respiratory,

nervous systems, and many others to function optimally in vertical positions. In perioperative care, verticality plays several crucial roles. Preoperatively, maintaining vertical posture and mobility helps optimize the physiological function. During the immediate preoperative period, enabling surgical clients to walk to the operating theater and self-transfer, when possible, can help to maintain autonomy and sense of control, reduce anxiety, and preserve functional capacity. Postoperatively, early mobilization (when safe) is crucial not only because it reduces the risk of complications like deep vein thrombosis, respiratory infections, and muscle mass loss but also because it promotes psychological well-being through maintained independence and perceived sense of recovery and capacity. So, beyond physical benefits, verticality supports identity and autonomy, key components of a holistic recovery. Standing and walking represent independence and capability, directly impacting on motivation and engagement of the person through the perioperative journey (Dijkstra et al. 2022; Fried et al. 2001; Inouye et al. 1999, 2015; Kehlet and Wilmore 2008; Niemitz 2010; Partridge et al. 2012).

20.2.2 Sensory Capture

Sensory capture is one of the most valuable contributes of Humanitude care methodology to the professionalization of the caregiving relationship. It comprises a structured sequence of care procedures designed to establish and maintain meaningful human connections during healthcare interactions. This evidence-based procedure consists of five distinct stages that build upon each other to create a comprehensive framework for relationship-centered care (Gineste and Pellissier 2007; Melo et al. 2017a, b; Henriques et al. 2019).

Pre-preliminaries is the first stage of any human interaction, which establishes spatial awareness and consent, signaling an approaching human interaction while allowing the person to prepare for engagement. This initial stage fundamentally respects personal space and autonomy. Moving into the second stage, the preliminaries, the healthcare professional obtains explicit relational and care consent, building trust and rapport, through the sequential introduction of the Humanitude relational pillars. During the third stage, the sensory circle, the staff maintains a positive connection throughout the care delivery through multisensory and multimodal relational engagement. This promotes active participation in care procedures while sustaining well-being during interventions. The fourth stage, the emotional consolidation, then creates a positive emotional memory of the interaction, strengthening neural pathways associated with trust and facilitating future care interactions, while reinforcing the person's ability, the care value, and the importance of such therapeutic relationship. Finally, the re-encounter stage establishes clear continuity of care, prevents feelings of abandonment, and facilitates care acceptance. This final phase creates explicit commitment for future interactions and/or care interventions while maintaining relational connection between care episodes. Each stage in this sequence respects both neurobiological principles and fundamentals of human dignity, creating a foundation for effective operationalized, relationship-centered care (Gineste and Pellissier 2007; Henriques et al. 2019, 2022; Inácio 2022; Melo et al. 2017a, b, 2020).

Let us see how this could unfold in a post-anesthesia care unit:

1. Pre-preliminaries: Before entering the person's space, Sarah takes a moment to announce her presence. This can be done either by knocking on the bed footrest, giving a proprioceptive and auditory stimulus to the person, or wave inside the person's field of vision at a distance longer than an arm's length, to proactively engage with the person. By smoothly opening the relational channels of the person, Sarah is promoting the sense of control and respect on the person's space and privacy and therefore reducing the sense of surprise and threat provoked by a sudden invasion of private space.
2. Preliminaries: Sarah enters the person's field of vision with a smile, making eye contact for 3 s, lowering the level of the gaze to reduce the perception of threat and vulnerability, caused by vertical gaze. She introduces herself with a low melodic voice and introduces a gentle touch in a socially accepted area. This is intentionally done to obtain relational consent, to promote a sense of trust and well-being, before initiating a more invasive intervention or more intimate conversation.
3. Sensory Circle: As Sarah performs necessary care tasks, she maintains a positive connection through a permanent gentle touch; maintains a calm tone of voice using validating words, to induce a sense of trust; and recurrently searches the person's gaze to induce the sense of recognition. She explains each step, involving the person as much as possible to reduce the fear of the unknown. Sarah tries to engage intentionally with the person as much as she can with this multisensory approach and promote participation during care with the verticality, as much as possible.
4. Emotional Consolidation: After the care task is completed, Sarah takes a moment to reinforce the positive benefits of the task and of the interaction, to value the care and the trusting relationship with the caregiver.
5. Re-encounter: Before leaving, Sarah plans the next interaction, giving the person the sense of continuity of care and trying to motivate the person for care. Something like: "I'll be back in an hour to help you sit up. We'll move at your pace, but getting upright is important for your recovery. Can I come back?"

20.2.3 Structured Sequence of Humanitude Care Procedures (SSHCP)

The operationalization of sensory capture has led to the development of the Structured Sequence of Humanitude Care Procedures (SSHCP), a validated 27-step compliance measurement instrument. This tool evaluates the professionalization of caregiving relationships and has revealed striking insights into care delivery. Research shows that healthcare professionals significantly overestimate their performance of relationship-centered care steps, with studies documenting discrepancies between perceived and actual practice as high as 83.4%. This led to the conclusion that even though therapeutic relationships are highly valued by healthcare professionals, they are often neglected, thus needing training and continuous monitoring for professional development (Henriques et al. 2019, 2022; Inácio 2022; Melo et al. 2017a, b, 2020).

SSHCP's significance is that it transforms seemingly intangible aspects of human interactions into quantifiable, improvable relational skills (Henriques et al. 2022; Inácio 2022). This is particularly crucial in healthcare environments where high time pressures and technical demands often overshadow essential human interactions. While we develop interaction rituals through lifelong social experiences, their application in clinical settings requires specific training and deliberate practice (Cocker and Joss 2016; Fukuyasu et al. 2021; Kobayashi et al. 2021; Meier et al. 2001; Melo et al. 2020).

In perioperative settings, the SSHCP enables teams to track specific relational behaviors such as maintenance of appropriate eye contact, clear procedure explanations, and effective therapeutic touch. This systematic approach to measuring care interactions drives continuous improvement while ensuring the consistent application of Humanitude techniques. Most importantly, it supports the professionalization of therapeutic relationships, elevating perioperative care beyond technical excellence to include skilled human connection (Melo et al. 2020; Henriques et al. 2019, 2022; Honda et al. 2016; Giang et al. 2023).

20.2.4 Personalized Care Prescription

The personalized care prescription is another distinctive Humanitude tool that complements traditional medical charts and care plans. It addresses the common challenges of perioperative care, while reducing the wasted capacity of misaligned interventions among healthcare professionals, who may have different and perhaps conflicting care goals, interventions, and priorities throughout the care journey (Gineste and Pellissier 2007; Marescotti and Gineste 2011).

Effective perioperative care requires systematic evaluation, prescription, execution, and monitoring. The personalized care prescription establishes a common care goal that addresses core challenges recognized by the entire team, family, and surgical client, focusing on nonpharmacological interventions to improve or maintain the person's well-being. This structured approach ensures consistency in care delivery and enables the monitoring of care outcomes across different healthcare disciplines (Henriques et al. 2017, 2019, 2021; Marescotti and Gineste 2011; Melo et al. 2017a, b; Santana et al. 2018).

The prescription comprises several essential elements to ensure fidelity: person identification, verticality profile assessment, and both primary and alternative care goals that remain non-discipline specific. It includes discipline-specific objectives while maintaining focus on personalized care conditions and required resources to optimize the care quality. Specific interventions and relational strategies are detailed, alongside monitoring documentation to track progress and care outcomes (Gineste and Pellissier 2007; Henriques et al. 2021; Inácio 2022; Marescotti and Gineste 2011).

The prescription follows a systematic review process: it should be established on admission, revised after sudden health changes, after three unsuccessful intervention attempts, or at regular intervals established by the protocol. The first revision of the care prescription focuses on adjusting the care conditions. The second revision focuses on revising the care goal itself, requiring a reassessment and perhaps a referral to specialty (Henriques et al. 2019, 2021; Inácio 2022; Marescotti and Gineste 2011; Melo et al. 2017a, b).

The success of this approach fundamentally depends on thorough care evaluation. This evaluation considers the person's functional and cognitive capacity, their personal expectations and care preferences, the team's care plans, and the resources required and available for care delivery. It also incorporates individualized relational techniques, such as using preferred names or specific engagement strategies that work best for each person. Through this comprehensive approach, the entire team works cohesively toward common perioperative care goals while maintaining a truly personalized care delivery (Chou and Gaysynsky 2023; Henriques et al. 2021; Inácio 2022; Marescotti and Gineste 2011; Santana et al. 2018).

How could this help during a preoperative moment? Imagine if Sarah knew that the person she is caring for was a retired music teacher who still plays piano regularly at her local church. Perhaps, Sarah could more easily connect with the person while preparing for surgery, by breaking the ice discussing favorite composers, forging a sense of trust more effectively.

By learning about the person's preferred name, favorite conversational topic, or cherished emotional memories, surgical staff can more effectively personalize and improve the care experience. This knowledge can also be used, for example, to distract and comfort the person, using it as a diversion strategy during stressful moments, such as the induction of anesthesia or the journey to the recovery room, to reduce stress and perception of pain. Also, by establishing a common care goal with the person, all surgical interventions can be aligned toward that goal, promoting its achievement in a more efficient manner, while involving the person on the care process and fostering motivation for recovery (Altamirano et al. 2022; Henriques et al. 2019, 2021; Inácio 2022; Mancini et al. 2015; Marescotti and Gineste 2011; Paget et al. 2011; Petrescu et al. 2022; Wang et al. 2024).

20.2.5 Effects of Humanitude

Published research has demonstrated that Humanitude care can have significant positive effects on both clients and healthcare providers. Two scoping reviews found that Humanitude reduces neuropsychiatric symptoms in people with dementia and improves their acceptance of and participation in care. Moreover, people with dementia were found to be more relaxed and calmer without psychotropic medication when receiving Humanitude care, with improved functional and well-being scores (Giang et al. 2023; Honda et al. 2016; Kobayashi et al. 2024; Won et al. 2024).

For healthcare providers, evidence indicates that Humanitude improves care quality, communication and empathy skills, and job satisfaction while reducing burnout. Studies identified that healthcare providers who received Humanitude training demonstrated higher average percentages on essential care communication elements like eye contact, verbal communication, and touch compared to conventional care. Studies also demonstrated that healthcare providers trained in SSHCP showed progressive improvement in their relational competency scores across multiple observation points (Fukuyasu et al. 2021; Henriques et al. 2019; Inácio 2022; Kobayashi et al. 2021; Melo et al. 2017a, b, 2020).

By implementing evidence-based Humanitude practices in perioperative care, we can potentially improve both client outcomes and provider satisfaction while maintaining the fundamental human connection that is essential to quality healthcare delivery. Future research should explore Humanitude's effects on surgical outcomes like length of hospital stay, readmission rates, and posthospitalization recovery (Giang et al. 2021, 2023; Honda et al. 2016; Sugimoto et al. 2018).

20.3 Relationship-Centered Care in Perioperative Setting

20.3.1 Understanding Relationship-Centered Care

The surgical practice involves much more than technical excellence—it requires understanding the person behind the surgical case. Relationship-centered care acknowledges that surgical outcomes depend not just on technical skill but also on the quality of care and the interactions between healthcare providers, clients, and their support networks (Beach et al. 2006; Soklaridis et al. 2016). Figure 20.2 proposes a model of relationship-centered care that highlights the therapeutic alliance among healthcare providers, persons receiving care, support networks, and healthcare systems.

In perioperative care, relationship-centered care means seeing beyond the immediate surgical needs to understand the person's broader life context. As Charon (2001) argues, this narrative competence—the ability to absorb, interpret, and respond to clients' stories—is crucial for effective medical care. This includes their fears and hopes, their social support systems, and the impact surgery might have on their daily lives. A person facing surgery brings a lifetime of experiences, relationships, expectations, fears, and circumstances that influence their surgical journey. Not identifying them, considering them, or addressing them might ultimately compromise the surgical outcome (Dewar and Nolan 2013; Kelm et al. 2014; Ko et al. 2021; Paget et al. 2011; Ross 2021; Soklaridis et al. 2016).

While many assume that building relationships comes naturally, research consistently shows that these skills must be developed through deliberate practice and training. Just as surgeons spend years perfecting their technical abilities, healthcare providers need structured learning and practice to build effective relationship skills, especially in environments where time and efficiency set the pace (Altamirano et al. 2022; Bauchat et al. 2016; Kelm et al. 2014;).

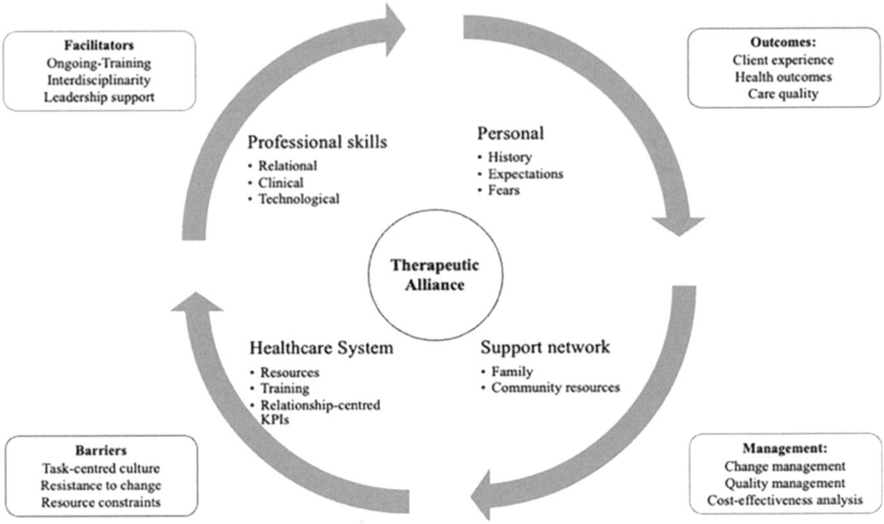

Fig. 20.2 Proposed relationship-centered care model (Source: Original work by author)

20.3.2 Evidence Supporting Relationship-Centered Care

The impact of relationship-centered care may extend throughout the surgical journey, though implementing this approach presents both opportunities and challenges. When people feel understood and supported, their surgical experience tends to improve (Beach et al. 2006; Derksen et al. 2013; Dewar and Nolan 2013; Paget et al. 2011; Santana et al. 2018; Soklaridis et al. 2016).

For healthcare providers, building meaningful connections with clients can bring renewed purpose to their work. However, establishing these connections within the constraints of busy surgical settings presents significant challenges. Time pressures, high patient turnover, and system-level barriers such as rigid schedules and documentation requirements can make it difficult to cultivate deeper relationships. Additionally, providers must balance emotional involvement with professional boundaries, which requires skill and ongoing support (Meier et al. 2001; Cocker and Joss 2016; Gleichgerrcht and Decety 2014; Kelm et al. 2014).

Despite these challenges, the effects of positive relationships may manifest in practical ways throughout the care process (Chou and Gaysynsky 2023; Altamirano et al. 2022; Ko et al. 2021). When positive relationships facilitate communication, assessments often become more efficient. For example, pain evaluation may be more accurate when trust exists between the provider and client. Informed consent can evolve from a legal requirement into a more meaningful dialogue about care choices. Care management may improve when providers understand not just the physical symptoms but also the person's experience and broader biopsychosocial needs (Paget et al. 2011; Santana et al. 2018; Sinclair et al. 2016).

20.3.3 Key Elements of Relationship-Centered Care

Building effective positive relationships in perioperative care requires specific skills and approaches (Kelm et al. 2014; Bearman et al. 2015). The ability to be mindfully present with each person despite the busy surgical environment may require setting aside distractions and giving complete attention to the person (Dewar and Nolan 2013; Paget et al. 2011; Soklaridis et al. 2016).

Active listening goes beyond hearing words to understand their deeper meaning. It involves noticing the tone of voice, observing body language, and picking up on unspoken concerns. Through active listening, providers can detect fears about recovery, worries about family obligations, or uncertainty about the surgical process itself (Derksen et al. 2013; Sinclair et al. 2016).

Nonverbal communication plays a crucial role in building trust. The way providers make eye contact, use their speech, and employ appropriate touch can either create connection or reinforce distance. Small gestures—sitting down during conversations, maintaining eye contact, and offering a reassuring touch when appropriate—can significantly impact the quality of relationships (Hertenstein et al. 2006; Melo et al. 2017a, b, 2020; Ko et al. 2021).

These elements do not work in isolation but come together in a structured approach. Healthcare providers should learn to establish initial connections effectively, since they set the tone for the entire clinical journey (Bauchat et al. 2016; Altamirano et al. 2022). Perhaps, more importantly, the development of these skills for building and maintaining trust through each interaction promotes professionalism in healthcare (Beach et al. 2006; Dewar and Nolan 2013; Fukuyasu et al. 2021; Kobayashi et al. 2021).

20.3.4 Barriers to Relationship-Centered Care

Building relationships in perioperative care faces numerous challenges. In today's healthcare environment, system-level barriers often work against meaningful human connection. Fast-paced surgical units prioritize efficiency, leaving little time for understanding each person's unique situation. When healthcare providers must care for many clients in quick succession, they may default to task-focused interactions rather than relationship building (Cocker and Joss 2016; Meier et al. 2001).

The physical environment itself can work against relationship-centered care. Many surgical units lack quiet spaces for private conversations. Shared rooms, busy corridors, and clinical environments designed for technical efficiency and safety rather than human interaction make it difficult to have meaningful discussions about fears, concerns, and preferences (Petrescu et al. 2022; Soklaridis et al. 2016).

Professional barriers also play a significant role. Healthcare education emphasizes mastery of technical skills and procedures, often overlooking the vital importance of relationship building. Many providers lack formal training in communicating with older adults, in particular older adults with cognitive impairment, or managing complex family dynamics. When faced with challenging situations, they may not have the tools or confidence to engage effectively (Bearman et al. 2015; Kelm et al. 2014; Ko et al. 2021).

The growing reliance on technology creates its own set of barriers. Electronic health records and digital monitoring systems, while valuable for data collection, can create a physical and psychological barrier between providers and clients. Providers often find themselves interacting more with screens than with people (Paget et al. 2011; Ko et al. 2021).

Emotional barriers significantly impact relationship building. Healthcare providers experiencing burnout may emotionally distance themselves as a coping mechanism. The emotional toll of caring for people facing serious health challenges can lead to compassion fatigue, making it harder to maintain empathetic connections (Gleichgerrcht and Decety 2014).

Organizational culture can also hinder relationship-centered care. When institutions prioritize throughput and technical outcomes over relationship quality, providers may feel pressured to limit time spent on building connections. Performance metrics rarely capture the quality of relationships, making it harder to justify investing time in this aspect of care (Chou and Gaysynsky 2023).

Communication barriers extend beyond simple language differences. Healthcare providers and clients may have different cultural understandings of illness, recovery, the role of social support networks, and healthcare professionals. These differences become especially challenging when working with people who have difficulties communicating, who have cognitive impairments, or come from cultural backgrounds that view healthcare differently from the predominant culture (Beach et al. 2006; Santana et al. 2018).

Power dynamics in healthcare settings can also create additional barriers. The inherent power imbalance between providers and clients can make it difficult to establish genuine partnerships. Clients may feel intimidated or hesitant to express their needs and preferences, while providers may unconsciously adopt authoritative communication styles and assume the decision-making process, as the specialist, neglecting or disregarding the persons will (Kelm et al. 2014; Ko et al. 2021).

Systemic issues like staff shortages and high turnover rates also impact relationship building. When teams are understaffed or constantly changing, it becomes harder to maintain continuity of relationships. New team members may lack context about clients' personal situations and preferences, which might constitute yet another barrier to relationship-centered care (Sinclair et al. 2016).

20.3.5 Moving Forward

Making relationship-centered care work requires treating it as essential rather than optional. Organizations need to provide time and space for staff to build relationships with clients. Regular training and practice monitoring help staff develop and maintain these skills (Beach et al. 2006; Bearman et al. 2015; Dewar and Nolan 2013; Kelm et al. 2014; Soklaridis et al. 2016).

Current evidence points to the value of relationship-centered approaches in surgical care. Future research should examine specific outcomes like recovery times, client satisfaction, and staff well-being. Meanwhile, healthcare organizations can work on creating environments that support meaningful relationships between providers and clients (Altamirano et al. 2022; Chou and Gaysynsky 2023; Derksen et al. 2013; Ko et al. 2021; Santana et al. 2018).

20.4 Particular Complexities of Geriatric Perioperative Care

Geriatric perioperative care presents a unique set of challenges associated with aging-related frailty and vulnerability. While conditions like sarcopenia, frailty, and multimorbidity undoubtedly complicate surgical outcomes (Cruz-Jentoft et al. 2019; Partridge et al. 2012), this chapter focuses specifically on the relational and psychological aspects of geriatric surgical care. Some of these challenges, which include care refusal, postoperative delirium, immobility syndrome, and failure to thrive, significantly impact older adults' surgical experiences and recovery trajectories.

Care refusal and postoperative delirium represent two of the most prevalent and consequential relational challenges in geriatric surgery. Both conditions emerge from a complex interplay of factors. Understanding their determinants is crucial for developing effective prevention and management strategies that prioritize the older adults' well-being. Recent research emphasizes the importance of comprehensive approaches to preventing and managing delirium, highlighting the need for personalized interventions (Araújo et al. 2025; Inouye et al. 1999, 2015; Petrescu et al. 2022; Ross 2021).

Immobility syndrome and failure to thrive further complicate the picture, highlighting the profound impact of psychological and social factors on surgical recovery (Morales-Cariño et al. 2012; Vázquez Pedrazuela et al. 1995). These conditions often manifest as behavioral changes, such as withdrawal or heightened defensiveness, signaling deeper issues that require interdisciplinary attention (Boechat et al. 2012). The underlying mechanisms are complex, involving physical decline, psychological distress, and social isolation (Aguilera et al. 2004; Fried et al. 2001; Roubenoff and Harris 1997).

This chapter explores these particular four challenges, examining their impact on surgical outcomes, client–provider relationships, and the broader healthcare system. It presents a relationship-centered approach to addressing these challenges, emphasizing the importance of positive human interactions, effective communication, and environmental modifications in promoting optimal recovery for older surgical clients.

20.4.1 Care Refusal in Geriatric Surgery

Care refusal represents one of the most challenging aspects in perioperative care of older adults. When a person refuses necessary care, it creates immediate risks to their health and recovery, while also straining relationships with healthcare providers and family members. Studies indicate that care refusal rates in older adults range from 9 to 59.8% in institutional settings, but it is far from being fully understood. The impact extends beyond the refused care itself—it can delay access to care, recovery, increase health complications, compromise surgical outcomes, and in some cases, lead to the cancellation of planned procedures (Araújo et al. 2025).

Care refusal in older surgical clients emerges from a complex interplay of personal, relational, environmental, and organizational determinants. Understanding these determinants and intentionally modifying them are crucial for effective perioperative care (Araújo et al. 2025; Ko et al. 2021; Altamirano et al. 2022).

Personal determinants include cognitive impairment, communication difficulties, unmet needs like pain, and neuropsychiatric symptoms such as anxiety or depression. Many older adults facing surgery experience vulnerability that manifests as care refusal when their personal needs are not properly understood or addressed.

Relational determinants are the way that healthcare providers approach, communicate, and engage with clients. Patronizing or infantilizing communication styles often trigger refusal behaviors. When providers fail to build trust or use inappropriate communication approaches, older adults may refuse care as a way to maintain control over their situation.

Unfamiliar and overstimulating environments can be a determinant for care refusal. The loss of routine and perceived threats to dignity from a cold, fast-paced, and perceived hostile environment all contribute to resistance. The technical and fast-paced nature of surgical units can overwhelm older adults, leading to exacerbated defensive responses, which can translate into care refusal.

Organizational determinants include staffing ratios, lack of training, inflexible routines, and workplace culture which can also influence care refusal.

Care refusal has significant implications. It can compromise health outcomes, disrupt care provision, and increase risks to both clients and providers. When older adults refuse essential care, it can lead to compromised interventions, delayed recovery, increased complications, and extended hospital stays. For healthcare providers, managing care refusal increases stress and can affect job satisfaction. It is needed to conduct ongoing assessments that consider not only physical readiness for surgery but also psychological preparedness, cultural factors, and social support systems. Preventing and managing care refusal requires understanding its complex and dynamic determinants (Altamirano et al. 2022; Araújo et al. 2025).

20.4.2 Postoperative Delirium: A Relationship-Centered Approach

Postoperative delirium is one of the most common and serious complications in geriatric surgery (Partridge et al. 2012). Affecting up to 50% of older surgical clients, it significantly impacts recovery outcomes and represents a major source of distress for clients, families, and healthcare providers (Inouye et al. 1999, 2015).

Despite its high prevalence and serious consequences, which include increased mortality rates, longer hospital stays, and higher risk of institutional care, postoperative delirium remains under-recognized and undertreated (Ross 2021). The condition often manifests as acute changes in attention and awareness, but its impact goes far beyond cognitive symptoms—it affects the person's ability to participate in their recovery, disrupts essential relationships, and can lead to long-term functional loss and decline (Aguilera et al. 2004).

Care approaches to delirium have traditionally focused on pharmacological management. However, growing evidence suggests that nonpharmacological, relationship-based interventions can play a role in both prevention and management of this phenomenon. Understanding delirium through this lens shifts the focus from merely treating symptoms to maintaining the person's connection with their environment and support system throughout their surgical journey (Beach et al. 2006; Ko et al. 2021; Santana et al. 2018).

Nonpharmacological interventions focused on human connection form the foundation of delirium prevention and management. These include maintaining ongoing positive human connections through regular interaction, ensuring consistent and appropriate communication, reducing environmental triggers, preserving familiar routines, and promoting family involvement. As shown by Japanese studies, simple actions like obtaining spatial consent before approaching, explaining each care procedure, maintaining leveled eye contact, and using a calm voice can help reduce anxiety and confusion and therefore reduce delirium incidence (Inouye et al. 1999, 2015; Sugimoto et al. 2018; Honda et al. 2016).

The presence of familiar faces plays a vital role in postoperative care for older adults. Family members and trusted caregivers may serve as important anchors to reality, particularly for those at risk of delirium. Their presence can help maintain the person's orientation, comfort, and sense of security during the vulnerable postoperative period. Healthcare providers should consider facilitating family presence and participation in care when appropriate, while recognizing that family members may need support to engage effectively. This often requires providing family caregivers with clear guidance about their role, basic training in supportive techniques, and ongoing support from healthcare professionals who are skilled in relationship-centered care approaches. However, it is important to note that family dynamics vary, and care plans should be tailored to each person's specific circumstances and preferences (Altamirano et al. 2022; Bauchat et al. 2016; Chou and Gaysynsky 2023; Paget et al. 2011; Watson 2008).

A timely assessment and recognition of delirium's different presentations is crucial. While hyperactive delirium with agitation is easily noticed, hypoactive delirium—characterized by withdrawal and decreased responsiveness—often goes unrecognized. Both types require careful attention to the person's behavioral changes and level of engagement. Healthcare providers need to establish baseline behavior and cognition before surgery and monitor subtle changes afterward (Inouye et al. 1999, 2015; Partridge et al. 2012; Ross 2021).

The relationship-centered approach to delirium includes individual interactions and environmental modifications. Reducing noise, maintaining appropriate lighting that supports normal day–night cycles, and creating a more slow-paced prosthetic environment can help prevent and manage delirium. These modifications work best when combined with consistent, supportive human interactions (Beach et al. 2006; Inouye et al. 1999, 2015; Santana et al. 2018).

Prevention and early recognition of delirium require the entire healthcare team's involvement. From surgeons to environmental services staff, everyone plays a role in maintaining the person's orientation and comfort. Regular training in delirium recognition and management helps staff understand their role in prevention and creates a more supportive care environment. Clear in services protocols and updated evidence-based guidelines are fundamental to ensure best practice in perioperative care for older adults with risk of post-op delirium (Bauchat et al. 2016; Inouye et al. 1999, 2015; Ko et al. 2021; Partridge et al. 2012).

20.4.3 Immobility Syndrome

When older adults become immobile after surgery, they face risks that extend beyond muscle weakness or pressure injuries. The immobility syndrome can affect up to 65% of hospitalized older adults, creating a cascade of complications that can turn a routine surgical recovery into a complex journey marked by functional decline and loss of independence (Vázquez Pedrazuela et al. 1995; Boechat et al. 2012).

The barriers to mobility before and after surgery are not only physical but also psychological. Fear of falling, loss of confidence, demotivation, depression, and anxiety about pain can keep older adults from moving, even when medically appropriate. These psychological barriers are particularly powerful in unfamiliar hospital environments where older adults may feel vulnerable and unsure (Dijkstra et al. 2022; Morales-Cariño et al. 2012). Moreover, the experience of functional loss and newly acquired dependency can profoundly affect the person's self-image. This often leads to a state of acute demotivation and, in extreme cases, depression, where the person loses the will to engage in self-care and refuses to participate in recovery activities or interact with others. The relationship between healthcare provider and client becomes crucial in overcoming these complex barriers, as they affect not just mobility but also the person's entire interest and personal investment in rehabilitation and recovery (Araújo et al. 2025; Fried et al. 2001; Roubenoff and Harris 1997).

This approach recognizes that successful mobilization depends not just on physical capability but also on the person's confidence and willingness to move. Healthcare providers need to understand each person's unique concerns and motivations. For some, the goal might be returning home independently; for others, it might be attending a cultural or family event. These personal goals become powerful motivators for mobility (Cruz-Jentoft et al. 2019; Santana et al. 2018).

Social support plays a vital role in preventing immobility syndrome. Family and other members of the social support network and caregivers can provide encouragement and continuity in mobility efforts. Their presence often helps older adults feel more secure and confident in movement and motivated for recovery. Healthcare providers should actively involve family in mobility programs, teaching them how to provide safe assistance and encouragement (Dijkstra et al. 2022; Morales-Cariño et al. 2012).

Maintaining dignity during mobility assistance requires particular attention. Many older adults feel embarrassed or vulnerable when needing help with movement. Healthcare providers must balance safety requirements with the person's need for comfort, autonomy, and self-respect. Simple actions like asking permission before touching, explaining movements in advance, using tender touch techniques, and respecting privacy can make mobility assistance more effective (Figueiredo et al. 2018; Gineste and Marescotti 2010; Henriques et al. 2017).

20.4.4 Failure to Thrive in the Surgical Setting

Failure to thrive in older surgical clients represents a complex syndrome where physical decline intersects with psychological and social factors, leading to unexpected deterioration in health status. This condition affects postoperative recovery prognosis, manifesting as a progressive decline that affects multiple domains of well-being. While medical complications may initiate the decline, the progression typically involves cascading losses in functional autonomy, emotional engagement, and social participation (Aguilera et al. 2004; Roubenoff and Harris 1997; Tsui et al. 2020).

The clinical presentation of failure to thrive in surgical settings often follows two distinct patterns. The hyperactive pattern may manifest through behavioral changes such as increased agitation, expressions of frustration toward staff, defensive responses, or active resistance to care interventions. Without appropriate intervention, this pattern may progress to a decline in both physical strength and psychological resilience. Alternatively, the hypoactive pattern presents as diminished participation in care, reduced nutritional intake, social withdrawal, and decreased motivation for recovery activities. Notably, either pattern can emerge even when surgical outcomes are technically successful and prognosis appears favorable, yet the outcomes are not. Healthcare providers should recognize these behavioral changes as potential indicators of underlying biopsychosocial distress requiring specialized assessment and intervention (Araújo et al. 2025; Cruz-Jentoft et al. 2019; Fried et al. 2001; Roubenoff and Harris 1997; Tsui et al. 2020).

Early recognition and intervention may help prevent or mitigate the progression of failure to thrive. Strong positive therapeutic relationships with healthcare providers, combined with sustained family involvement and appropriate support systems, appear to help maintain the person's sense of identity and purpose during recovery. When these connections deteriorate, older adults may become increasingly vulnerable to both physical and psychological decline. Therefore, healthcare providers must systematically work to preserve and strengthen these vital social connections throughout the surgical journey (Altamirano et al. 2022; Beach et al. 2006; Partridge et al. 2012).

The development and maintenance of comprehensive support networks becomes essential for recovery. This network should integrate both family caregivers and healthcare professionals who possess specialized relational skills and can establish meaningful emotional connections aligned with the person's needs and preferences. Regular, purposeful interactions help preserve the individual's sense of self and connection to their life goals. Healthcare professionals should intentionally facilitate these connections within the perioperative setting, despite operational constraints (Chou and Gaysynsky 2023; Gineste et al. 2008; Melo et al. 2017a, b).

Intervention strategies should be individualized based on comprehensive interdisciplinary assessment of each person's interests, capabilities, and goals, with specific personalized interventions documented in the care prescription. Effective care plans often incorporate familiar daily routines into the hospital setting while creating structured opportunities for family involvement. The implementation of Humanitude principles in daily interactions might provide a framework for meaningful engagement, which can be enhanced through purposeful activities throughout the perioperative journey. These strategies require regular assessment and adjustment to ensure they continue to meet the person's evolving needs and support their recovery goals (Giang et al. 2023; Honda et al. 2016; Melo et al. 2020).

Success in preventing and addressing failure to thrive requires a coordinated approach that recognizes the interconnected nature of physical recovery, psychological well-being, and social engagement. Healthcare providers must move beyond viewing failure to thrive as simply a physical decline and instead address it as a complex syndrome requiring multifaceted, relationship-centered interventions (Beach et al. 2006; Santana et al. 2018; Tsui et al. 2020).

20.5 Conclusion

The surgical care of older adults implies technical excellence, human connection, and specialized geriatric knowledge. Throughout this chapter, we have explored how the integration of Humanitude care methodology, a relationship-centered care model, and understanding of specific perioperative geriatric challenges can transform the surgical experience for older adults (Giang et al. 2023; Partridge et al. 2012).

The Humanitude care methodology offers a structured, evidence-based approach to human connection through its four pillars—gaze, speech, touch, and verticality. When combined with tools like the Structured Sequence of Humanitude Care Procedures (SSHCP) and personalized care prescriptions, it provides healthcare professionals with concrete ways to professionalize and improve their caregiving relationships. This systematic approach transforms seemingly intangible aspects of human connection into measurable, improvable skills that directly impact care outcomes (Gineste and Marescotti 2010; Henriques et al. 2021; Honda et al. 2016; Melo et al. 2020).

Relationship-centered care emerges as a crucial framework for addressing the unique challenges of geriatric surgery. By seeing beyond immediate surgical needs to understand the person's broader life context, healthcare providers can better address the complex interplay of physical, psychological, and social factors that influence surgical outcomes. This approach becomes particularly vital when managing some geriatric challenges like care refusal, postoperative delirium, immobility syndrome, and failure to thrive (Araújo et al. 2025; Beach et al. 2006; Ko et al. 2021).

The evidence presented throughout this chapter demonstrates that successful surgical care of older adults requires more than technical surgical expertise. It demands a sophisticated understanding of how to maintain human connection in clinical settings, prevent psychological deterioration, and support perioperative care through meaningful engagement. The integration of Humanitude principles with relationship-centered care provides a much-needed framework for achieving these goals (Altamirano et al. 2022; Giang et al. 2023; Santana et al. 2018).

Looking forward, several key priorities emerge for improving the surgical care of older adults:

1. Training and Education: Healthcare providers need systematic training in relationship-centered care techniques and methodologies like Humanitude, with particular emphasis on managing geriatric syndromes in the surgical setting (Fukuyasu et al. 2021).
2. Organizational Support: Healthcare institutions must create environments that support meaningful provider–client relationships, allowing time and space for connection while providing necessary resources and training (Henriques et al. 2019).
3. Research and Development: Further investigation is needed to quantify the impact of relationship-centered approaches on specific surgical outcomes (Won et al. 2024).
4. Care Integration: Surgical teams need to better integrate interdisciplinary geriatric expertise into their practice, recognizing that technical surgical success alone does not guarantee optimal outcomes for older adults (Partridge et al. 2012).

As our population ages and surgical interventions become more common in older adults, the importance of these approaches will only grow. By combining technical excellence with specialized relationship-centered care strategies, we can work toward perioperative care that truly addresses the complex needs of older adults, promoting better outcomes and maintaining human dignity throughout the surgical journey (Cruz-Jentoft et al. 2019; Melo et al. 2017a, b).

The success of surgical interventions in older adults ultimately depends on our ability to see beyond the immediate technical challenges to address the whole person. Through intentional application of Humanitude care methodology and relationship-centered care principles, we can create surgical experiences that not only resolve medical issues but also support the overall well-being and dignity of older adults in our care (Beach et al. 2006; Giang et al. 2023).

References

Aguilera A, Pi-Figuews M, Arellano M, Torres RM, García-Caselles MP, Robles MJ, Miralles R, Cervera AM (2004) Previous cognitive impairment and failure to thrive syndrome in patients who died in a geriatric convalescence hospitalization unit. Arch Gerontol Geriatr 9:7–11. https://doi.org/10.1016/j.archger.2004.04.004

Altamirano J, Kline M, Schwartz R, Fassiotto M, Maldonado Y, Weimer-Elder B (2022) The effect of a relationship-centered communication program on patient experience and provider wellness. Patient Educ Couns 105(7):1988–1995. https://doi.org/10.1016/j.pec.2021.10.025

Araújo JP, Melo R, Luz HA, Van Son C, Giang TA, Henriques L, Noor S (2025) Care refusal by older adults with dementia receiving professional care: a scoping review. J Appl Gerontol 44(7):1158–1171. https://doi.org/10.1177/07334648241298660

Bales KL, Witczak LR, Simmons TC, Savidge LE, Rothwell ES, Rogers FD, Manning RA, Heise MJ, Englund M, Arias del Razo R (2018) Social touch during development: long-term effects on brain and behavior. Neurosci Biobehav Rev 95:202–219. https://doi.org/10.1016/j.neubiorev.2018.09.019

Bauchat JR, Seropian M, Jeffries PR (2016) Communication and empathy in the patient-centered care model—why simulation-based training is not optional. Clin Simul Nurs 12(8):356–359

Beach MC, Inui T, Relationship-Centered Care Research Network (2006) Relationship-centered care: a constructive reframing. J Gen Intern Med 21:3–8

Bearman M, Palermo C, Allen LM, Williams B (2015) Learning empathy through simulation: a systematic literature review. Simul Healthc 10(5):308–319

Boechat JCDS, Manhães FC, Gama Filho RVD, Istoe RSC (2012) A síndrome do imobilismo e seus efeitos sobre o aparelho locomotor do idoso [The immobility syndrome and its effects on the elderly locomotor system]. Revista Cientifica Internacional 1(22):89–193

Charon R (2001) Narrative medicine: a model for empathy, reflection, profession, and trust. JAMA 286(15):1897–1902

Chou WS, Gaysynsky A (2023) A relationship-centered approach to addressing mistrust. J Commun Healthc 16(4):320–323. https://doi.org/10.1080/17538068.2023.2258683

Cocker F, Joss N (2016) Compassion fatigue among healthcare, emergency and community service workers: a systematic review. Int J Environ Res Public Health 13(6):Article 618

Cruz-Jentoft AJ, Bahat G, Bauer J, Boirie Y, Bruyère O, Cederholm T, Cooper C, Landi F, Rolland Y, Sayer AA, Schneider SM, Sieber CC, Topinkova E, Vandewoude M, Visser M, Zamboni M (2019) Sarcopenia: revised European consensus on definition and diagnosis. Age Ageing 48(1):16–31

Derksen F, Bensing J, Lagro-Janssen A (2013) Effectiveness of empathy in general practice: a systematic review. Br J Gen Pract 63(606):e76–e84

Dewar B, Nolan M (2013) Caring about caring: developing a model to implement compassionate relationship centred care in an older people care setting. Int J Nurs Stud 50(9):1247–1258. https://doi.org/10.1016/j.ijnurstu.2013.01.008

Dhabhar FS (2014) Effects of stress on immune function: the good, the bad, and the beautiful. Immunol Res 58(2–3):193–210

Dijkstra F, van der Sluis G, Jager-Wittenaar H, Hempenius L, Hobbelen JSM, Finnema E (2022) Facilitators and barriers to enhancing physical activity in older patients during acute hospital stay: a systematic review. Int J Behav Nutr Phys Act 19(1):Article 99

Figueiredo AMG, Melo RCCP, Ribeiro OP (2018) Humanitude care methodology: difficulties and benefits from its implementation in clinical practice. Revista de Enfermagem Referência 4(17):53–62. https://doi.org/10.12707/RIV17063

Fried LP, Tangen CM, Walston J, Newman AB, Hirsch C, Gottdiener J, Seeman T, Tracy R, Kop WJ, Burke G, McBurnie MA (2001) Frailty in older adults: evidence for a phenotype. J Gerontol Ser A Biol Med Sci 56(3):M146–M157

Fukuyasu Y, Kataoka HU, Honda M, Iwase T, Ogawa H, Sato M, Watanabe Y, Fujitani T, Yamamoto K, Gonnella JS (2021) The effect of Humanitude care methodology on improving empathy: a six-year longitudinal study of medical students in Japan. BMC Med Educ 21(1):1–8. https://doi.org/10.1186/s12909-021-02773-x

Giang TA, Koh JEJ, Cheng LJ, Tang QC, Chua MJ, Liew TM, Lee CN, Yap PLK, Wong CH (2023) Effects of Humanitude care on people with dementia and caregivers: a scoping review. J Clin Nurs 32(13–14):2969–2984

Giang TA, Ling Jie C, Min Jia C, Yap P (2021) Humanitude care on patients with dementia and delirium in acute hospital improves outcomes [Conference presentation]. 2021 IPA International Congress

Gineste Y, Marescotti R (2010) Interest of the philosophy of humanitude in caring for patients with Alzheimer's disease. Soins Gerontol 15(85):26–27

Gineste Y, Marescotti R, Pellissier J (2008) L'humanitude dans les soins [Humanitude in care]. Rech Soins Infirm 3:42–55. https://doi.org/10.3917/rsi.094.0042

Gineste Y, Pellissier J (2007) Humanitude: Comprendre la vieillesse, prendre soin des hommes vieux [Humanitude: understanding old age, caring for old men]. Armand Colin

Gleichgerrcht E, Decety J (2014) The relationship between different facets of empathy, pain perception and compassion fatigue among physicians. Front Behav Neurosci 8:Article 243

Henriques L, Melo R, Martins A (2017) Metodologia de Cuidado Humanitude: Contributo para a dignificação da pessoa nos cuidados de higiene e conforto [Humanitude care methodology: contribution to the dignification of the person in hygiene and comfort care]. Servir 55(1–2):30–37

Henriques LVL, Dourado MARF, Melo RCCP, Tanaka LH (2019) Implementation of the humanitude care methodology: experience reports in a health service. Rev Bras Enferm 72(3):825–829. https://doi.org/10.1590/0034-7167-2017-0363

Henriques LVL, Melo RCCP, D'Espiney LMCA (2022) Sequência Estruturada de Procedimentos Cuidativos Humanitude: Validação por peritos [Structured sequence of humanitude care procedures: validation by experts]. Revista Investigação em Enfermagem 39:23–36

Henriques LVL, Pereira RC, Pereira MO, Martins MA, Alves RE (2021) Desafios no cuidar dos idosos: Contributo da metodologia de cuidado humanitude na redução da ansiedade dos cuidadores [Challenges in caring for the elderly: contribution of the humanitude care methodology in reducing caregiver anxiety]. In: Ciências Humanas: Afeto, Poder e Interações 2. Atena Editora, pp 236–247

Hertenstein MJ, Keltner D, App B, Bulleit BA, Jaskolka AR (2006) Touch communicates distinct emotions. Emotion 6(3):528–533

Honda M, Ito M, Ishikawa S, Takebayashi Y, Tierney L (2016) Reduction of behavioral psychological symptoms of dementia by multimodal comprehensive care for vulnerable geriatric patients in an acute care hospital: a case series. Case Rep Med 2016:4813196. https://doi.org/10.1155/2016/4813196

Inácio MSC (2022) (Re)construção da autonomia da pessoa idosa com dependência no autocuidado de higiene: Contributo da Metodologia de Cuidado Humanitude (MCH®) [(Re)construction of the autonomy of the elderly person with dependence on hygiene self-care: contribution of the humanitude care methodology (MCH®)]. Doctoral dissertation, University of Lisbon, University of Lisbon Repository. http://hdl.handle.net/10451/58258

Inouye SK, Bogardus ST Jr, Charpentier PA, Leo-Summers L, Acampora D, Holford TR, Cooney LM Jr (1999) A multicomponent intervention to prevent delirium in hospitalized older patients. N Engl J Med 340(9):669–676

Inouye SK, Robinson T, Blaum C, Busby-Whitehead J, Boustani M, Chalian A et al (2015) Postoperative delirium in older adults: best practice statement from the American Geriatrics Society. J Am Coll Surg 220(2):136–148e1

Kehlet H, Wilmore DW (2008) Evidence-based surgical care and the evolution of fast-track surgery. Ann Surg 248(2):189–198

Kelm Z, Womer J, Walter JK, Feudtner C (2014) Interventions to cultivate physician empathy: a systematic review. BMC Med Educ 14:Article 219

Ko CJ, Kim R, Fortin AH 6th, Spak JM, Hafler JP (2021) Relationship-centered care in the physician-patient interaction: improving your understanding of metacognitive interventions. Cutis 107(6):320–324. https://doi.org/10.12788/cutis.0266

Kobayashi M, Ito M, Iwasa Y, Motohashi Y, Edahiro A, Shirobe M, Hattori M, Sugai Y, Honda M (2021) The effect of multimodal comprehensive care methodology training on oral health care professionals' empathy for patients with dementia. BMC Med Educ 21(1):315–322. https://doi.org/10.1186/s12909-021-02760-2

Kobayashi M, Une S, Hara H, Honda M (2024) The impact of training in multimodal communication skills on psychotropic medication use in dementia care. Cureus 16(6):e63413

Liljencrantz J, Olausson H (2014) Tactile C fibers and their contributions to pleasant sensations and to tactile allodynia. Front Behav Neurosci 8:Article 37

Mancini F, Beaumont AL, Hu L, Haggard P, Iannetti GD (2015) Touch inhibits subcortical and cortical nociceptive responses. Pain 156(10):1936–1944

Marescotti R, Gineste Y (2011) Debout jusqu'au bout, c'est possible! [Standing until the end, it's possible!]. La Revue Francophone de Gériatrie et de Gérontologie 18(178)

McGlone F, Uvnäs Moberg K, Norholt H, Eggart M, Müller-Oerlinghausen B (2024) Touch medicine: bridging the gap between recent insights from touch research and clinical medicine and its special significance for the treatment of affective disorders. Frontiers in Psychiatry 15:1390673. https://doi.org/10.3389/fpsyt.2024.1390673

Meier DE, Back AL, Morrison RS (2001) The inner life of physicians and care of the seriously ill. JAMA 286(23):3007–3014

Melo RCCP, Fernandes DSC, Albuquerque JS, Duarte MN (2017a) Methodology of care Humanitude in promoting self-care in dependent people: an integrative review. In: Duffy VG, Lightner N (eds) Advances in human factors and ergonomics in healthcare. Springer International Publishing, pp 187–193. https://doi.org/10.1007/978-3-319-41652-6_18

Melo RCCP, Queirós PJP, Tanaka LH, Salgueiro NRM, Alves RE, Araújo JP, Rodrigues MA (2017b) State-of-the-art in the implementation of the Humanitude care methodology in Portugal. Revista de Enfermagem Referência 4(13):53–62. https://doi.org/10.12707/RIV17019

Melo RCCP, Queirós PJP, Tanaka LH, Henriques LVL, & Neves HL. (2020). Nursing Students' Relational Skills with Elders Improve through Humanitude Care Methodology. International journal of environmental research and public health, 17(22), 8588. https://doi.org/10.3390/ijerph17228588

Morales-Cariño EM, Jiménez-Herrera BL, Serrano-Miranda TA (2012) Evaluación del colapso del cuidador primario de pacientes adultos mayores con síndrome de inmovilidad [Evaluation of the primary caregiver syndrome when caring for elderly adults with immobility syndrome]. Revista de Investigacion Clinica 64(3):240–246

Niemitz C (2010) The evolution of the upright posture and gait—a review and a new synthesis. Naturwissenschaften 97(3):241–263

Nilsson U (2009) Soothing music can increase oxytocin levels during bed rest after open-heart surgery: a randomised control trial. J Clin Nurs 18:2153–2161. https://doi.org/10.1111/j.1365-2702.2008.02718.x

Paget L, Han P, Nedza S, Kurtz P, Racine E, Russell S, Von Kohorn I, Theirry J, Gruman J, Davis K, Schwartzberg J (2011) Patient-clinician communication: basic principles and expectations. NAM Perspect 1(6):1–7. https://doi.org/10.31478/201106a

Partridge JS, Harari D, Dhesi JK (2012) Frailty in the older surgical patient: a review. Age Ageing 41(2):142–147

Petrescu MD, Popa F, Purcărea VL (2022) How could perioperative anxiety be addressed via surgical team communication approaches? Findings from a scoping review. Hosp Pract 50(3):159–169. https://doi.org/10.1080/21548331.2022.2059979

Ross IR (2021) Through the fog. N Engl J Med 384(20):1882–1883. https://doi.org/10.1056/NEJMp2033891

Roubenoff R, Harris TB (1997) Failure to thrive, sarcopenia and functional decline in the elderly. Clin Geriatr Med 13(4):613–622

Santana MJ, Manalili K, Jolley RJ, Zelinsky S, Quan H, Lu M (2018) How to practice person-centred care: a conceptual framework. Health Expect 21(2):429–440

Sato W, Nakazawa A, Yoshikawa S, Kochiyama T, Honda M, Gineste Y (2023) Behavioral and neural underpinnings of empathic characteristics in a Humanitude-care expert. Front Med 10:1059203. https://doi.org/10.3389/fmed.2023.1059203

Sinclair S, Norris JM, McConnell SJ, Chochinov HM, Hack TF, Hagen NA, McClement S, Bouchal SR (2016) Compassion: a scoping review of the healthcare literature. BMC Palliat Care 15:Article 6

Soklaridis S, Ravitz P, Adler Nevo G, Lieff S (2016) Relationship-centred care in health: a 20-year scoping review. Patient Exp J 3(1):130–145. https://doi.org/10.35680/2372-0247.1111

Sugimoto C, Fukuda K, Honda M (2018, June) Multimodal comprehensive care methodology reduced incidence of delirium and restraints in ICU [Poster presentation]. American Delirium Society Annual Meeting, San Francisco, CA, United States

Tsui C, Kim K, Spencer M (2020) The diagnosis "failure to thrive" and its impact on the care of hospitalized older adults: a matched case-control study. BMC Geriatr 20:1–7

Uvnäs-Moberg K, Handlin L, Petersson M (2015) Self-soothing behaviors with particular reference to oxytocin release induced by non-noxious sensory stimulation. Front Psychol 5:1529

Vázquez Pedrazuela C, Lázaro del Nogal M, Verdejo Bravo C, Royuela Arte T, Torrijos Torrijos M, Ribera Casado JM (1995) Síndrome de inmovilidad en pacientes atendidos en una unidad de ayuda a domicilio [Immobility syndrome in patients being care for in a home care unit]. An Med Interna 12(10):489–491

Verghese A (2011, July) A doctor's touch [Video]. TED Conferences. https://www.ted.com/talks/abraham_verghese_a_doctor_s_touch

Wang X, Liu H, Tang G, Sun F, Wu G, Wu J (2024) The effect of distraction techniques on pain, fear, and anxiety in children undergoing circumcision: a meta-analysis of randomized controlled trials. Am J Mens Health 18(1):15579883241230166

Watson J (2008) Nursing: the philosophy and science of caring. University Press of Colorado

Won KA, Yun S, Lee MA, Kim H, Song B, Kim J, Chung S (2024) Effects of Humanitude care on dementia patients and caregivers: a scoping review. J Korean Gerontol Soc 44(3):357–380. https://doi.org/10.31888/JKGS.2024.44.3.357

MIX
Papier aus verantwortungsvollen Quellen
Paper from responsible sources
FSC® C105338

If you have any concerns about our products,
you can contact us on
ProductSafety@springernature.com

In case Publisher is established outside the EU,
the EU authorized representative is:
Springer Nature Customer Service Center GmbH
Europaplatz 3, 69115 Heidelberg, Germany

Printed by Libri Plureos GmbH
in Hamburg, Germany